Physical Examination and Diagnostic Skills for Nurses and Allied Health Professionals

Chrysi Leliopoulou • Lily Holman

Physical Examination and Diagnostic Skills for Nurses and Allied Health Professionals

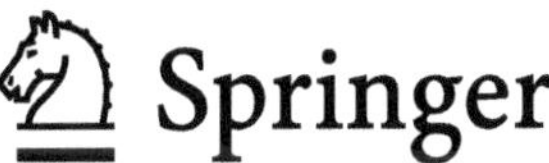

Chrysi Leliopoulou
Faculty of Medicine and Health Sciences
University of East Anglia, Health Sciences
Norwich, UK

Lily Holman
Department of Natural Sciences,
The Burroughs, Hendon
Middlesex University
London, UK

ISBN 978-3-032-26538-8 ISBN 978-3-032-26539-5 (eBook)
https://doi.org/10.1007/978-3-032-26539-5

This Springer imprint is published by the registered company Springer Nature Switzerland AG
The registered company address is: Gewerbestrasse 11, 6330 Cham, Switzerland

If disposing of this product, please recycle the paper.

Preface

This book was written as an introductory text for registered nurses and other health professionals embarking on advanced clinical assessment courses. Early on in my career as an academic, I taught clinical skills, nursing sciences, and simulation long before I got involved in clinical and physical examination courses. I taught registered nurses and other health professionals on these modules and courses for over 20 years, and I always found our conversations with students in these sessions inspirational.

Before I joined academia, I worked as a senior adult haemato-oncology nurse at UCL (University College London) and Royal Free Hospital, and later on as a research assistant at the Royal Free Medical School for the Marie Curie Research Centre. Part of the research assistant role was to deliver communication skills training for senior cancer nurses, which allowed me to explore pertinent issues around clinical practice and clinical assessment. This experience sparked my interest in clinical assessment, physical examination, and diagnosis. For over 20 years I taught physical examination modules, courses, and CPD (Continuous Professional Development) study days at Middlesex University, London. Over the course of my 30 years of career I have come to understand that physical examination is not simply about performing tasks but it is more about observing patterns, communicating them to others, and picking up cues on the way to understand disease development and progression, but also what the patient is really saying about their symptoms and their disease.

The idea of a book came about when my colleague and co-author, Dr Lily Holman, and I were looking through notes and cross-references to create further student activities and workbooks. At the time we were teaching together at Middlesex University and planning teaching materials for courses and study days. We then realized we had enough notes between us to write a book; we joked about it, but also the idea of this book was born.

I also noticed over the years how clinical practice steadfastly was shifting and reshaping towards advanced clinical practice and broadening the scope of professional practice to a more effective, person-centred clinical care and decision-making model.

The new NHS long-term plan "Fit for the Future" (2025) clearly opens a huge opportunity to rethink our clinical practice for the benefit of patients and their families. This book has several special features which I hope will appeal to registered nurses, other health professionals, students, and lecturers interested in developing their physical examination skills and knowledge.

We have deliberately started with a chapter introducing the role of communication and consultation models, and a chapter on general examination skills to put the book in context, and the choice of further topics was governed by our conception of the role of the body systems in physical examination and clinical assessment. Chapters focus on how professionals may apply their physical examination skills and knowledge to aid their decision-making process and use their findings from the physical examination to aid diagnose or differentiate a diagnosis and make a decision to refer or start on a treatment plan. The book presents concise and focused nuggets of knowledge we collected over many years of observing and working with students in clinical practice, and we used scenarios and student activities to facilitate transfer of their knowledge and understanding in a classroom situation. Over the years, we also had discussions and debates with students and colleagues on instances and cases presented in class for discussion to illuminate or pinpoint significant complexity. With this in mind, we have concluded each chapter with a series of case studies and student activities to enable the professional to apply and test their knowledge so far. With their increased knowledge, we hope students can transfer and apply their findings from the physical examination and produce an evidence-based decision for a treatment plan.

By using a systematic approach, we have made it possible for students to dip in at a particular point to supplement lecture materials or to find guidance for further study and reading. But the student will soon become aware from the extensive notes and learning points offered in this book that the topics are interdependent. I also hope that the student will get personal satisfaction from drawing on their own knowledge and experience assessing patients and from knowing that this book can help them explore their own speciality.

No book of this kind could possibly be written without the help and encouragement of others. Among these I particularly want to thank my mentor, Kate Ambrose, who introduced me to this area of clinical practice; Maggie Malik, a dear friend and colleague, for her positive outlook and encouragement; Harry Oliver, for her belief in me and her support in the classroom; and of course my dear colleague and co-author Dr Lily Holman for her motivation and clear vision. To students and colleagues, past and present, I owe a debt of gratitude for their participation in sharpening my thinking, and lastly to my husband Christopher Paraschidis and our three beautiful children, who have been patiently supporting and encouraging me throughout the writing of this book! I would also like to dedicate this to my beloved father, who passed away in 2022, for his tremendous courage and love and for being my motivation for this book.

Norwich, UK   Chrysi Leliopoulou
London, UK   Lily Holman
10 April 2026

Contents

Assessing and Diagnosing Using the Calgary-Cambridge Communication-Based Model (CCCM)

1

Learning Objectives

In this part of the chapter, the use of the Calgary-Cambridge Communication-based Model is explained and discussed with the view to assess and diagnose conditions, diseases, and disorders before the healthcare professional can proceed with the physical examination.

> **Learning Objectives**
> *By the end of this chapter, the student will be able to:*
>
> *Undertake a safe and effective history taking before physically examining the patient using a consultation model*
> *Advocate a patient-centred care plan*
> *Build a trusting relationship and rapport with the patient*
> *Communicate effectively and collaborate with the patient, their family/carer, and other healthcare professionals*

1.1 Part 1: Exploration of Consultation Models in Clinical Practice

Consultation models are used in clinical practice to interview patients on admission and before a treatment plan is formulated. These models such as the CCCM can enhance communication and streamline information gathered during the patient interview but also allow to understand patients' diverse needs. The CCCM model guides carefully the healthcare professional to interact with the patient to ensure that the patient is engaging with the process.

© The Author(s), under exclusive license to Springer Nature Switzerland AG 2026
C. Leliopoulou, L. Holman, *Physical Examination and Diagnostic Skills for Nurses and Allied Health Professionals,*
https://doi.org/10.1007/978-3-032-26539-5_1

1.1.1   The Calgary-Cambridge Model (CCCM)

The Calgary-Cambridge Model (CCCM) is used in clinical practice widely and involves stages the clinician is expected to go through during the consultation. Each of the following stages below promotes a collaborative approach that respects patient autonomy and fosters shared decision-making. This structured interaction not only enhances patient satisfaction but also improves documentation, continuity of care, and clinical safety.

Learning Point
This model consists of five stages as follows:

Stage 1: Initiating the session
   This stage involves greeting the patient, introducing oneself, and ensuring that the patient feels comfortable and respected. Initial rapport building is crucial for setting a positive tone for the consultation. Clarifying the purpose of the consultation is also critical at this stage of the consultation.
Stage 2: Gathering information
   The model underscores the importance of skilled questioning and active listening. It encourages healthcare professionals to employ open-ended questions that prompt patients to express their concerns freely, thus facilitating a comprehensive understanding of their issues. Employing both open and closed-ended questions facilitates the accumulation of data regarding symptoms, medical history, lifestyle, and concerns, leading to a more informed assessment.
Stage 3: Building the relationship
   Establishing trust is paramount in healthcare interactions. The model highlights the significance of empathetic communication and picking up non-verbal cues, which contribute to a sense of safety for the patient during discussions about sensitive topics. Demonstrating empathy, respect, and a genuine interest in the patient's perspective fosters a sense of connection that underlies effective healthcare delivery.
Stage 4: Explaining and planning
   This stage focuses on discussing the findings, laying out management options, and collaboratively developing a care plan with the patient. It promotes patient participation in decision-making, reinforcing their engagement in care. Communicating findings clearly, discussing options, and actively involving patients in the decision-making process enhances the likelihood of adherence to care plans.
Stage 5: Closing the session
   Summarizing the key points discussed and addressing any remaining questions ensures that both the clinician and patient are aligned on the care plan, leaving the patient feeling heard and valued. Also, at this stage we can verify the patient's understanding, and ensure that the patient feels informed and supported, which can solidify the consultation experience.

The Calgary-Cambridge model, through structured communication, can improve patient satisfaction and care outcomes. One of the notable strengths of this model is its emphasis *on viewing the healthcare interaction from the patient's perspective*. It encourages healthcare professionals to explore not only the biomedical aspects of illness, but also the psychological, emotional, and social dimensions that influence their health. This model is reported to translate the patient's understanding, beliefs, and concerns regarding their conditions through shared decision-making, and the assessment commences from the moment the patient walks in by actively observing the patient's gait, posture, facial expressions, and behaviours, all of which can provide insightful indicators of the patient's health status.

A central tenet of the Calgary-Cambridge model is to foster a trusting relationship that encourages openness, alleviates anxiety, promotes collaboration, and prevents the potential for conversational drift by enabling the patient to focus on the relevant information while also respecting the patient's narrative.

The healthcare profession can reflect on what has been asked in each part of the consultation by asking the following questions:

- Where am I in this assessment?
- What do I want to achieve?
- What are my objectives and envisioned outcomes?
- How will I arrive at those outcomes?

This reflection can enable the clinician keep track of the significant aspects of the patient's health that may not be readily visible through clinical observations alone. The models also allow the clinician to advocate for the patient's unique context.

1.1.2   Stage 1: Initiating the Patient Interview

This part of the patient interview aims to understand the patient's concerns and ensure their safety. This can be achieved by creating a trusting and fulfilling atmosphere to actively engage the patient in discussing their individual needs and preferences. Such preparation enables the patient to assume an active role in their consultation, facilitating a collaborative process in the development of a tailored management plan.

Learning Point
The initiation of the consultation session involves four distinct areas:

- Preparation
- Establishing rapport
- Identifying the reasons for the consultation
- Negotiating the agenda

Each area contributes to a smoother consultation process, fostering both trust and collaboration between the clinician and the patient.

A. **Preparation**

Preparation is a critical stage that requires the clinician to set aside distractions and focus on the upcoming consultation.

- *Setting aside last tasks and attending to self-comfort.*

  It is essential for the clinician to mentally disengage from previous responsibilities and emotional stressors from their own life that could hinder their ability to engage effectively with the patient.
- *Self-care.*

  A healthcare professional can deliver compassionate and focused care during the consultation if they feel both physically and emotionally ready to undertake the consultation.
- *Focusing attention on the consultation.*

  Preparation extends to familiarizing oneself with the patient's medical history, including recent notes and records.
- *Questions must be considered in the consultation, including*:

  What potential biases or feelings might affect the way I approach the patient?

  How previous experiences with similar patients may influence my expectations or behaviour towards the patient?
- *Reviewing this information.*

  This can help approach the patient in an informed manner, allowing for a more objective and empathetic interaction.

B. **Establishing Initial Rapport**

Building rapport with the patient within the first few moments of the consultation is crucial to alleviating any anxiety they may have. Effective rapport can be established through the following strategies:

- *Greeting the patient.*

  A warm greeting sets a positive tone. This should include confirming the patient's name and ensuring respectful acknowledgment before commencing further discussion.
- *Introducing yourself and clarifying your role.*

  The clinician should introduce their name and qualifications, clarifying their role in the consultation process.
- *Attending to physical comfort.*

  Addressing the patient's physical comfort, such as adjusting their seat or offering water, can significantly contribute to a relaxed atmosphere. Demonstrating interest through appropriate eye contact and attentive body language reinforces respect and care.
- *Time to think and reflect.*

  Consider how you greet a patient using non-verbal skills?

What strategies can you employ to make the patient feel more at ease?

Non-verbal gestures, such as a genuine smile or maintaining appropriate eye contact, serve to establish a welcoming environment for the patient. Additional actions, like assisting the patient with their belongings, can further enhance the initial rapport.

C. Identifying the Reasons for the Consultation

Identifying the primary reasons for the patient's visit is essential for targeted and effective assessment:

- *Opening question.*

  The initial question should facilitate dialogue. Phrasing such as "What would you like to discuss today?" encourages the patient to express their concerns freely. Open questions are effective in eliciting detailed responses from patients.

  Examples include:

  "Can you describe what you have experienced regarding your symptoms?"

  "What brings you in today?"

  One should carefully avoid leading questions that may bias the patient, such as "You've been feeling well, haven't you?" or "Your symptoms aren't too bothersome, are they?" This type of questioning can inadvertently influence the patient's responses, preventing a full understanding of their issues

- *Active listening.*

  Listen attentively to the patient's opening statements without interjecting. This practice fosters trust and allows the patient to convey their narratives in their own words.

- *Screening for additional issues.*

  After the patient has shared their concerns, you may summarize what has been discussed and inquire if there are other issues to address: "So, we have talked about headaches and tiredness. Is there anything else you would like to cover in today's consultation?"

- *Time to think and reflect.*

  How does one distinguish between open and closed questions?

  Explore and list potential opening questions for your consultations.

D. Active Listening

Active listening is a skill that requires focus and intention; it allows you to pick up on verbal and non-verbal cues from the patient. This skill is fundamental for achieving a true understanding of the patient's concerns.

- *Open questions.*

  Utilizing open questions to further explore patient issues is vital:

  "You mentioned feeling fatigued. Could you elaborate more on that?"

- *Facilitation.*

    Enabling the patient to express themselves without interruption encourages openness. Non-verbal affirmations, such as head nodding and appropriate facial expressions, convey attentiveness.

- *Reflecting back.*

    When the patient shares information, reflecting back reinforces that you are engaged:

    "You mentioned feeling overwhelmed. What specifically is causing that feeling?"

- *Additional active listening strategies.*

    Strategies that enhance active listening may include:

    (a) Avoiding interruptions and distractions.

    (b) Encouraging patient responses with subtle verbal affirmations (e.g. "mm-hmm," "I see").

    (c) Reflecting on the content of what has been said instead of fixating on the speaker.

    (d) Examples of techniques to encourage patient contribution.

        (i) *Open Questions*: "What concerns would you like to share today?"

        (ii) *Clarifying*: "Can you explain what you mean by…?"

        (iii) *Repetition*: "How do you think you will manage?"

        (iv) *Reflecting*: "How do you feel looking back on that experience?"

        (v) *Screening*: "Is there anything else that has been on your mind?"

        (vi) *Summarizing*: "So, just to confirm, you've mentioned experiencing headaches and dizziness, is that correct?"

E. **Negotiating and Agenda Setting**

In the negotiation and agenda-setting phase, you are actively inviting the patient to prioritize their issues. This collaborative approach not only fosters respect but also empowers the patient, allowing them to feel valued in the assessment process.

- *Allowing the patient to drive the assessment.*

    Encouraging the patient to convey their priorities helps remove uncertainty for both parties. It also cultivates an environment where the patient feels free to voice concerns without fear of judgment.

- *Recognizing patient priorities.*

    Establishing the agenda through negotiation provides you with the opportunity to understand what is most pressing for the patient.

- *Setting the conversation agenda.*

    Listening to the first problem and begin by allowing the patient to express their primary concern: "What is the first issue you would like to address?"

> • ***Summarizing and acknowledging problems.***
>   Regularly summarize and confirm the patient's listing of concerns to demonstrate understanding. "Let's review the issues together to ensure I have captured everything accurately."
> • ***Prioritizing issues.***
>   Anticipate asking: "Which is the most significant issue for you today?" This question enables the patient to guide subsequent assessment and discussion, which can facilitate a more effective and efficient interaction.

Engaging in this manner transforms the consultation from a mere task into a collaborative dialogue that prioritizes the patient's needs, ensuring that the care provided aligns with their expectations and concerns. Initiating the nursing consultation interview is a multifaceted process that is foundational to establishing a therapeutic relationship. By effectively preparing, establishing rapport, identifying patient concerns, implementing active listening techniques, and negotiating the agenda collaboratively, you can foster an environment conducive to open communication and trust. This comprehensive approach not only enhances patient satisfaction but also contributes significantly to the accuracy of assessments and the quality of care delivered. Developing these skills through practice and reflection will empower you to perform with greater confidence, ultimately leading to better health outcomes for your patients.

1.1.3   Stage 2: Gathering Information

• ***Information gathering.***
Information gathering influences diagnostic accuracy but also helps bolster our therapeutic relationship with the patient. Collecting relevant information allows us to understand the complexities of the patient's condition and open the dialogue about meaningful care and management which may enhance the patient's sense of value and trust, leading to a more collaborative care experience. The objectives at this stage include explaining the process, providing information, and arriving at a mutually agreeable management plan that considers the patient's preferences, concerns, and input. To achieve these goals, we must employ a strategic approach in structuring the interview, facilitating patient involvement, and attentively listening to the patient's perspectives.

• ***The importance of patient perspectives.***
During the consultation interview, it is vital we invite the patient to share their personal experiences and concerns they may have. Gathering substantial clinical information can also reinforce our commitment to listen and validate the patient's experiences. By asking open-ended questions such as, "Can you describe what it is like living with your condition?" or "What concerns do you have about your

current treatment?" we invite the patient to offer richer narratives that illuminate the patient's illness and its significance to their lives.

- ***Time to think and reflect.***

    How can you explore and understand the patient's illness framework and the meaning of the illness for the patient?

    How can you foster a sense of being listened to while ensuring that the patient's information and views are welcomed and valued?

    In what ways can you promote a supportive and collaborative environment involving the patient and their family?

    How can you structure the assessment interview to ensure efficient and effective information gathering?

    How can you clarify the direction of the assessment interview to enable the patient to understand their involvement in the process?

Learning Point

Skills for effective information gathering.

Through careful planning and active engagement, we can utilize a variety of skills designed to facilitate not only the gathering of information but also to ensure a collaborative atmosphere. The following outlines several important techniques and strategies we can employ throughout the consultation interview:

Question style.

- Open Questions: Open questions allow the patient to elaborate and provide more detailed responses.

    Examples include:

    "How can I help you today?"
    "Could you tell me more about that?"
    "Is there anything else you have noticed?"

- Closed Questions: Closed questions, while limited in scope, can clarify specific details when needed.
- For example:

    "When you say vomiting, do you mean that you actually threw up, or did you just feel sick?"

    By employing a balanced mix of open and closed questions, we can create an engaging dialogue that elicits comprehensive information while also pinpointing particular issues.

Active listening.
Active listening encourages a therapeutic interaction by showing the patient that they are being heard. Strategies include:

- Facilitative responses: Non-verbal affirmations, such as nodding and utilizing verbal cues (e.g. "I see," "Uh-huh"), indicate to the patient that they are being actively engaged.
- Reflecting back: Reiterating key statements or using hanging sentences can prompt the patient to expand on their thoughts.

For example, "You mentioned earlier that ... could you tell me more?"
Picking up cues.
We can enhance our assessments by picking up on verbal and non-verbal cues from the patient:

- "You sound tired; is that how you feel?"
- "You seem anxious. Can you elaborate on that?"

Doing this enables you provide tailored support while validating the patient's emotions.
Clarification.
Ensuring mutual understanding is essential during the consultation:

- "We've covered a lot of information so far; is there anything you would like me to clarify?"

Such inquiries help verify that you and the patient are aligned and that information has been accurately understood.
Time-framing.
Effective time management during the consultation ensures that all necessary subjects are addressed within a reasonable timeframe, while also respecting the patient's needs.
Summarizing.
Summarizing the main points discussed helps consolidate the information gathered during the interview:

- "To make sure I've understood correctly, you have mentioned headaches and fatigue. Is that accurate?"

Summarizing not only clarifies understanding but also shows the patient that their contributions have been valued.
Use of appropriately simple language.
We should communicate in plain language, avoiding jargon that may confuse the patient. This enables clarity and ensures that the patient understands the information discussed.

Understanding the patient's perspective.

To fully appreciate the patient's experience, we must consider several elements:

- Patient ideas and concerns:
  "What does this diagnosis mean to you?"
- Patient expectations:
  "What are your thoughts on the next steps moving forward?"
- Effects on life:
  "How has this condition impacted your daily life or work?"
- Patient feelings:

  "How are you coping with all of this?"

These questions facilitate a deeper understanding of the patient's context and allow for a holistic approach to care delivery.

Time to think and reflect.

How would you incorporate these skills into your practice while considering your personality and how it influences your development of these skills?

What broad areas should be taken into account to meet patient needs? For instance, using plain English or engaging the patient collaboratively in care planning.

In navigating the conversation, we must take an active role to maintain control over the structure of the interview. While interpersonal interactions can develop spontaneously, a well-considered framework for the assessment process is fundamentally important for its success.

Learning Point

The way to build a strong relationship with the patient depends on the following four areas:

- How we phrase it in the way our patient understands what we are asking.
- How we make sure that we are developing and maintaining a continuous relationship over time with our patient.
- How we use non-verbal communication to enable the patient to feel understood, valued, and supported.
- How can we phrase our management plan in a way the patient understands.

By involving the patient:
e.g. "How do you feel about that plan?"
By sharing our thoughts we share our thinking with the patient to encourage the patient's involvement
e.g. "What I'm thinking now is...."

By providing a rationale:
We explain the rationale for questions we ask or parts of physical examination we undertake.
e.g. "So your ... is very likely to be related to the ... you were telling me about earlier."

By examination:
During physical examination, we explain the process and we ask for permission.
e.g. "Is it okay for me to examine your chest?"
- How can we make sure that we are maintaining a continuing relationship over time?

There are three non-verbal communication skills we can employ here to ensure this to happen.

Acceptance: we acknowledge the patient's views and feelings; accept legitimacy, by being not judgmental.
Empathy and support: we express concern, understanding, willingness to help; acknowledge coping efforts and appropriate self-care.
Sensitivity: we deal sensitively with embarrassing and disturbing topics and physical pain, including when associated with physical examination.
- Finally, how can we use non-verbal communication to enable the patient to feel understood, valued, and supported?

We can achieve this by:

Demonstrating appropriate non-verbal behaviour.
e.g. eye contact, posture and position, movement, facial expression, use of voice.
Use of notes.
If reads, writes notes or uses computer, we do in a manner that does not interfere with dialogue or rapport.
Picks up the patient's non-verbal cues.
e.g. Body language, speech, facial expression, affect, we check them out and acknowledge as appropriate.

1.1.4   Stage 4: Explanation and Planning

Explanation and planning are of utmost importance to a successful consultation, but we need to ensure that a joint management plan is drawn together with the patient. That way the patient feels comfortable with the plan, understands it, and is prepared to adhere to. Patient adherence to the treatment is invaluable in any care management setting.

We can achieve this by ensuring that we:

- Give the correct amount and type of information to each individual patient.
- Provide explanations that the patient can remember and understand.
- Provide explanations that relate to the patient's medical case.
- Clarify any concerns and questions for the patient can ensure a shared understanding of the problem with the patient.
- Involve the patient and plan together to increase the patient's commitment and adherence to the plans made.

Learning Point
- How can we make sure that we are providing the right amount and type of information?

Chunk and check: give information in assimilable chunks, check understanding, use the patient's response as a guide for how to proceed
e.g. "The type of headache you are describing is called a migraine, migraines is …. Does that make sense to you?"

Assess the patient's starting point: ask for the patient's prior knowledge early on when giving information and find out how much information the patient wants.
e.g. "I don't know how much you know about …, It would be good if you could tell me what you already know so that I might be able to fill in the gaps"

Ask patient what other information it would be helpful (i.e. aetiology, prognosis):
e.g. Ask them if they have any questions they'd like us to answer or any points that we may haven't covered?

Give explanation at appropriate times: avoid giving advice, information, or reassurance prematurely
e.g. Pt: "I think I've got a chest infection and needs some antibiotics."
You: "Would you mind if I put that on hold just for a second and come back to it after I've asked you a bit more about …?"

- How can you make information easier for the patient to remember and understand?

Clarify any concerns and question the patient may have to ensure a shared understanding of the problem with the patient.

We can ensure this from happening by:

Organize explanation logically.

Using explicit categorization or signposting:

e.g. "There are two important things I'd like to explain. First ... Second ..."
"Now I'm going to move on to the treatment."

Use repetition and summarizing to reinforce information.

e.g. "So, just to recap, you think your headaches are called migraines. To help make you better it would be good if...."

Provide them with leaflets and visual aids where appropriate.

Use language concisely and easily understood statements; avoid jargon.

Use visual methods for conveying information such as diagrams, models, written information, and instructions.

Check patient's understanding of information given or plans made, ask the patient to restate in own words what has been said, clarify as necessary.

e.g. "It would help me if you could repeat back to me what we've agreed so far so I can make sure we're both on the same track."

Clarify any concerns and questions the patient may have to ensure a shared understanding of the problem with the patient.

Involve the patient and plan together to increase the patient's commitment and adherence to the plans made.

We need to provide explanations that:

Relate to the patient's view of the problem

e.g. "You've obviously been thinking about this a lot recently. It would help me to know what you were thinking it might be?"

e.g. "Is there anything in particular that was worrying you about it?"

e.g. "What were you hoping that I might be able to do for you today?"

- Help find out the patient's thoughts and feelings about the information given?

For example, by picking up on verbal and non-verbal cues, e.g. Does the patient need to ask questions to avoid information overload; distress

By checking out verbal cues.
   e.g. "You said earlier you have…, can you expand on that?"
By clarifying verbal cues.
   e.g. "So you said these … have really been preying on your mind. What's been worrying you about them?"
By repetition on verbal cues.
   e.g. "You feel down?"
By checking out non-verbal cues.
   e.g. "I can see you look worried about that."

Encourage interaction rather than one-way transmission:
   For example, provide opportunity and encouragement for the patient to contribute and seek clarification or express doubts and respond appropriately. Elicit the patient's beliefs, reactions, and feelings about the information given and the terms used, acknowledge and address feelings if necessary
   e.g. "Tell me about your thoughts and feelings"
   • We can check the patient's understanding of both diagnosis and management by asking the following questions about.

Understanding of diagnosis:
   e.g. "I don't know whether that makes sense, is there anything you want me to clarify on or to ask me?"
   "What are you going to say when your husband asks you about what the problem is when you get back home?"

Understanding of treatment/management plan:
   e.g. "How do you feel about that plan?"
   "Is there anything I haven't covered or explained?"

Noticing the patient's non-verbals. If a patient looks confused during your explanation, STOP and say what you see:
   e.g. "Am I right in sensing that you're still worried about something?"
   "If you don't mind me saying, it looks like there's still something bothering you?"
   "You look a bit confused to me. What would help to get rid of the confusion?"

1.1.5 Stage 5: Closing the Session

Closing the session with the patient is also a critical point in the consultation interview because it confirms the agreed management plan of care. At this stage of the consultation interview it is important that we clarify the next steps. It also allows us and the patient to establish contingency plans and alternatives if the management plan does not work. That way we maximize patient adherence which can produce better health outcomes for the patient. This last part of the interview assessment also offers an opportunity to make efficient use of time in the interview and allows the patient to feel part of a collaborative process and to build trust.

In summary, we need to

Confirm the established plan of care:
e.g. Summarize & ask "Does that sound about right"?
Clarify the next steps for the patient:
e.g. "Just to check that I've explained things clearly, how are you going to take … or what are you going to do?"
Establish contingency plans:
e.g. "Just to check that I have explained things clearly, can you tell me what you're going to do/how you're going to take your medication and what to look out for in terms of side effect?"
Maximize patient adherence and health outcomes by offering alternative options to the patient to choose from:
e.g. "There are a number of options: …, and … Which do you prefer?"
Continue to allow the patient to feel part of the consultation interview and build on the relationship for the future:
e.g. "So where do we go from here? We could …. What do you think?"
"Just so I know that I have explained things right, do you want to summarize what we have agreed to do today?"

Finally, we need to employ a set of skills to conclude our consultation interview by

Summarizing the session briefly and clarifying the plan of care.
e.g. "So, just to recap, I think that what you getting is … and that to try and help relieve it we should…"
Agreeing with the patient the next steps in the management plan for patient.
e.g. "Can I see you again in 2 weeks, but sooner if you are worried or if you get …"
Safety-netting appropriately and explain possible unexpected outcomes, what to do if the plan is not working, when and how to seek help
e.g. "What I mean when I say if it's not improving is if you start to develop…"
Final checking that the patient agrees and is comfortable with the plan and feels free to ask any questions or if there are any other issues to discuss.
e.g. "Now, are there any outstanding things you wanted to talk about or things I haven't fully explained?"

In a nutshell, it is important that we build a trusting relationship to continuously build rapport with the patient and establish a caring relationship during the consultation interview. Using appropriate non-verbal behaviour, we can demonstrate confidence and rapport as advocators for patients to ask questions or express doubts. This can facilitate a mutually accepted understanding between the professional and the patient. We and the patient may have a different world view and perspectives on a situation. However, if they respect each other's view and understand what is important for the patient at the time of the consultation interview then it is more likely that you can successfully convey the message to the patient.

1.2 Part 2: Student Activities

Despite the best preparations, there will be instances when the assessment interview does not unfold smoothly. Reflecting on such situations can uncover areas for growth and improvement. For instance, consider a recent patient interaction that felt uneasy; what insights emerged from that experience?

Reflecting on this scenario allows one to analyse:

Information discovered:
What was learned from the conversation? Where did clarity emerge?
Missing information:
What additional details might have benefited the consultation?
Barriers to effective assessment:
Consider potential obstacles that might have hindered the assessment.
Comprehensive assessment:
Was there inadequacy in clinical knowledge about the specific issue presented by the patient?
Did personal anxieties or tiredness from other responsibilities affect focus?
Were there deficiencies in skills for delving further into responses when the patient expressed negative sentiments?
Did previous patient interactions cast a shadow on your ability to remain fully present with the current patient?

Understanding the dynamics at play during these challenging assessments serves as an opportunity for personal and professional development, guiding you towards improved interaction strategies in future consultations.

Effectively gathering information is a cornerstone of the consultation interview, pivotal for diagnosing patient needs and fostering supportive relationships. Employing a structured framework that promotes open communication, active listening, and validation not only enhances the quality of patient assessments but also empowers patients, allowing them to contribute meaningfully to their care plans.

Activity 1

Read the case students below and plan your patient interviews using the Communication Cambridge-Calgary model (CCCM) to start the conversation with the patient (Initiating session), make sure you greet, identify reason for visit, and gather information, i.e. explore history and symptoms related to their signs.

Finally, look for features as shown in Table 1.1 to exam systematically the patients. Explain findings, i.e. link to possible causes clearly and plan, i.e. order some investigation and offer a differential diagnosis.

Table 1.2 details clinical information you may gather at each stage of the consultation interview. Table 1.3 contains information about different case studies you required to apply the CCCM to plan their care.

Table 1.1 This shows what you should be looking out for involving the hands, nails, eyes, and mouth

General clinical features—hands, nails, eyes, mouth			
	Clinical feature	Common/uncommon	What it may indicate
Hands			
Hands—temperature & texture			
	Abnormally hot/sweaty	Uncommon	Pyrexia, liver disease, hyperthyroidism
	Clammy	Common	Acute coronary syndrome, myocardial infarction
	Cold	Common	Hypothermia
	Localized cool areas	Uncommon	Impaired circulation, Raynaud's phenomenon
	Localized hot areas	Uncommon	Inflammation, infection
	Very dry skin	Common	Hypothyroidism, ageing, dehydration, skin disease
	Poor skin turgor	Common	Dehydration
	Peripheral cyanosis	Uncommon	Low cardiac output
	Palmar erythema	Uncommon	Liver disease, pregnancy
Hands—deformities & features			
Dupuytren's contracture	Uncommon	Liver disease, diabetes, anticonvulsant use	Gathering information → Ask about alcohol use, medication
Heberden's nodes	Common	Osteoarthritis	Clinical reasoning → Degenerative joint disease
Osler's nodes/ Janeway lesions	Uncommon	Infective endocarditis	Safety netting → Discuss need for urgent investigations
Joint deformity	Common	Arthritis (RA, OA)	Explanation and planning → Discuss chronic management
Muscle wasting	Uncommon	Neurological disease, trauma, arthritis, ageing	Building relationship → Explore functional impact
Nails			
Pitting	Uncommon	Psoriasis, autoimmune/ connective tissue disease	Gathering information → Ask about rash or joint pain
Splinter haemorrhages	Uncommon	Trauma, endocarditis, vasculitis, melanoma	Clinical reasoning → Check for systemic features

(continued)

Table 1.1 (continued)

General clinical features—hands, nails, eyes, mouth

	Clinical feature	Common/uncommon	What it may indicate
Nicotine staining	Common	Cigarette smoking	Health promotion → Discuss smoking cessation
Koilonychia (spoon nails)	Uncommon	Iron deficiency anaemia, folate deficiency	Explanation → Advise dietary sources, investigation
Onycholysis	Uncommon	Fungal infection, thyroid disease, psoriasis, Raynaud's	Problem solving → Check for systemic features
Clubbing	Uncommon	Hereditary, cardiac (endocarditis, congenital), pulmonary (CA, ILD), IBD	Clinical reasoning → Identify systemic cause
Eyes			
Conjunctival rim pallor	Common	Iron deficiency anaemia	Explanation → Investigate cause of anaemia
Yellow sclera	Common	Jaundice (liver disease, haemolysis)	Clinical reasoning → Assess for liver tenderness
Corneal arcus (young patient)	Uncommon	Hyperlipidaemia	Health promotion → Lipid management counselling
Xanthelasma	Uncommon	Hyperlipidaemia	Shared decision-making → Discuss lifestyle change, statin use
Mouth			
Dry mucous membranes	Common	Dehydration	Examination → Check hydration status
Angular stomatitis	Uncommon	Iron deficiency anaemia	Clinical reasoning → Investigate for nutritional cause
Central cyanosis	Uncommon	Hypoxia (respiratory/cardiac)	Safety netting → Oxygen, urgent review
Poor dental hygiene	Common	Risk for infective endocarditis	Health promotion → Advise oral hygiene
Mouth ulcers	Common	Crohn's, coeliac, HIV	Gathering information → Ask about bowel symptoms
Gum/tongue abnormalities	Uncommon	Vitamin deficiencies, systemic disease	Explanation → Investigate deficiencies
Neurological sign			
Asterixis (flapping tremor)	Uncommon	CO_2 retention (COPD), liver failure	Clinical reasoning → Assess for hepatic/respiratory cause

Table 1.2 This table details clinical information you may gather at each stage of the consultation interview

CCCM stage	Example clinical features	Common/ uncommon	What they may indicate	Clinical approach/key skills
1. Initiating the session	Fever, chest pain, cough	Common	Infection, cardiac, or respiratory causes	Establish rapport, identify reason for visit, open-ended questions ("Can you tell me more about what's been happening?")
2. Gathering information	Weight loss, night sweats, fatigue	Common/ uncommon	Malignancy, TB, depression, endocrine disorders	Explore presenting complaint (SOCRATES), full history (HPC, PMH, DH, SH, FH), screen for red flags
3. Physical examination	Pallor, jaundice, clubbing, cyanosis, oedema	Common/ uncommon	Anaemia, liver disease, chronic lung disease, heart failure	Perform focused exam guided by symptoms; interpret signs systematically
4. Explanation and planning	Discuss findings like "You have symptoms suggestive of anaemia"	–	–	Explain diagnosis in lay terms, confirm understanding, discuss investigations & management collaboratively
5. Closing the session	Summarize key findings and next steps	–	–	Safety-netting ("If your symptoms worsen, come back immediately"), ensure patient satisfaction, clarify follow-up
6. Building the relationship (*continuous*)	Empathic response to distress, fatigue, pain	–	May indicate underlying psychosocial distress	Use active listening, show empathy, validate feelings
7. Providing structure (*continuous*)	Managing complex features (e.g. multiple complaints like cough + weight loss + haemoptysis)	–	Could indicate lung cancer or TB	Keep consultation organized, use signposting ("Let's discuss your cough first...")
8. Clinical reasoning/ problem solving	Haematuria, ascites, focal weakness	Uncommon	Kidney disease, liver disease, stroke	Integrate history, exam, and investigations; prioritize differential diagnoses
9. Shared decision-making	Long-term conditions (e.g. diabetes, hypertension)	Common	Chronic disease management	Discuss lifestyle, medications, patient preferences; encourage autonomy

(continued)

Table 1.2 (continued)

CCCM stage	Example clinical features	Common/ uncommon	What they may indicate	Clinical approach/key skills
10. Safety netting and follow-up	Red flag symptoms (e.g. haematemesis, chest pain radiating to jaw)	Uncommon but urgent	GI bleed, acute coronary syndrome	Give clear advice on when to return, document plan, ensure continuity of care

Table 1.3 This table contains information about different case studies you required to apply the CCCM to plan their care

Case Study 1

Mohammad is a 22-year-old male presented with weakness, weight loss, and low appetite for few months. He has a past history of tuberculous spondylitis, but he was successfully treated with anti-tuberculous drugs.

However, Mohammed experienced a severe backache since then and became dependent on narcotics for pain management. He is currently living alone after his mother's death and is suffering from depression. Since then, Mohammad received several courses of parenteral iron therapy and he is currently presenting with pallor, glossitis, angular stomatitis, and shortness of breath.

His nails are brittle, ridged, and spoon-shaped (koilonychias) and his BMI is 17.58 kg/m^2 indicating mild thinness. Complete blood counts showed a low haemoglobin (8.1 g/L) and a low haematocrit (26.4). Subsequent tests showed serum ferritin of 2 ng/mL and an upper GI endoscopy was advised but refused by the patient.

Case Study 2

Layla is widowed, 60 years of age, and a retired post office clerk. Her main complaint is breathlessness after moderate exertion, unable to walk more than 100 m without stopping due to breathlessness. Layla has a cough that produces yellow sputum (particularly in the mornings) and an intermittent wheeze. Her symptoms have worsened over the last 6 months, and she feels anxious leaving the house alone because of her breathlessness and reduced exercise tolerance.

Layla smokes 10 cigarettes a day, but she has not experienced any haemoptysis (coughing up blood) or chest pain, and her weight is stable; a body mass index of 40 kg/m^2 meaning she is classified as obese. She has had three exacerbations of COPD in the previous 12 months, each managed in the community with amoxicillin, prednisolone, tiotropium, and salbutamol. Her predicted FEV1 (Forced expiratory volume for the first minute) is 57%.

Layla admitted to only using the inhalers, despite also being prescribed a combined Beclomethasone and formetrol inhaler.

Case Study 3

Barbara is an 80-year-old lady living on her own with a past medical history of type 2 diabetes, hypertension, and depression. Barbara has also reduced mobility due to a previous fall which resulted in a total hip replacement.

Barbara has been generally feeling unwell over the past week and was admitted to hospital with a recurrent productive cough. On admission Barbara's bloods showed a rise in CRP, WCC, and an x-ray showed right lower lobe consolidation. She was started on Tazocin 4.5 g and admitted to a respiratory ward for further management of right lower lobe pneumonia.

On admission to the ward Barbara's observations and blood results were as follows: Temperature 38.5 °C, BP 90/50 mmHg, HR 110/min, O2Saturations 90% on room air, bloods and ABG, CRP >10 mg/L, WCC 14.7, PaO2 7.0 kPa, PaCO2 7.0 kPa.

(continued)

Table 1.3 (continued)

Case Study 4

Stan is an 18-year old, Afro-Caribbean, who lives with parents and has a past medical history of sickle cell anaemia. He recently complained of dyspnoea, and feeling tired, sleeping most of the day with little or no appetite and nausea. Stan also mentioned he is in pain in his legs and arms (VAS score 8). Stan was eventually prescribed Diamorphine 5 mg IM, oxygen, and planned exchange transfusion.

His blood results were: Haemoglobin was 7.5 g/dL, mean corpuscular volume (MCV) under 70 fl., Haematocrit: 0.26, Ferritin: 128 mg/L.

Case Study 5

Helen is a 28-year-old asthmatic who suffers from a cough that is worse at night and is having to take a few days off work each month due to her asthma symptoms. Helen smokes mainly at weekends when she is out with friends but would like to give up.

She admits sometimes forgets to take her inhalers. She is keen to get her asthma under control as it is beginning to affect his life.

Bibliography

1. Arkowitz, H., Miller, W. R., & Rollnick, S. (Eds.). (2015). *Motivational interviewing in the treatment of psychological problems*. Guilford Publications.
2. Baniaghil, A. S., Ghasemi, S., Rezaei-Aval, M., & Behnampour, N. (2022). Effect of communication skills training using the Calgary-Cambridge model on interviewing skills among midwifery students: A randomized controlled trial. *Iranian Journal of Nursing and Midwifery Research, 27*(1), 24–29.
3. Dayasiri, K., Krishnapradeep, S., Caldera, D., Wijayasinghe, H., & Mudiyanse, R. (2025). Effectiveness of a Calgary-Cambridge model-based communication skills training for paediatric trainees in Sri Lanka: A nationwide pre-post intervention study using observed practices. *Patient Education and Counseling, 133*, 108635.
4. Kurtz, S. M. (2002). Doctor-patient communication: Principles and practices. *Canadian Journal of Neurological Sciences, 29*(S2), S23–S29.
5. Kurtz, S. M., & Cooke, L. J. (2017). Communication training. In *Oxford textbook of communication in oncology and palliative care*. https://doi.org/10.1093/med/9780198736134.001.0001. Oxford University Press.
6. Kurtz, S., Silverman, J., Benson, J., & Draper, J. (2003). Marrying content and process in clinical method teaching: enhancing the Calgary–Cambridge guides. *Academic Medicine, 78*(8), 802–809.
7. McCance, T., & McCormack, B. (2017). The person-centred practice framework. In *Person-centred practice in nursing and health care: Theory and practice* (pp. 36–64). Wiley.
8. Miller, W. R., & Rollnick, S. (2012). *Motivational interviewing: Helping people change*. Guilford Press.
9. Miller, W. R., & Rollnick, S. (2012). Meeting in the middle: Motivational interviewing and self-determination theory. *International Journal of Behavioral Nutrition and Physical Activity, 9*(1), 25.
10. Ricci, L., Villegente, J., Loyal, D., Ayav, C., Kivits, J., & Rat, A. C. (2022). Tailored patient therapeutic educational interventions: A patient-centred communication model. *Health Expectations, 25*(1), 276–289.

Clinical History Taking **2**

Learning Objectives

In this part of the chapter, we revisit the Calgary-Cambridge Communication Model (CCCM) with an emphasis on information gathering and differential diagnosis.

Learning Objectives

By the end of this chapter, you will be able to:

Develop and apply a clear structured approach to information gathering from a patient.

Demonstrate a systematic approach to history taking to gain an accurate patient history.

Understand and demonstrate a clear and structured approach to the physical, social, and psychological assessment of the patient using the clinical skill of history taking followed by clinical examination.

Undertake a full assessment of the patient's main problem(s) by gathering accurate information from the patient's history.

Demonstrate taking a patient history of a simple disease.

Common Medical Terms

The list of medical terms below is cited for easy reference and the reader is expected to understand these medical terms before they proceed to read this chapter.

CCCM
History taking
Patient interview

© The Author(s), under exclusive license to Springer Nature Switzerland AG 2026
C. Leliopoulou, L. Holman, *Physical Examination and Diagnostic Skills for Nurses and Allied Health Professionals*,
https://doi.org/10.1007/978-3-032-26539-5_2

Presenting complaint
MJTHREATS
SOCRATES

2.1 Part 1: The Role of History Taking in the Calgary-Cambridge Communication Model (CCCM)

The Calgary-Cambridge Communication Model enables professionals to collect an accurate patient history. The model directs the healthcare professional to ask skilfully the reason why the patient has come to see them. Moreover, the model helps the professional establish rapport with the patient because they are prompted to ask open-ended questions and explore sensitive or personal information with ease. Effective use of verbal and non-verbal communication is at the heart of this model, such as maintaining appropriate eye contact, using affirmative nods, and providing empathetic responses, which all can reinforce rapport and validate the patient's feelings and concerns. Approximately 70–80% of diagnoses can be derived solely based on the patient's history provided that the professional deploys key verbal and non-verbal communication skills to facilitate the patient's articulation of their concerns in their own words. Professionals should be attuned to the patient's body language, tone of voice, and facial expressions, which can provide valuable insights into their emotional state and level of discomfort. By being observant, healthcare professionals can better tailor their questioning and approach to meet the needs of the patient. This becomes especially significant in situations where patients may be reluctant or hesitant to disclose information due to fear, embarrassment, or misunderstanding.

Assumptions should be avoided and the patient's narrative should be directly received instead. This can be facilitated by gathering through open-ended questioning to understand the patient's experiences and comprehensively evaluate the patient and their presenting complaint. This skilful assessment empowers the patient to take an active role in their health assessment and underscores the importance of their contribution to the process. Precise questioning can facilitate a conducive environment for the patient before proceeding to undertaking the physical examination. It is important to note that initial impressions often hold significant accuracy during the history taking process.

Understanding a patient's cultural background, including their beliefs, values, and communication styles, is necessary for achieving an accurate and comprehensive history. A culturally sensitive approach allows professionals to avoid biases and assumptions that may distort the patient's narrative and can lead to inaccuracies in diagnosis and treatment. Engaging in discussions about cultural preferences and practices can empower patients and create a more inclusive healthcare environment.

As the history taking process unfolds, it is beneficial for the clinician to employ a systematic approach to ensure that all relevant aspects of the patient's experience are explored. This may include gathering information about the patient's medical history, family history, and psychosocial factors that could influence their current condition. Each of these components contributes to forming a holistic view of the patient and facilitates a more thorough assessment, ultimately leading to more accurate diagnoses and effective treatment plans.

The CCCM framework underscores the essential role of patient history taking in clinical practice. By harnessing effective communication skills, fostering rapport, and accounting for cultural sensitivities, healthcare professionals can facilitate a meaningful exchange of information that elevates the standard of care provided. The active involvement of patients in their assessment not only enhances the accuracy of findings but also promotes their autonomy and reinforces their role as partners in the healthcare process. This collaborative approach is pivotal for informing subsequent diagnostic considerations and optimizing treatment strategies.

> **Learning Point**
> **What is history taking?**
>
> *The process allows the patient to present their account of the problem*
> *It allows the practitioner to gathering data by questioning the patient*
> *It provides essential information to aid diagnosis*
> *Allows the generation of differential diagnosis*
> *Allows the practitioner to evaluating change in the patient's condition*
> *Allows the practitioner to evaluating the impact of a specific disease process*

During history taking you should:

- Explain the reason of the assessment to the patient.
- Establish the reason why the patient seeks medical help.
- Identify with the patient what is the main complaint or presenting problem.
- Explore with the patient when and how the patient realized they had a problem, what they did about it, how they felt about it, and what treatment they had to date.
- Identify any other illnesses they may have had prior to this problem (past medical history, family history, and systems review are all part of the history taking).
- Find out with whom the patient lives and have a meaningful relationship (satisfaction with their sexual relationship, if appropriate) and the extent of support they receive, patient's home conditions and ability to cope with chores, their hobbies and activities, whether they are in work or not, what is their job, do they have any dependents (social assessment).
- Establish the patient's present mood state, in terms of how the illness is affecting them. Pick up cues as to how the patient has been feeling in terms of anxiety and depression (psychological assessment).
- Summarize and prioritize patient's concerns, invite questions, and discuss plan of action and close assessment.

Learning Point

A healthcare professional should take a patient history using a history taking sequence as follows:

1. Presenting compliant/illness (PC)
2. History of the present compliant/illness
3. Past medical history
4. Medication history
5. Family history
6. Social history
7. Occupational history
8. Systemic review
9. Further information from a third party
10. Summary

The Calgary-Cambridge Communication Model (CCCM) is used in clinical practice widely and involves a structured interaction that aims to enhance patient satisfaction, improve documentation, continuity of care, and clinical safety. Within the Calgary-Cambridge Model (CCCM) at stage two under gathering information, the patient is asked about their illness and their presenting complaint.

2.2 Presenting Complaint (PC)

The ability to elicit a detailed and accurate account of the patient's presenting complaint at the beginning of the history taking interview is strategically beneficial, as it allows patients the opportunity to express their concerns freely and in their own words.

Encouraging patients to articulate their symptoms or concerns without interruption is crucial. This approach not only acknowledges the patient's perspective but also mitigates the risk of biasing their narrative with preconceived notions or leading questions. By employing active listening techniques, clinicians can create an environment that fosters trust, thereby enabling patients to disclose sensitive information that may be critical for an accurate diagnosis.

Furthermore, while patients may initially present with a single symptom or issue, it is essential for clinicians to remain attentive to any additional concerns that may arise during the consultation. Patients might present multiple complaints, sometimes prioritizing one over others. Clinicians should remain flexible and adaptive, allowing the discussion to evolve naturally, which can surface underlying issues that might be interrelated or reflective of a broader health concern.

As the patient shares their narrative, it is imperative that clinicians document their accounts verbatim, capturing the essence of the patient's descriptions and using their own words as much as possible. Such documentation not only serves to validate the patient's experience but also enhances the accuracy of recorded information. This practice enriches the clinical picture, providing a nuanced understanding of the patient's condition that can inform subsequent diagnostic and therapeutic decisions.

Moreover, the interaction should be a collaborative dialogue, whereby the clinician intermittently summarizes or paraphrases the patient's statements to confirm understanding and demonstrate engagement. This practice is not only respectful of the patient's narrative but also serves as a mechanism for ensuring clarity and allowing for any necessary corrections or additional details to emerge. By actively involving the patient in this process, the clinician also empowers the patient, thereby promoting a shared decision-making framework that is central to contemporary healthcare practice.

The aim of the history taking is to identify the chief presenting complaint the patient suffers from or think they suffer so we need to ask a direct and open question to the patient. Identifying the main reason(s) why the patient came in is the first step and needs to be recorded the complaint as briefly as possible using patient's own words if possible. The history taking interview usually starts with the open-ended question such as: How can I help you today? What is the reason you came to see me today?

Learning Point

Some example questions we can ask to identify the presenting complaint may include:

- When were you last completely well?
- When did it start and was it gradual or sudden in onset?
- How has it progressed?
- What makes it better and what makes it worse?
- Are there any associated problems?
- Have you had this problem before?

Below there are example questions regarding the presenting complaint which enables the patient to express in their own words what is happening to them.

Example questions you may ask a patient regarding the presenting complaint

- How can I help you today?
- What seems to be the problem?
- What has the problem been?
- What made you go to your doctor?
- Can you tell me the background to how you came to be in hospital?

In the process of history taking, we formulate questions that delve deeper into the history of the presenting complaint and explore relevant associated symptoms. This approach not only enhances the clinician's understanding of the primary issue but also aids in identifying any potential red flags that may indicate more serious underlying conditions. Red flags can include alarming symptoms such as unexplained weight loss, persistent fever, significant changes in bowel or bladder habits, or neurological deficits. Recognizing these indicators early in the assessment is important for timely intervention and appropriate referrals.

Additionally, understanding the impact of the presenting complaint on the patient's daily activities and quality of life is crucial in forming a comprehensive clinical picture. Clinicians should inquire how the symptoms have affected the patient's ability to perform daily tasks, participate in social activities, or fulfil occupational responsibilities. Questions such as "How has your condition affected your daily life?" or "Are there specific activities you are now unable to perform?" can offer insights into the functional limitations imposed by the complaint. This information is essential not only for diagnosing the condition but also for developing a management plan that addresses both medical and psychosocial needs.

Moreover, gathering information about the onset, duration, and progression of symptoms can help clinicians begin to formulate differential diagnoses. Effective questioning should include aspects such as "When did you first notice the symptoms?" and "Have they been consistent, or do they come and go?" Understanding the temporal pattern of symptoms can guide clinicians in distinguishing between acute and chronic conditions and may provide clues to potential aetiologies.

It is also helpful to ask about any associated symptoms that may co-occur with the primary complaint. For instance, if a patient presents with chest pain, inquiring about symptoms such as shortness of breath, nausea, or radiating pain can help the clinician assess the situation with greater accuracy. The interplay of various symptoms often provides critical context that can narrow down the differential diagnosis.

In addition, a thorough exploration of the patient's medical history, including any previous diagnoses, treatments, or surgeries, is instrumental in informing the current clinical assessment. Understanding any pre-existing health conditions or ongoing treatments may reveal connections with the presenting complaint and guide further evaluation.

In conclusion, effective history taking encompasses a multidimensional approach that explores the presenting complaint in depth, assesses potential red flags, and evaluates the impact on the patient's daily life. By employing targeted questioning to elicit relevant details, clinicians can initiate a differential diagnosis framework that not only prioritizes immediate concerns but also considers the holistic well-being of the patient. This thorough practice ultimately enhances clinical decision-making and improves patient outcomes.

2.3   Red Flags

Understanding and identifying red flags may warrant urgent or specialized medical treatment. Red flags can sometimes be underestimated by both patients and clinicians, leading to complications and delays if not addressed promptly. By systematically exploring these symptoms and employing targeted questioning, healthcare professionals can better assess the severity and implications of the presenting complaint.

The outlined questions provide a structured approach to gathering relevant information regarding red flag symptoms, enabling clinicians to gauge their impact effectively. Each inquiry serves to elicit comprehensive responses that illuminate the nature of the complaint:

- **When did the problem start?**
  Understanding the timeline of symptom onset can help differentiate between acute and chronic conditions, guiding the clinician in forming an appropriate differential diagnosis.
- **Is it a new or old problem?**
  Clarifying whether the symptoms are recent or long-standing can inform the clinician's understanding of disease progression and potential causing factors.
- **What did it feel like?**
  Eliciting a description of the symptom helps clinicians assess its characteristics (e.g. sharp, dull, throbbing, or aching) and inform their diagnostic considerations.
- **How often does it occur?**
  Frequency of episodes can illuminate patterns that may be diagnostic cues, contributing to the identification of cyclical conditions or exacerbations of chronic diseases.
- **What starts it off?**
  Identifying triggers or precipitating factors can offer critical insights into the pathology of the symptoms and inform management strategies.
- **How long does it last?**
  The duration of symptoms is crucial for understanding the potential seriousness and management of the condition; transient versus persistent symptoms can suggest different clinical paths.
- **What makes it worse?**
  Understanding aggravating factors can clarify the nature of the condition, furnishing clues that may elucidate whether the issue is mechanical, inflammatory, or systemic.
- **What makes it better?**
  Effective treatments or interventions identified by the patient can inform management strategies and provide insights into the underlying pathology.

- **Does anything else happen to you at the same time, before, or after?**
  Exploring associated symptoms can uncover relationships that provide a broader
  context, enhancing the clinician's diagnostic perspective and leading to more
  accurate assessments.

Incorporating these questions into the patient interview ensures a thorough
assessment of potential red flag symptoms but also promotes a patient-centred
approach by actively engaging patients in their care. This dialogue encourages
patients to articulate their experiences, and further refine the clinician's understanding of the presenting issue.

2.3.1   Red Flag Symptom: Pain

Assessment of pain is a crucial component in the clinical evaluation process, particularly when assessing for red flag symptoms that may indicate serious underlying
pathology. The SOCRATES mnemonic serves as an invaluable tool for healthcare
professionals to systematically gather pertinent information regarding a patient's
pain experience. Each component of the SOCRATES acronym provides a framework for thorough exploration, leading to a comprehensive understanding of the
pain's nature and context.

- **Site:** Precise localization of pain is essential, as it can help in narrowing down
  potential causes. Clinicians should ask, "Where is the pain?" and "Does it radiate?" Understanding whether the pain is localized to a specific area or if it radiates to other parts of the body can guide differential diagnoses, particularly in
  cases of referred pain.
- **Onset of Pain:** Gaining insight into when the pain started for assessing the
  acuity of the condition. Questions such as "When did it start?" can elucidate
  the timeline, aiding in distinguishing between acute and chronic pain
  syndromes.
- **Character:** The quality of pain provides essential diagnostic clues. Clinicians
  might ask, "What type of pain is it?" and "Can you describe it?" Options like
  sharp, dull, throbbing, or burning can indicate different underlying pathologies. Additionally, determining whether the pain is accompanied by other
  symptoms (e.g. nausea, vomiting, or sweating) can be critical in differential
  diagnosis.
- **Precipitating factors:** Identifying triggers that initiate the pain can offer
  insights into its aetiology of the pain and you should inquire about circumstances or activities that precede the onset of pain to uncover potential causative
  factors.
- **Radiation:** Understanding whether the pain radiates to other body parts can be
  pivotal in diagnosing specific conditions. For instance, cardiac pain can often
  present as discomfort radiating to the left arm or jaw, making this inquiry particularly important.

- **Alleviating factors:** Exploring what relieves the pain can provide additional context. And you may ask, "Have you noticed anything that alleviates the pain?" This can include medication, rest, or specific positions that ease discomfort, which may help guide you diagnose.
- **Timing:** Inquiring about the temporal nature of the pain enhances understanding of its pattern. Questions such as "When does it come and go?" and "How long does it last?" can reveal whether the pain is constant or intermittent. This exploration may further inform the clinician's understanding of the patient's condition.
- **Exacerbating factors:** Identifying activities or factors that worsen the pain is also a part of the interview. This information can illuminate the behaviours that may need modification to manage the patient's discomfort effectively.
- **Severity:** Quantifying the pain's intensity help us develop a treatment plan. You can ask, "How severe is the pain?" and encourage patients to use a numerical scale from 1 to 10, with 10 being the worst pain imaginable. In addition, understanding how the pain impacts the patient's daily activities, such as whether it disrupts sleep or prevents them from performing their regular tasks, provides critical insight into the functional implications of their condition.
- Severity: What is the pain like? How bad is it? Can you score your pain from 1 to 10, 10 being worse pain ever? How severe is the pain? Does it wake you at night? Does it stop you doing what you are doing at the time?

2.3.2 Past/Previous Medical History (PMH)

Gathering a comprehensive past medical history helps form an accurate diagnosis and treatment plan. Understanding a patient's previous health issues can provide insight into their medical background and potential risk factors, patterns, and predispositions to certain conditions. Therefore, you must inquire systematically about a patient's past illnesses, hospitalizations, surgical interventions, and treatments received.

When exploring the patient's past medical history, you should elicit details about:

- Serious childhood diseases: Inquiring about significant childhood illnesses, such as rheumatic fever, chickenpox, or other infectious diseases, can help you diagnose as these can have long-term implications on health. For example, certain childhood illnesses may predispose individuals to future complications or affect their immune responses.
- Previous hospital admissions: This information can help you weight up or down the severity and nature of past health issues and asking patients to provide information regarding the reasons for hospital admissions can inform current clinical considerations. For instance, a history of repeated admissions for respiratory conditions may guide further your evaluation for potential underlying causes.
- Surgical history: Previous surgical interventions should be clearly documented, including the type of surgery, dates performed, and any complications that may

have arisen. This information helps us anticipate potential risks in the current clinical context, especially if the patient is presenting with symptoms related to the area that was surgically treated. For example, prior abdominal surgery could influence our approach to a patient presenting with gastrointestinal complaints.

- Treatments received: Documenting any treatments (pharmacological and non-pharmacological) associated with past illnesses should be explored and details about what medications were prescribed, the response to those treatments, and any side effects experienced at the time.

In addition, you should request the dates when diagnoses were made and any follow-up treatments or interventions took place as this information helps you assess the progression of disease, and facilitates a better understanding of the patient's current complaints and overall health trajectory. Moreover, documentation of any chronic conditions, such as hypertension, diabetes, or asthma, should be meticulously maintained, as these comorbidities significantly influence the management of present health issues.

It is important we approach the collection of past medical history with sensitivity and nuance, as some patients may have difficulty recalling specific details or may feel apprehensive about discussing previous health challenges.

Learning Point
The information on past diagnosis should include:

- The actual past medical diagnosis.
- The date the diagnosis was made.
- The sequence of events prior and after the diagnosis in patient's own words.
- The management plan given for patient's illnesses and problems.
- Any current prescribed medication including the name of the drug, the reason for taking it, its dosage and frequency of administration and for how long the patient has been taken it.
- Note any allergies including environmental factors and foods.
- Note any over-the-counter medication the patient may have been taken such as herbal remedies. Here we also need to include the name of the drug, the reason for taking it, its dosage and frequency of administration and for how long the patient has been taken it.
- Check whether the patient is up to date with immunizations for example, patients with co-morbidities to have had their pneumococcal and covid-19 booster jab.
- Find out whether the patient has ever used any illicit drugs in the past.
- It is also important that the nurse assesses patient's compliance with treatment. Some of the questions we need to ask the patient during history taking are:
- Have you experienced any side effects or problems with medication?

- Have you ever had a drug reaction due to an allergy? If yes, what happened? How long did it last? How did they manage their symptom? For example, their rash.
- List of all patients' drugs and doses. Any recent changes in medication, such as increase or decrease in dose or change in the amount of times the patient takes the medication.

Examples of alternative questions you may ask to gain information about patient's past medical history include:

- Have you had any similar problems in the past?
- Have you had any admissions to hospital?
- Have you had any recent illnesses?
- Have you had any chronic conditions?
- Have you had any investigations or operations?

Examples of alternative questions you may ask to gain information about patient's drug allergies include:

- What other medication are you currently taking?
- Have you notice any problems or side effects with your medicines?
- Have you had in the past any side effect with your medicines?

2.3.3   Medical Conditions—MJAMTHREADS

The MJAMTHREADS mnemonic serves as a practical tool to elicit information regarding specific medical conditions that may significantly impact a patient's health status. This structured approach aids comprehensive assessment by asking the patient about specific medical conditions. These questions can be phrased as:

Learning Point
Mnemonic—MJAMTHREADS

- **J—jaundice**
  Have you ever suffered from jaundice?
- **A—anaemia and other haematological conditions**
  Do you suffer from anaemia or other haematological conditions?
- **M—myocardial infarction**
  Have you ever suffered from a Myocardial Infraction?

- **T—tuberculosis**
  Have you ever suffered from tuberculosis?
- **H—hypertension and heart disease**
  Do you suffer from high blood pressure or any cardiac problems?
- **R—rheumatic fever**
  Have you ever suffered from Rheumatic fever?
- **E—epilepsy**
  Have you ever suffered from epilepsy?
- **A—asthma and COPD**
  Have you ever suffered from asthma or COPD?
- **D—diabetes**
  Have you ever suffered from diabetes?
- **S—stroke**

  Have you ever suffered from stroke?

2.3.4 Family History

Finding out about our patient's parents' health and illnesses can give us clues to any predisposition the patient may have to any illnesses. It is also an opportunity for us to find out about any hereditary conditions within the family. At this point in the history taking the patient may raise a concern in relation to family's history about a certain disease or condition within the family. We may also ask whether their parents are alive and well. If they have died, then we need to ask what their parent(s) died from and at what age. We also need to ask for each parent about their diagnosis, age of onset, and, if appropriate, age and cause of death.

Example of questions to gain information about your patient's family history include:

- Are your parents alive and well?
- If they have died, how did they? What age were they? What did they die from?
- Have you got any brothers and sisters? How old are they? Any health problems?
- Is this a disease running through the family or not?
- Has anyone else in the family been diagnosed with this illness?

2.3.5 Systems Review

At this point of the interview, you will have some idea of what the problem is but there is still scope for further review to eliminate any other potential diagnoses. This can be achieved by undertaking a general review of the main body systems on top of MJAMTHREAD screening. We may also offer the patient a "head to toe" assessment because illnesses can affect different parts of the body and many illnesses may be multi-system. Therefore, it is important to ask about connected symptoms.

- *Review of the nervous system and neurological symptoms*: This system can be hard to assess as some of the symptoms can be shared across different illnesses across systems. Some example questions you can ask are:
  - Have you had any headaches? This is a symptom with wide diagnostic range from head injury to brain tumours.
  - Have you experienced any altered sensation? Changes in the sense of smell can result from head injury or following a viral upper respiratory tract infection.
  - Have you noted any visual disturbances or dizziness? Have you had any fits? Or experience any fainting? Here we need to establish when it happened and any warning symptoms or any seizure activity may have taken place.
  - Have you noticed a hearing loss, tinnitus (ringing), dizziness or vertigo? Changes in hearing can result from aging, infections and tumour compression.
  - Have you notice any muscle weakness, pins and needles? Stroke can lead to muscle weakness and sensory changes. Motor neurone disease usually lead to muscle weakness without sensory changes. On the other hand, diabetes can cause sensory changes.
  - Have you ever experienced loss of consciousness or blackouts? Establish the situation when it occurred and if they had any witness to this.
  - Have you ever experienced any mood swings? They can be related to menopause or other hormonal changes.
  - Have you ever experienced any disturbances in your memory and/or concentration? This is common symptom in menopause.
    Have you noticed any changes in your vision? Altered vision can be due to optic nerve damage or can be due to lesions of the oculomotor, trochlear, and abducens nerves. This is an important part of the body which often is overlooked hence a systematic approach to assessing symptoms associated with the eyes is vital in making a diagnosis.
- *Review of the endocrine system*. Have you had any swelling in the neck? This could be a clinical sign for thyroid enlargement. Have you noticed you can't tolerate easily heat and/or cold? This symptom is associated with thyroid dysfunction.
- *Review of the cardiovascular system*. Have you experienced any chest pain? Cardiovascular system. Shortness of breath (dyspnoea) after exertion is caused by poor heart function or pulmonary oedema. Exercise tolerance history is also important to be taken from the patient. Have you got any palpitations? Palpitations refer to awareness of heart beat but it could mean different things to different people. Thus, we should carefully ask patient to describe their heartbeat. Have you noticed your ankles swelling? Swelling of the ankles can be associated with right side heart failure, decreased levels of albumin and certain drugs (calcium

channel blockers). Do you have calf swelling? This can be due to deep vein thrombosis thus it is important we assess this for patients who had surgery recently, immobility and people who travel long haul flights. Do you usually have cold hands and feet? This can indicate poor peripheral circulation in the patient.

- *Review of the respiratory system*. Have you got any shortness of breath? What do you think cause your shortness of breath? When does it happen more often at rest, on exertion, on lying flat at night? Have you got any chest pain? You need to establish the nature of the chest pain in respiratory system this pain is usually associated with pleuritic conditions (pneumothorax, pneumonia, pulmonary embolism). A screening tool may help assess chess pain such as the Mnemonic—SOCRATES

  1. Have you got any shortness of breath?
  2. Assess the severity of the shortness of breath and any associated symptoms with it.
  3. Have you got any cough? Cough is an important respiratory symptom caused by a number of pathologies and associated symptoms can help make a differential diagnosis.
  4. Have you got any wheeze in your chest? Wheezes are caused by airway obstructions and can be heard on expiratory phase of patient's breathing.
  5. Have you got any sputum? How much? What colour was it? Did you cough up any blood? Sputum can be yellow, green in colour which can be due to infection in the lungs. Pink frothy sputum is found in pulmonary oedema. Blood stained sputum is usually found in lung cancer, pulmonary embolism, and pneumonia.

- *Review of gastrointestinal system*. Some example questions can be:
  - How is your appetite? Change in appetite can be noted at different stages of a disease (cancer, diabetes).
  - Have you got any abdominal pain? You need to establish the nature of the abdominal pain in the gastrointestinal system, this pain is usually associated with gastric ulcer to oesophageal or stomach cancer. A screening tool may help assess chess pain such as the Mnemonic—SOCRATES (Talley & O'Connor 2010)
    - Site—Where is the pain?
    - Onset—When did the pain start, and was it sudden or gradual?
    - Character—What is the pain like? An ache? Stabbing?
    - Radiation—Does the pain radiate anywhere?
    - Associations—Any other signs or symptoms associated with the pain?
    - Time—Does the pain follow any pattern?
    - Exacerbating/Relieving factors—Does anything change the pain? Severity—How bad is the pain?
  - Have you noticed any dysphagia (difficulty in swallowing)? Where things get stuck? Is there a difficulty with fluid, solid, or both? If there are mechanical

obstruction (cancer) dysphagia will be for solids first and later on for fluids. If dysphagia is caused by neuromuscular disease then the patient will experience difficulties with swallowing fluids at onset.

Have you noticed any change in bowel habit? Have you seen any stool change (blood in stool is called melena)? You should also ask about patient having any diarrhoea and constipation or alternating with each other and for the presence of rectum bleeding with or without mucus. You should also observe or find out from the patient about the colour and texture of the faeces (bloody, too pale, too dark).

Some example questions related to the GI system are:

- Have you lost or put any weight in the past 6 weeks? Was it intentional to lose or put on weight? How much did you lose or put on during this period? Weight lost can have multiple causes but it can also be the first sign of malignant tumour.
- Have you been feeling nauseous? Have you been vomiting? Any blood? What colour was your vomit? Vomiting red blood is a sign of upper gastrointestinal bleeding. Coffee brown colour vomit indicates old upper gastrointestinal bleeding.
- Have you been suffering with indigestion and/or flatulence? How often? Indigestion (heartburn) is due to gastric acid reflux into the oesophagus and usually is associated with burping and belching.
  Have you noticed any jaundice or itching of the skin (yellowish of the skin)? Jaundice may indicate liver function impairment and built up of bile in the liver can cause itchiness which is a feature of obstructive jaundice.

- *Review of the genitourinary system.* Some example questions can be:
  - Have you got any difficulty passing urine or a burning sensation when passing urine? This is known as dysuria due to urinary tract infection.
  - Have you noticed an increase in frequency in passing urine? How badly do you need to go (urgency) to pass urine? Frequency and urgency in passing urine can be associated with bladder irritation caused by infection, tumour, and kidney stones. Other causes of increased frequency and urgency can be outflowing obstruction of the bladder such as prostatic hypertrophy and neurological causes such as multiple sclerosis. However, decreased frequency in passing urine can be due to dehydration or kidney failure.
  - Do you notice any blood in urine (haematuria)? Is your urine clear or cloudy? Red colour in the urine may be caused by certain types of food such as beetroots. Blood in urine should be further investigated. Cloudy urine could be due to infection.
  - Have you had loin pain? This pain can be found in kidney conditions such pyelonephritis and Reynold calculus.
    Have you experienced any symptoms such as difficulties in starting and stopping or poor stream? This is a feature of prostatic enlargement clinical presentation and it could be benign or indicate carcinoma of the prostate gland.

- *Review of the musculoskeletal review.* Some example questions can be:
    - Have you got any joint pain and/or stiffness? Any swelling? These symptoms can help diagnose conditions such as arthritis but further investigation needed to exclude other conditions.
      Have you ever had backache? This is a common musculoskeletal symptom caused by a number of diseases and conditions such as bad posture, osteoporosis, and ankylosing spondylitis.
- *Review of the skin.* Some example questions can be:
      Have you got any rashes or skin conditions? Distribution and character of rashes, lumps and bumps can help determine the diagnosis. Skin rashes can vary from anaphylactic to infection rashes. Changes in moles need to be further investigated. Any changes in moles can be a first sign of skin cancer.

2.3.6 Social Assessment

Social History

This part of the interview is also crucial to gathering information about the patient as a person. It gives insight into how the illness affects the patient and their family and what are their home circumstances.

Learning Point

Example questions you can use during social history include:

- What do you do for living?
- Do you have a partner? Is your partner fit and well? Do you have children?
- Where do you live? What is your home life like?
- Do you have any hobbies?
- How have you been in general?
- Do you exercise regularly? What type of exercise do you take? How often?
- How is your social life? Do you go out? How often?
- Do you smoke? Do you drink? How much? How often? How long have you been drinking? What type of drinks? Asking about alcohol and drug use can sometimes be difficult, it is easier to be very open and direct. If you suspect a patient has an alcohol or drug problem, then more detailed questioning can occur.
- Are you using any recreational drugs?
- How much do you weight? Any dietary requirements? Any allergies?

2.3.7   Mental Health Assessment

Mental Health History
The use of skilful interviewing techniques includes responding to emotional cues such as "this must be difficult for you", showing understanding of patient's feelings for example, "I understand why you feel upset". Most importantly you should always respect patient's efforts "you did your best under the circumstances".

Learning Point
Example questions you can use during mental health history include:

- How are you today?
- How have you been feeling recently?
- Tell me more about…Have you felt low, depressed, or hopeless at any time?
- Do you usually enjoy doing things?
- Are you interested in things?
- How have you been sleeping?
- How has your mood been recently?
- What is your diet at the moment?
- How do you feel about yourself?
- Have you ever felt the same way before?
- Do you have any past mental illness?
- Are you currently taking any prescribed medication or over the counter treatments?

In this last part of history taking you should summarize and prioritize patient's concerns, invite questions, discuss the management plan of action, and close the history taking.

Example phrases you can use to close the history taking include:

- So, to sum up in the past week/month/year you ….
- The plan of action is ….
- Any questions?
- Thank the patient for their time.

2.4   Part 2: Student Activities

Focused Learning
Case Study

Kathy is a 48-year-old teacher with four children and works at the local college. She is a single parent but her mum lives nearby and helps her with the younger kids. Kathy is vegetarian and recently has been diagnosed with asthma and arthritis. She drinks 4 units of alcohol per week and is vegetarian. She exercises regularly and loves rowing. In the past few months Kathy has been feeling dizzy and very tired, but she thought it was due to her hectic life as a single parent and working mum. Last week she felt so dizzy that she collapsed on a tiled floor and hurt her left hip.

Learning Activity 1

Kathy, a 48-year-old teacher, presents with complaints of dizziness and fatigue, which have significantly worsened over the past few months. Her recent episode of dizziness culminated in a collapse where she sustained an injury to her left hip.

(a) Can you assess Kathy's presenting complaint?

Answer

1. *Dizziness:*
   - *Onset: When did you first notice dizziness?*
   - *Nature: Can you describe the dizziness? Is it spinning (vertigo) or just a feeling of light-headedness?*
   - *Duration: How long does the dizziness last? Is it constant or intermittent?*
   - *Triggers: Have you noticed any specific activities or positions that exacerbate the dizziness?*
2. *Fatigue:*
   - *Onset: When did you start feeling excessively tired?*
   - *Characteristics: Is the fatigue affecting your ability to perform daily activities, including work and parenting?*
   - *Sleep: How are you sleeping? Do you feel rested in the morning?*
3. *Hip Injury:*
   - *Details of the fall: How did it happen? Were there any preceding symptoms?*
   - *Current symptoms: Is there ongoing pain, swelling, or reduced mobility in the hip?*
   - *Previous injuries: Have you had any similar incidents or falls in the past?*
4. *Asthma and Arthritis:*
   - *Control of asthma symptoms: Do you have an asthma action plan? Have you had any recent exacerbations?*
   - *Arthritis management: What treatments or medications are you currently using? Are you experiencing joint pain that affects your daily life?*

Learning Activity 2

(b) What treatment plans are you suggesting for Kathy?

Answer

- *Management of anaemia:*
  - *Education on anaemia: I will explain anaemia in simple terms, focusing on symptoms like tiredness and dizziness. I'll also explain any prescribed ferrous sulphate treatment (1× daily for 3 months) and potential side effects (e.g. stomach upset, constipation).*
  - *Encourage adherence to the medication plan and monitor for any side effects.*
- *Dietary assessment:*
  - *Kathy follows a vegetarian diet but also check eating habits.*
  - *I'll provide education on how to improve intake and highlight iron-rich foods (e.g. lentils, beans, spinach, tofu, fortified cereals).*
  - *Discuss practical suggestions for including these foods in her diet despite her busy lifestyle (e.g. ready-to-eat meals from stores like Tesco or M&S, joining peer vegetarian groups).*
  - *I'll also address the importance of combining iron with vitamin C to aid absorption (e.g. oranges, tomatoes).*
- *Physical activity:*
  - *Encourage her to engage in regular, light physical activity to combat fatigue (e.g. 10–15-min daily walks, using stairs instead of the lift, walking the dogs).*
- *Stress and sleep hygiene:*
  - *Discuss the impact of stress and poor sleep on her symptoms, considering her full-time job and busy family life.*
  - *Encourage prioritizing rest and ensuring adequate sleep.*
- *Referral to dietitian:*
  - *Given her busy lifestyle and dietary challenges, I will refer her to a dietitian to support her in making sustainable dietary changes.*

Learning Activity 3

(c) Can you take Kathy's history using the CCCM?

Answer

Presenting Complaint/Illness: Kathy presents with dizziness and fatigue that have been worsening over the past few months. She experienced a significant episode where she collapsed after feeling very dizzy, resulting in a hip injury.

History of the Present Complaint/Illness:

- ***Dizziness:*** *Kathy reports that her dizziness started several months ago. Initially, she attributed it to the demands of being a single parent and working. The dizziness has increased in severity, culminating in a fall last week.*

- *Fatigue:* Kathy has been experiencing excessive tiredness, which she initially dismissed as a consequence of her hectic lifestyle. The fatigue is impacting her daily life and ability to engage in activities with her children.
- *Recent Episode:* Kathy describes the incident last week where she felt overwhelmingly dizzy and collapsed, hitting her left hip on the tiled floor. She has pain, a bruise, and some mobility issues since the fall.

Past Medical History:
- *Asthma:* Recently diagnosed; need details on management and control.
- *Arthritis:* Also a recent diagnosis; need to clarify the type and management.
- *Other Illnesses:* No additional details provided; further inquiry needed regarding any significant past medical conditions, especially childhood illnesses.

Medication History:
- Need to clarify if Kathy is currently prescribed any medications for asthma or arthritis. She may also take over-the-counter medications or supplements related to her vegetarian diet. Inquiry into past medication responses and any side effects is necessary.

Family History:
- Inquire about any family medical history relevant to chronic conditions such as asthma, arthritis, cardiovascular diseases, and other significant health issues that may suggest a genetic predisposition.

Social History:
- *Diet:* Kathy is a vegetarian; it is essential to explore her dietary habits to ensure she is obtaining adequate nutrients, particularly iron and vitamin B12.
- *Alcohol Consumption:* Kathy consumes approximately 4 units of alcohol per week; inquire if this has changed recently.
- *Lifestyle:* Kathy exercises regularly and enjoys rowing. Explore how her fatigue and dizziness affect her ability to maintain her usual level of activity and her parenting responsibilities.

Occupational History:
- Kathy works as a teacher at a local college. Inquire about her work environment, hours, and any stressors related to her job that may contribute to fatigue or health issues.

Systemic Enquiry:
- *Cardiovascular:* Assess for any chest pain, palpitations, or shortness of breath.
- *Respiratory:* Given her asthma, inquire if she has experienced any exacerbations or respiratory symptoms.
- *Gastrointestinal:* Check for any changes in appetite, digestion, or bowel habits.

- *Neurological: Assess for headaches, visual disturbances, or other neurological symptoms.*
- *Musculoskeletal: Document any joint pain or limitations related to her arthritis, especially concerning her left hip after the recent fall.*

Further Information from a Third Party:
- *If needed, gather additional insight from Kathy's mother, who is nearby and may have observed changes in Kathy's health or lifestyle affecting her ability to care for her children. This can provide context on any recent developments in her physical or mental wellbeing.*

Summary: Kathy is a 48-year-old vegetarian teacher who is a single parent of four children. She recently experienced a worsening of dizziness and fatigue, leading to a collapse and injury to her hip. Her past medical history includes newly diagnosed asthma and arthritis. A comprehensive review of her health, dietary habits, and socioeconomic factors will be essential for diagnosing potential nutritional deficiencies, assessing the management of her chronic conditions, and addressing any contributing factors to her symptoms. This holistic approach will aid in developing an effective treatment plan tailored to her specific needs and lifestyle. Further investigation of her dietary intake and potential referrals to specialists may be necessary based on the gathered information.

Learning Activity 5
(d) What are the differential diagnoses for Kathy?

Answer

Based on Kathy's symptoms and history, several differential diagnoses can be considered for her presenting complaints of dizziness and fatigue, as well as her recent collapse and hip injury. The following differential diagnoses encompass a variety of potential underlying conditions that may require further investigation:

Orthostatic hypotension:
Kathy's dizziness could be related to orthostatic hypotension, where a significant drop in blood pressure occurs upon standing or changing positions, leading to light-headedness or fainting.

Anaemia:
Given Kathy's vegetarian diet, she could be at risk for iron deficiency anaemia or vitamin B12 deficiency anaemia, both of which can cause fatigue and dizziness. Blood tests would be necessary for confirmation.

Vestibular disorders:
Conditions such as benign paroxysmal positional vertigo (BPPV) or vestibular neuronitis can lead to episodes of dizziness or imbalance. These conditions are

characterized by symptoms that may occur suddenly and typically worsen with certain head movements.

Chronic fatigue syndrome:

If Kathy's fatigue is persistent and disproportionately severe compared to her activity levels, chronic fatigue syndrome could be considered. This condition is often accompanied by unexplained fatigue that is not improved by rest.

Hypothyroidism:

Fatigue and dizziness can be symptoms of an underactive thyroid. A thyroid function test would be necessary to rule out thyroid dysfunction.

Psychological factors:

Stress, anxiety, or depression can manifest as physical symptoms, including fatigue and dizziness. A thorough mental health assessment may be beneficial to determine if psychological factors are contributing.

Cardiovascular issues:

Conditions such as arrhythmias or other cardiovascular abnormalities may present with dizziness, especially if there is a history of heart disease in her family. An evaluation of cardiovascular health, potentially including ECG monitoring, might be warranted.

Medication side effects:

If Kathy is taking any new medications for her recently diagnosed asthma or arthritis, side effects could include dizziness or fatigue. A review of her medication history is essential.

Inner ear problems:

Conditions affecting inner ear function, which plays a crucial role in balance, may lead to dizziness or balance issues. Meniere's disease or labyrinthitis could also be considered.

Dehydration or electrolyte imbalance:

Particularly with a busy lifestyle, dehydration or disruptions in electrolyte balance can cause dizziness and fatigue. Assessing fluid intake and potential dietary insufficiencies is important.

Neurological conditions:

Although less likely, certain neurological conditions could lead to dizziness and fatigue. These may include multiple sclerosis or transient ischemic attacks (TIAs). A neurological assessment would be appropriate in the context of significant red flags.

Underlying infections:

Any acute or chronic infections, such as a urinary tract infection or respiratory infection, can manifest with systemic symptoms like fatigue and dizziness.

Bibliography

1. Arkowitz, H., Miller, W. R., & Rollnick, S. (Eds.). (2015). *Motivational interviewing in the treatment of psychological problems.* Guilford Publications.
2. Baniaghil, A. S., Ghasemi, S., Rezaei-Aval, M., & Behnampour, N. (2022). Effect of communication skills training using the Calgary-Cambridge model on interviewing skills among

midwifery students: A randomized controlled trial. *Iranian Journal of Nursing and Midwifery Research, 27*(1), 24–29.

3. Bickley, L. (2012). *Bates' guide to physical examination and history taking.* Lippincott Williams & Wilkins.

4. Dayasiri, K., Krishnapradeep, S., Caldera, D., Wijayasinghe, H., & Mudiyanse, R. (2025). Effectiveness of a Calgary-Cambridge model-based communication skills training for paediatric trainees in Sri Lanka: A nationwide pre-post intervention study using observed practices. *Patient Education and Counseling, 133*, 108635.

5. Kurtz, S. M. (2002). Doctor-patient communication: Principles and practices. *Canadian Journal of Neurological Sciences, 29*(S2), S23–S29.

6. Kurtz, S. M., & Cooke, L. J. (2017). Communication training. In *Oxford textbook of communication in oncology and palliative care.* https://doi.org/10.1093/med/9780198736134.001.0001 Oxford University Press.

7. Kurtz, S., Silverman, J., Benson, J., & Draper, J. (2003). Marrying content and process in clinical method teaching: enhancing the Calgary–Cambridge guides. *Academic Medicine, 78*(8), 802–809.

8. McCance, T., & McCormack, B. (2017). The person-centred practice framework. In *Person-centred practice in nursing and health care: Theory and practice* (pp. 36–64). Wiley.

9. Miller, W. R., & Rollnick, S. (2012). *Motivational interviewing: Helping people change.* Guilford Press.

10. Miller, W. R., & Rollnick, S. (2012). Meeting in the middle: Motivational interviewing and self-determination theory. *International Journal of Behavioral Nutrition and Physical Activity, 9*(1), 25.

11. Ricci, L., Villegente, J., Loyal, D., Ayav, C., Kivits, J., & Rat, A. C. (2022). Tailored patient therapeutic educational interventions: A patient-centred communication model. *Health Expectations, 25*(1), 276–289.

12. Talley, N. J., & O'connor, S. (2010). Clinical examination: a systematic guide to physical diagnosis. Elsevier Australia.

13. Wieling, W., Kaufmann, H., Claydon, V. E., et al. (2022). Diagnosis and treatment of orthostatic hypotension. *Lancet Neurology, 21*(8), 735–746. https://doi.org/10.1016/S1474-4422(22)00169-7

Learning Objectives

In this part of the chapter, we revisit basic anatomy and physiology of the respiratory system and identify the clinical signs and symptoms diagnostic of respiratory disease and disorders.

Learning Objectives
By the end of this chapter, you will be able to:

Identify the key points to note on seeing the patient for the first time.
Assess the mobility and posture to explain the common disorders of gait.
Describe and explain distinctive physical changes associated with specific diseases.
Assess the state of hydration (dehydration and oedema) and nutrition.
Explain the general features of common vitamin deficiencies.
Identify and explain abnormal skin colour changes.
Inspect and palpate the sites associated with lymph node enlargement.
Describe and explain ways in which the body temperature may be assessed.

Common Medical Terms

The list of medical terms below is cited for easy reference and the reader is expected to understand these medical terms before they proceed to read this chapter.

Angular stomatitis
Atrophic glossitis
Ataxic gait
Clubbing

© The Author(s), under exclusive license to Springer Nature Switzerland AG 2026

C. Leliopoulou, L. Holman, *Physical Examination and Diagnostic Skills for Nurses and Allied Health Professionals,*
https://doi.org/10.1007/978-3-032-26539-5_3

Corneal arcus
Cyanosis
Foot-drop
Gait
Goitre
Hypoalbuminaemia
Jaundice
Koilonychia
Kyphosis
Leukonychia
Lymphadenopathy
Lordosis
Parkinsonian gait
Posture
Scoliosis
Spastic gait
Thyrotoxicosis
Xanthelasmata
Oedema
Waddling-Myopathic gait

3.1   Part 1: Seeing the Patient for the First Time

Our first impressions of patients during general examinations are vital in determining the overall approach to care and can significantly influence clinical assessment. These impressions are formed through careful observation and communication, succinctly capturing essential components of the patient's overall health and demeanour. Observing closely the patient's body can help assess and diagnose illnesses and diseases. This observation may involve looking (inspection), feeling (palpation), tapping (percussion), and listening (auscultation) during physical examination. In cardiovascular, respiratory, and abdominal assessment, all four physical examination skills (inspection, palpation, percussion, and tapping) are used to varying degrees. In musculoskeletal and neurological systems, we normally involve only inspection and palpation. Differentiating between normal and abnormal parameters across each system can help identify subtle changes and spot pathologies.

> **Learning Point**
> As the healthcare professional undertaking physical examination, you may consider the following prior:
>
> - Use of appropriate communication skills to suit the patient's condition and behavioural responses. Attentive listening to what the patient has to say,

clear articulation of their concern, and an empathetic response to their issues may foster a supportive environment, allowing patients to express their concerns comfortably. Adapting your tone, language complexity, and non-verbal communication techniques can enhance rapport between you and the patient.

- During history taking you should evaluate whether the patient exhibits signs of illness such as pallor, diaphoresis, or distress suggesting they may suffer from underlying medical issues requiring immediate attention. Patient's overall demeanour can provide important clues about their illness.
- Spot diagnoses immediately recognizable through physical signs. For example, in Herpes Zoster infection (Shingles) there is a distinctive vesicular rash along a dermatome so you may note this in their notes, or with Parkinson's disease often you may denote a distinctive shuffling gait, bradykinesia, and tremors or in Cushing's syndrome you may spot a rounded, red facial appearance (moon facies) and fatty tummy.
- Also understanding the patient's emotional state such as signs of anxiety, depression, distraction, or anger can provide insights into their psychological well-being which may inform how mental health may be affecting their physical health.
- Observation of obvious physical abnormalities such as limb asymmetry, skin lesions, or joint deformities. Documenting these abnormalities during the general examination at initial assessment helps establish baseline data and may influence further diagnostic evaluations.
- The patient's attire, grooming, personal hygiene, and any noticeable body odour can reflect their health status and psychosocial conditions. Poor hygiene or inappropriate dress may indicate depression, neglect, or socio-economic factors affecting them.
- The patient's posture and mobility provide insights into their musculoskeletal and neurological conditions. Assessing gait can reveal issues related to balance, strength, and coordination, which are essential for understanding their functional capabilities.
- Also, taking measurements of height and weight helps for calculating body mass index (BMI) and understanding their overall health. Observing body shape can indicate potential nutritional issues or metabolic conditions that may warrant further exploration.

A gentle handshake upon first meeting the patient can yield valuable clinical information. Through this action, you can assess hand deformities or joint issues that may indicate underlying health problems; their grip strength, which can reflect general muscle function and the temperature of the hands, which can suggest circulatory health or systemic conditions.

3.2   Mobility, Posture, and Gait

Assessing their mobility, posture, and gait may give you an insight into their overall physical health, functional abilities, and potential underlying conditions. Mobility assessment involves observing the patient's ease of movement in various contexts, including how they sit, stand, and walk.

Learning Point

Key aspects to consider include:

- Ease of Movement: Note how effortlessly the patient transitions between sitting and standing, and their ability to manoeuvre in space. Utilize non-verbal cues to assess any visible struggle or hesitation.
- Observe whether the patient uses a walking stick, cane, or wheelchair, and assess how they utilize these aids. The presence of assistive devices can indicate reduced mobility and related health issues.
- Reduced mobility can significantly affect a patient's quality of life, particularly in older adults, and they may increase the risk of falls and associated complications, including mortality.
- Assessing a patient's posture and gait provides crucial information about their musculoskeletal and nervous systems. Alterations in posture and gait can be important indicators of conditions affecting mobility, especially in older adults.
- Postural changes also should be noted in this first meeting with the patient. Physical abnormalities such as kyphosis, scoliosis, and lordosis can lead to altered posture and consequently impact gait. A careful history should be taken to discern potential causes of these abnormalities.

Learning Point

- Kyphosis: *Increased flexion* of the spine leading to a *hunchback appearance*, associated with loss of height and characterized by forward bending postures.
- Scoliosis: *Lateral curvature* of the spine that may present with *uneven shoulders and hips*, significantly altering the patient's centre of gravity and stability.
- Lordosis: *Increased extension* of the spine, which can be either congenital or a result of prolonged poor posture, *affecting alignment and movement*.

3.2.1 Gait Assessment

Differentiating normal gait from abnormal gait is key in diagnostics because gait requires coordination between the musculoskeletal and nervous systems, and changes can provide insights into neurological or muscular disorders. Many diseases can impact a person's ability to walk.

Assessment of normal gait typically includes:

- Natural gait: The ability to walk and turn smoothly and in a coordinated manner, with natural upper extremity movements complementing the walking cycle.
- Tandem gait: This involves asking the patient to walk heel-to-toe in a straight line, which tests balance and strength in the distal lower extremities. The patient should be able to perform this without losing balance or deviating to the side.

Learning Point
Assessment of abnormal gait recognition typically includes five primary types of abnormal gaits:

- Spastic gait: Characterized by dragging feet while walking, with stiff and slow movements. This gait type signifies weakness and stiffness, often associated with cerebrovascular disorders such as stroke.
- Foot-drop gait: The individual flexes the leg at the hip excessively to prevent the toes from catching while walking, creating a stamping action when the foot strikes the ground. Typically caused by peripheral neuropathy or motor neuron disorders that lead to weakness and sensory loss.
- Ataxic gait: This gait is marked by an unsteady stance and broad base, with the patient lurching from side to side when walking. This condition often arises from cerebellar diseases, such as tumours affecting the cerebellum.
- Parkinsonian gait: Indicates a stooped posture and difficulty in initiating movement, often leading to small, shuffling steps. This gait is commonly associated with Parkinson's disease.
- Waddling-myopathic gait: Described by an inability to tilt the pelvis appropriately when swinging each leg through during walking, leading to exaggerated lateral trunk movements. This gait is associated with proximal muscle disorders, such as those seen in thyrotoxicosis.

Assessing mobility, posture, and gait during a general examination can identify potential health issues and inform significant patient care. By understanding normal and abnormal gait patterns and the underlying conditions associated with these variations, as a healthcare professional can facilitate early detection and intervention, and ultimately enhance patient safety.

A detailed history taking can pinpoint any abnormalities in posture or gait because it may provide information on the patient's prior medical conditions, lifestyle habits, and any relevant familial trends which can help discern possible causes of observed changes. A detailed and precise history taking can inform the physical examination by reinforcing the general examination skills employed to isolate the physical examination findings and put the presenting complaint into context.

As expected, changes in posture and gait are significant findings during the musculoskeletal examination of the patient as both muscle tone, structure, and density can affect movement, and they can be important cues to conditions and illnesses particularly with older adults. Patient's medical history should be taken carefully to uncover possible causes of abnormal gait and posture. Some common abnormal postures such as kyphosis, scoliosis, and lordosis are responsible for altered posture. Differentiating normal gait from abnormal gait and noting this information is important as many diseases can alter a person's gait and lead to abnormal walking.

3.2.2   Physical Features Associated with Specific Conditions

Certain diseases can manifest through specific combinations of subtle and overt physical characteristics, while gross abnormalities are often noticeable, subtle physical changes can be equally significant and should not be overlooked. Distinctive physical features include:

Recognizing *subtle changes* such as:

- Alcoholism usually characterized by a round, plethoric (red) face reminiscent of Cushing's syndrome, alongside a glowing red nose, visible dilated veins, red conjunctivae, and the distinct smell of alcohol.
- Smoking includes the smell of cigarettes, increased skin wrinkling in heavy smokers (though sun exposure can also cause similar effects), and nicotine-stained fingers.
- Self-inflicted trauma can indicate underlying mental health issues, particularly in young adults and adolescents.
- Solvent abuse is linked to red sores around the nose and lips suggestive of solvent abuse in younger individuals.
- Intravenous drug abuse involves track marks on veins and noticeable scarring which are common signs of drug abuse, easily detected during a physical examination.
- Corneal arcus, a white ring around the cornea of the eye, can indicate normal age-related changes but may also suggest familial hyperlipidaemia in younger patients.
- Advanced depression may present with a withdrawn and expressionless face, while milder depression could appear similar to transient unhappiness.
- Menopause: Women may experience episodic hot flushes indicative of this natural phase in life.
- Significant wrinkling of the earlobes leading to deep clefts is a notable sign associated with the condition of coronary heart disease.

Recognizing _endocrine disorders_ such as:

- Thyroid disorders manifest as either hyperthyroidism or hypothyroidism, each presenting with distinct physical characteristics.
- Hyperthyroidism involves unintentional weight loss despite increased appetite, rapid heartbeat (tachycardia), often exceeding 100 beats per minute. Tremors are typically a fine trembling in the hands and fingers. Increased sweating and sensitivity to heat and enlargement of the thyroid gland appears as swelling at the neck's base (Goitre).
- Hypothyroidism includes fatigue, sensitivity to cold, constipation, weight gain, and a puffy face. Goitre may also occur alongside this condition.

Learning Point
Common facial and general body features associated with hyperthyroidism (overactive thyroid)
Hyperthyroidism:

- Unintentional weight loss, even when your appetite and food intake stay the same or increase
- Rapid heartbeat (tachycardia)—commonly more than 100 beats a minute
- Irregular heartbeat (arrhythmia)
- Pounding of your heart (palpitations)
- Increased appetite
- Nervousness, anxiety, and irritability
- Tremor—usually a fine trembling in your hands and fingers
- Sweating
- Changes in menstrual patterns
- Increased sensitivity to heat
- Changes in bowel patterns, especially more frequent bowel movements
- An enlarged thyroid gland (goitre), which may appear as a swelling at the base of your neck
- Fatigue, muscle weakness
- Difficulty sleeping
- Skin thinning
- Fine, brittle hair

Learning Point
Common facial and general body features associated with hypothyroidism (underactive thyroid) are:

- Fatigue
- Increased sensitivity to cold

- Constipation
- Dry skin
- Weight gain
- Puffy face
- Hoarseness
- Muscle weakness
- Elevated blood cholesterol level
- Muscle aches, tenderness, and stiffness
- Pain, stiffness, or swelling in your joints
- Heavier than normal or irregular menstrual periods
- Thinning hair
- Slowed heart rate
- Depression
- Impaired memory
- Enlarged thyroid gland (goitre)

Inspection of the anterior surface of the neck is important, and palpation should be carried out if an enlarged thyroid is suspected. If the patient has an enlarged thyroid gland (goitre). The term goitre describes a swelling of the neck resulting from enlargement of the thyroid gland. We need to find out the size, the consistency, and whether the surface is smooth or nodular, the mobility of the glands and whether the patient experiences any tenderness.

Learning Point
Types of Goitre

- ***Simple (Iodine) Goitre***: Develops from iodine deficiency, resulting in thyroid swelling.
- ***Toxic Goitre***: Associated with hyperthyroidism.
- ***Nontoxic Goitre***: Not resulting from inflammation or cancer, and no associated abnormal thyroid function.

Recognizing _adrenal disorders_ presenting as either _adrenal over-activity_ (Cushing's syndrome), which is most commonly due to prolonged, excessive steroid therapy, or _adrenal underactivity_. Adrenal underactivity is not very common, unless it results from suddenly stopping of steroid therapy.

Learning Point
Common facial and general body features associated with Cushing's syndrome are:

- Thinning of hair
- Acne, red cheeks
- Buffalo hump
- Moon face
- Supraclavicular fat pad
- Increased body and facial hair
- Purple striae
- Pendulous abdomen
- Ecchymosis (blood vessel rupture)
- Thin extremities with muscle atrophy
- Think skin and subcutaneous tissues
- Slow wound healing

Recognizing *pituitary disorders* such as:

These are not common, but you may see a condition called acromegaly, which is due to the *overproduction of growth hormone* by a pituitary tumour. Patients develop coarse, prominent facial features, protruding jaw, prominent nose and forehead, large tongue, spade-shaped hands, excessive sweating and a greasy skin, visual disturbances, and a kyphosis.

You may also occasionally see patients with features of *deficient production of pituitary hormones*. In men, this results in loss of libido, impotence, small testes, loss of secondary sexual characteristics. In women, there is loss of menstrual periods, decreased in vagina and breast size and loss of axillary and pubic hair. In children, there will be severe shortness of stature and delayed puberty.

Learning Point
Physical signs of Acromegaly

- Coarse facial features, including an enlarged jaw and nose.
- Spade-shaped hands with excessive sweating and oily skin.
- Visual disturbances and kyphosis may also be present.

Other pituitary deficiencies can lead to loss of libido in men, decreased secondary sexual characteristics in women, and delayed puberty in children.

Recognizing *familial hyperlipidaemia* (inherited excess lipids in the blood) characterized by recognizable physical features during examination, including:

- Corneal arcus: A white ring is clearly distinct in the outer part of the iris indicating possible hyperlipidaemia. Corneal arcus is usually associated with old age but is an indicator of hyperlipidaemia if found in younger people. In the picture below corneal arcus.
- Xanthelasmata (sing. = xanthelasma) are deposits of lipid (cholesterol) under the skin around the eyes, giving the appearance of yellow patches of lipid deposits around the eyes.
- Xanthomata (sing. = xanthoma) are similar deposits in the skin elsewhere and on the tendons of muscles.

Recognizing clubbing of fingers and toes, this condition is the enlargement of fingertips accompanied by a downward sloping of the nails, associated with low perfusion or oxygenation in the extremities.

The normally firm angle between the fingernail and nail bed is around 160 degrees. In clubbing, this angle increases. Upon palpation of the nail base, the nail appears to "float," and in severe cases, fingers may have a drumstick appearance, indicating more pronounced change.

3.3   The State of Hydration and Nutrition

Hydration is critical for maintaining health, and attention to fluid and electrolyte balance should be assessed to detect signs of dehydration such as dry mouth and skin to more severe manifestations of dehydration such as low blood pressure. Understanding the mechanisms of fluid movement in the body-related factors contributing to imbalances may aid healthcare professionals to recognize and address underlying conditions. Hydration serves as a critical aspect of numerous physiological processes within the body and maintaining a proper fluid balance may ensure the optimal functioning of organs and systems. The body constantly regulates its fluid and electrolyte levels, with intake meticulously matched to output (urine, faeces, and sweat). Any disturbance in this balance can lead to dehydration, a significant internal imbalance that adversely affects homeostasis.

Dehydration happens when the body loses more fluids than it takes in, leading to an insufficient amount of water to carry out normal physiological functions effectively. Excessive physical activity, exposure to high temperatures, inadequate fluid intake, and certain medical conditions that cause increased fluid loss (e.g. diabetes mellitus, fever, or gastrointestinal disorders) may induce dehydration manifested through a range of symptoms that vary in severity, such as:

- Dry mouth and lips: One of the earliest signs of dehydration is a parched feeling in the oral cavity due to reduced saliva production. The lack of moisture in the mouth can lead to discomfort, affecting the patient's ability to speak and eat.

- Dry skin: Skin turgor can serve as a vital indicator of hydration status. In dehydrated individuals, the skin may appear less elastic or develop a rough texture. Pinching the skin may demonstrate prolonged return time (a sign of reduced turgor), indicating dehydration.
- Dry eyes: Reduced tear production can lead to dryness and irritation in the eyes. This symptom is particularly concerning as it may affect vision and overall comfort.

Changes in vital signs: In more severe cases of dehydration, systemic effects can impact vital signs. A noticeable drop in blood pressure may occur due to decreased blood volume, leading to potential orthostatic hypotension when the patient transitions from a seated or supine position to standing. Heart rate may also increase as the body attempts to compensate for the reduced intravascular volume.

Learning Point
Fluid exchange between different compartments of the body is governed by pressure differences across semi-permeable membranes. Two fundamental forces play a role in this exchange:

- Hydrostatic pressure: This is the pressure exerted by a fluid at rest due to the weight of the fluid above. In the context of the cardiovascular system, hydrostatic pressure can drive fluid out of capillaries into the interstitial space, where it supports tissue perfusion.
- Osmotic pressure: This force is generated by the presence of solutes in solution. Osmosis refers to the movement of water across a semi-permeable membrane from an area of lower solute concentration to one of higher solute concentration. Osmotic pressure helps retain fluid within the intravascular space, counteracting hydrostatic pressure to maintain fluid balance.
- Capillary membrane permeability: The permeability of capillary membranes affects how easily fluids and solutes can pass from the bloodstream into surrounding tissues. Factors such as inflammation, injury, or pathology can alter this permeability, further complicating fluid dynamics.

The hydration status and fluid balance can be assessed by:

Monitoring fluid intake and output: Keeping a detailed record of fluid intake (oral and intravenous) and output (urine, faeces, sweating) allows clinicians to identify patterns of excess or deficit. This data can be vital for patients recovering from surgery or those necessitating careful fluid management, such as with renal impairment.

- Physical examination: A thorough physical examination should include assessment of skin turgor, mucous membranes, and vital signs. Moreover, evaluation of any signs of oedema or dehydration through clinical observation can guide further diagnostic testing or treatment plans.

- Laboratory tests: Routine laboratory evaluations, including serum electrolytes, blood urea nitrogen (BUN), and creatinine levels, can confirm dehydration or fluid overload and shed light on potential imbalances that may accompany fluid status changes.

If the hydrostatic pressure exceeds osmotic pressure significantly, excess fluid is forced out of capillaries and into opposing interstitial spaces, leading to oedema. Such a condition can affect various body areas and may present clinically as swelling in the extremities and abdomen (ascites). Oedema can occur when there is damaged capillary integrity, as seen in conditions like burns or anaphylaxis. In the case of burns, the damage to the skin disrupts the barrier function, compromising the ability of capillaries to maintain fluid homeostasis. Anaphylaxis, on the other hand, a severe allergic reaction, further enhances capillary permeability due to inflammatory mediators released during the response, leading to rapid fluid leakage into surrounding tissues and potentially resulting in systemic shock.

3.3.1 Fluid Overload

Fluid overload (interstitial oedema) is due to excess fluid movement from the intravascular into the extravascular compartments via the capillary walls because of the increase in hydrostatic pressure and decrease of the osmotic pressure. Interstitial oedema can be caused by the inflammatory response which will increase the permeability of capillary walls and fluid will leak into the extravascular tissues such as infections, injuries, or autoimmune diseases which trigger biochemical processes that promote vascular permeability. This leakage exacerbates fluid accumulation. Oedema can also be caused by obstruction in the lymphatic system due to returning excess interstitial fluid to the bloodstream. When lymphatic pathways are compromised, whether through surgical removal of lymph nodes, cancer, or infections, the result is fluid retention and swelling in the affected limbs, a condition referred to as lymphedema.

One of the most common forms of oedema is *pulmonary oedema*, characterized by the accumulation of fluid in the air sacs (alveoli) of the lungs. This condition often occurs as a complication of pulmonary hypertension, frequently seen in patients with heart failure. Symptoms of pulmonary oedema include shortness of breath (dyspnoea), which often worsens when the patient is lying down (orthopnoea). Patients may also present with tachycardia, a sensation of suffocation, and may cough up sputum that appears foamy or is occasionally tinged with blood. The presence of these symptoms necessitates immediate medical intervention, as pulmonary oedema can lead to respiratory distress and compromise oxygenation. *Pedal oedema*, another type of fluid accumulation, specifically affects the feet and lower legs. Patients with pedal oedema may experience restricted mobility and discomfort due to increased swelling in these extremities, impacting their overall quality of life. This condition may be especially pronounced in individuals with circulatory issues, diabetes, or prolonged periods of inactivity.

In contrast, *lymphoedema* presents as swelling in the arms or legs caused by impaired lymphatic circulation. This condition is frequently encountered following cancer treatments, particularly surgeries that involve the removal of lymph nodes. In these cases, the disruption of normal lymphatic drainage leads to fluid retention and swelling, which can be both uncomfortable and debilitating. *Cerebral oedema* is a more serious condition involving the accumulation of fluid within the cranial cavity, leading to increased intracranial pressure. This can occur due to various factors, including head injury, ruptured blood vessels, or the presence of tumours that either occupy space within the skull or obstruct blood flow. Additionally, increased permeability of cerebral capillaries, potentially resulting from allergic reactions or infections, can contribute to cerebral oedema. The consequences of this condition can be severe, including neurological deficits, impaired consciousness, and even potential loss of life.

Macular oedema occurs when fluid accumulates in the macula, the central part of the retina, often as a consequence of damaged blood vessels leaking fluid into the area, particularly in conditions such as diabetic retinopathy. This can lead to visual impairment and requires careful monitoring and management to prevent long-term damage to vision.

Several systemic conditions can predispose individuals to the development of oedema. One of the prominent contributing factors is congestive heart failure (CHF), characterized by increased venous pressure and subsequent back pressure in the venous capillaries. This rise in hydrostatic pressure encourages fluid extravasation from the intravascular space, resulting in oedema formation, particularly in the lower extremities and pulmonary regions.

Another significant condition is cirrhosis, a chronic liver disease in which the normal flow of blood through the liver is obstructed, leading to portal hypertension. The increased pressure in the portal vein, which brings blood from the intestines and spleen to the liver, can cause fluid to accumulate in the abdominal cavity (ascites) and also in the legs. Furthermore, the liver's decreased ability to synthesize proteins during cirrhosis results in reduced plasma colloid osmotic pressure, meaning that less fluid is reabsorbed at the venular ends of capillaries, contributing further to the formation of oedema.

Kidney disease also plays a significant role in the development of oedema. Dysfunction in the kidneys, particularly reduced glomerular filtration rate (GFR), compromises the body's ability to excrete salt and water. This salt and fluid retention leads to elevated hydrostatic pressure, and damage to the glomeruli can result in protein leakage into the urine. Consequently, decreased plasma colloid osmotic pressure means less fluid is reabsorbed from tissue back into circulation, promoting further oedema.

Healthcare professionals should take a thorough approach to evaluate and document the extent and nature of the fluid accumulation. In ambulant patients, the area behind the medial malleolus (the bony prominence on the inner side of the ankle) should be inspected for signs of ankle oedema. In recumbent patients, it is crucial to assess the sacral area and lower back for any indications of sacral oedema, especially in those who require prolonged bed rest.

3.4   Assessment of Nutritional Status

Nutritional status may indicate overall health, and the nutritional status of the patient may help determine the severity of serious diseases. Conversely, chronic illnesses can precipitate poor nutritional states, may impede healing, and adversely affect the immune response.

Learning Point

Furthermore, excessive obesity, indicative of poor nutritional choices, is also important to assess cardiovascular and other risks. This assessment typically comprises several key components:

- Examination of general appearance
- Measurement of weight and height, including assessment of muscle and fat bulk
- Assessment of haemoglobin levels and overall blood status
- Evaluation for vitamin and mineral deficiencies

Cachexia is a complex syndrome characterized by extreme weight loss and muscle wasting. This condition is the result of an intricate metabolic process associated with several chronic diseases, including cancer, chronic renal failure, HIV/AIDS, and multiple sclerosis. In cachexia, the body undergoes profound changes that affect nutritional status, resulting in significant health impacts. The management of cachexia involves addressing both dietary needs and the underlying disease processes that contribute to its development.

Learning Point

In addition to blood tests, healthcare professionals should observe physical features related to the eyes, mouth, tongue, and hands, which can provide valuable insights regarding nutritional deficiency-related anaemia or iron deficiency anaemia:

- Eyes: One of the first signs that may indicate an underlying nutritional deficiency is the colour of the conjunctivae, which should ideally present as a healthy red/pink. Changes from red to pale pink may suggest anaemia due to iron deficiency or other nutritional issues.

- Mouth: Inflammation and cracking at the corners of the mouth, known as angular stomatitis, commonly indicate deficiencies in the B vitamin complex. These cracks can cause discomfort and may reflect a broader issue of nutritional inadequacy.
- Tongue: Assessment of the tongue is critical; a smooth appearance lacking papillae indicates atrophic glossitis, often associated with iron deficiency and B vitamin deficiencies. This condition can impact a person's ability to taste and potentially result in further dietary challenges.
- Hands: Nail changes, such as the development of koilonychia, or spooning of the nails, can be a sign of iron deficiency anaemia.

Vitamins are classified into two primary categories: fat-soluble and water-soluble vitamins. Each type plays essential roles in various metabolic functions within the body, and deficiencies can lead to a range of clinical conditions. The following table summarizes the key vitamin deficiencies and their associated clinical features:

Vitamin deficiency	Clinical condition/features
A	Dry skin, dry eyes, thin cornea, night blindness
D	Bone softening, bone pain, proximal muscle weakness
K	Bruising, bleeding tendency
B1 (Thiamine)	Peripheral nerve damage, weakness
B2 (Riboflavin)	Angular stomatitis, inflamed oral mucous membranes, glossitis, anaemia
B3 (Niacin)	Skin rash (dermatitis), diarrhoea, dementia (pellagra)
B6 (Pyridoxine)	Peripheral nerve damage
B12	Anaemia, glossitis, spinal cord degeneration
Folic Acid	Anaemia, glossitis
C	Bleeding from gums, bleeding into joints, skin, muscles, anaemia (scurvy)

Beriberi, primarily caused by a deficiency of vitamin B1 (thiamine), presents in two forms: wet beriberi and dry beriberi. Wet beriberi affects the heart and circulatory system, leading to oedema and cardiovascular complications, while dry beriberi primarily affects the nervous system, causing peripheral nerve damage. Blood and urine tests are useful in measuring thiamine levels within the bloodstream, aiding in diagnosis. The physical examination may reveal additional neurological damage that may necessitate further investigation.

An important part of nutritional assessment revolves around the evaluation of blood status in order to identify causes of anaemia and recognize potential indicators of hypoalbuminemia (low plasma albumin levels). Anaemia can arise from various nutritional deficiencies, including inadequate intake of iron, vitamin B12, and folate. Low plasma albumin levels can be presented in various ways, including the appearance of white nails, known as leukonychia.

Learning Point

Finally, nutritional deficiencies can manifest through various clinical signs affecting multiple body systems:

- Vision impairments: Vitamin A deficiency can lead to night blindness and other visual disturbances.
- Skeletal weakness: Deficiencies in vitamins D, K, and calcium can contribute to conditions such as osteomalacia or osteoporosis.
- Dermatological symptoms: Deficiencies may lead to skin rashes or conditions like dermatitis.
- Mood disorders: Nutritional inadequacies can impact mental health, with certain B vitamins being linked to mood regulation and cognitive function.

3.5 Abnormal Skin Colour Changes

Skin discoloration is an important diagnostic indicator in clinical practice, providing essential clues to underlying health conditions. Among the most significant types of skin discoloration are jaundice, pallor, cyanosis, and hyperpigmentation. Each of these manifestations is associated with specific physiological processes and disease states.

Jaundice is characterized by the yellow or brownish discoloration of the skin, sclera (the white part of the eyes), and mucous membranes. This condition results from increased levels of bilirubin in the blood, known as hyperbilirubinemia. Bilirubin is a by-product of the normal breakdown of red blood cells (RBCs), particularly the haeme component of haemoglobin. In healthy individuals, bilirubin is processed by the liver, conjugated to make it water-soluble, and excreted into the bile. This process can be disrupted, and the bilirubin accumulates in the bloodstream, leading to the characteristic yellow discoloration associated with jaundice.

The sclera is typically the most reliable area for detecting jaundice, particularly in individuals with lighter skin pigmentation. In patients with darker skin tones, the yellow coloration may be more challenging to discern in the skin. Therefore, the examination of the conjunctivae and the abdominal wall provides critical adjuncts to help you assess for the presence of jaundice accurately. Numerous conditions can lead to jaundice, categorized broadly into pre-hepatic, hepatic, and post-hepatic causes:

Pre-hepatic jaundice: This type occurs due to increased bilirubin production stemming from haemolysis, which is the breakdown of red blood cells. Common causes include haemolytic anaemia, sickle cell disease, and certain infections:

- Hepatic jaundice: This condition results from liver dysfunction, which can occur for multiple reasons, such as hepatitis (viral, alcoholic, or autoimmune), cirrhosis, and hepatic tumours. The liver's impaired ability to process bilirubin leads to its accumulation in the bloodstream.

- Post-hepatic jaundice: This type arises from obstructions in the biliary tract affecting the flow of bile. Conditions like gallstones, tumours in the bile duct or pancreas, and strictures can inhibit bile's transport, resulting in bilirubin buildup.

Pallor refers to an abnormal paleness of the skin and mucous membranes, often an indicator of reduced blood flow, anaemia, or other systemic conditions. In assessing pallor, you focus on detecting changes in the colouration of the conjunctiva and mucous membranes, typically indicative of underlying blood dyscrasias. Pallor can manifest at different levels:

- Moderate pallor: Characterized by notable paleness of the conjunctiva or mucous membranes along with corresponding changes in the skin tone.
- Severe pallor: This condition involves significant paleness across the conjunctiva and mucous membranes in addition to pronounced paleness of the skin. It may also be associated with palmar pallor, where the palms of the hands appear unusually pale. Pallor can arise from a multitude of conditions, primarily linked to anaemia and reduced peripheral perfusion.

Common causes include:

- Anaemia: A reduction in the number of red blood cells (RBCs) or haemoglobin concentration leads to insufficient oxygen delivery to tissues, resulting in the pallid appearance. Nutritional deficiencies, such as a lack of iron, vitamin B12, or folate, significantly contribute to the development of anaemia.
- Hypovolemic shock: Severe blood loss or volume depletion, whether from trauma, haemorrhagic events, or dehydration, can cause generalized pallor due to decreased perfusion.
- Peripheral vascular disease: Conditions that impair blood flow to the extremities can lead to localized pallor, particularly in cases of obstruction.

Cyanosis, on the other hand, is characterized by a bluish or purplish discoloration of the skin and mucous membranes. This condition arises from an elevated concentration of deoxygenated haemoglobin in the blood. Cyanosis can be classified into two primary types: central and peripheral cyanosis:

- Central cyanosis: This type occurs when the arterial blood contains a high level of deoxygenated haemoglobin, typically when the saturation of oxygen falls below 85%. Central cyanosis is manifest across the entire body and particularly noticeable in visible mucosa such as the tongue, lips, and cheeks. Central cyanosis can be associated with significant hypoxemia and may indicate serious underlying respiratory or cardiac conditions.
- Peripheral cyanosis: Unlike central cyanosis, peripheral cyanosis often results from inadequate circulation, leading to a bluish discoloration localized to the extremities, such as fingertips, toes, and sometimes the ears and lips. This condition may not reflect overall oxygen saturation but rather localized issues such as low cardiac output, venous stasis, or vasoconstriction due to cold exposure.

Cyanosis can arise from various underlying conditions:

- Respiratory disorders: Conditions such as chronic obstructive pulmonary disease (COPD), pneumonia, or pulmonary embolism can lead to diminished gas exchange, resulting in childhood cyanosis.
- Cardiovascular disorders: Congenital heart defects presenting with right-to-left shunting often lead to cyanosis due to mixing deoxygenated blood with oxygenated blood. Conditions like tetralogy of Fallot may cause significant central cyanosis in affected individuals.
- Peripheral vascular disorders: Conditions like Raynaud's phenomenon, where blood vessels constrict in cold or stressful situations, can lead to peripheral cyanosis.

Differential cyanosis is observed in specific cases, such as coarctation of the aorta, where blood flow is impaired below the point of the narrowing. This results in the upper extremities being pink or normal while the lower extremities exhibit cyanosis due to decreased perfusion.

Hyperpigmentation is a condition characterized by darkened areas of skin resulting from an increase in melanin production. Various forms of hyperpigmentation may stem from different causes and have distinct clinical presentations.

Types of hyperpigmentation include:

- Melasma: Often referred to as the "mask of pregnancy," this condition is influenced by hormonal changes, particularly during pregnancy or with the use of certain contraceptives. Melasma presents as brown or grey-brown patches commonly appearing on the face, especially on the forehead, cheeks, and upper lip.
- Sunspots: Known as solar lentigines or liver spots, these flat, brown spots arise from chronic sun exposure and are prevalent in sun-exposed areas, such as the face and hands. They serve as a reminder of skin damage caused by ultraviolet light and the importance of sun protection.
- Post-inflammatory hyperpigmentation: This form of hyperpigmentation occurs after an inflammatory response, such as acne or dermatitis, leads to darkening of the skin and can persist long after the initial condition resolves.

Diffuse hyperpigmentation may be associated with systemic conditions such as:

Addison's disease: This adrenal insufficiency leads to an increase in adrenocorticotropic hormone (ACTH), which stimulates melanin production, resulting in increased pigmentation.

Haemochromatosis: This genetic disorder results in elevated iron levels in the body, which can lead to a slate-grey or bronze discoloration of the skin.

Thyroid dysfunction: Conditions involving hypothyroidism can also manifest with skin changes, including darker patches of skin in certain areas.

Recognizing and assessing skin discoloration as it often signifies underlying health conditions that may require further investigation. A comprehensive approach to evaluating skin colour changes includes:

- Visual inspection: Careful observation of skin colouring, particularly in areas frequently exposed to sunlight (e.g. face, back of hands) and other regions that may not receive light exposure (e.g. sclera and mucous membranes).
- Patient history: Obtaining a thorough history of the patient's medical conditions, medication use (as certain drugs can cause pigmentation changes), and lifestyle factors (like sun exposure and skin-care practices) will inform the clinical assessment.
- Dermatological Examination: In-depth examinations may involve dermatoscopy or skin biopsies to provide a clearer understanding of the changes seen in skin discoloration and rule out malignancies like melanoma.

3.6   Lymph Nodes Enlargement

Lymph nodes are an integral part of the body's immune system and overall homeostasis. These small, bean-shaped structures are distributed throughout the body and are an integral part of the lymphatic system. The functions of lymph nodes encompass several important processes, including the removal of excess fluid and debris, activation of immune cells, and the phagocytosis of pathogens. Understanding these functions is essential in appreciating the significance of lymph nodes in health and disease. One of the primary roles of lymph nodes is the filtration of lymph fluid that returns from the interstitial spaces to the bloodstream. This lymphatic fluid can contain excess interstitial fluid, cellular debris, and various organisms. Lymph nodes act as filters, trapping these substances and helping to prevent the spread of infections and diseases throughout the body. By doing so, they help to maintain fluid balance and prevent swelling in tissues.

Lymph nodes are critical for the activation of lymphocytes, when foreign substances, such as pathogens or antigens, are detected, lymph nodes help stimulate lymphocytes to react. This process begins when antigen-presenting cells (APCs) capture and process antigens, which they then present to naïve T-cells within the lymph nodes. As a result, the activated T-cells proliferate and differentiate into effector cells that can regenerate immune responses. Furthermore, B-cells within the lymph nodes undergo activation, leading to the production of antibodies that are pivotal for neutralizing harmful pathogens.

In addition to producing immune responses, lymph nodes contain macrophages, which are specialized cells that play a vital role in phagocytosis. These cells ingest and destroy pathogens, dead cells, and other debris found in lymph fluid. This cleansing function is essential for maintaining the body's defence system against infections and minimizing potential inflammatory responses. Macrophages also contribute to antigen presentation, further enhancing the immune response through their interaction with lymphocytes.

Lymphadenopathy is the condition when lymph nodes become enlarged, this condition is referred to as lymphadenopathy. Lymphadenopathy can be classified into localized and generalized enlargement, depending on the number of lymph nodes affected and their locations. *Localized lymphadenopathy*: Basic understanding of lymphadenopathy begins with recognizing localized conditions that can contribute to the enlargement of lymph nodes. Such enlargement typically suggests a pathological process, such as a localized infection or malignancy. For instance, swollen lymph nodes in the neck may indicate an upper respiratory infection, while masses under the arm may suggest a breast infection or malignancy. *Generalized lymphadenopathy*: Generalized enlargement refers to the swelling of multiple lymph node regions throughout the body. This condition can arise from systemic infections, haematological malignancies, or chronic inflammatory diseases. Some common causes for *generalized lymphadenopathy* include:

- Viral and bacterial infections: One of the leading causes of generalized lymphadenopathy includes infections like infectious mononucleosis (often caused by the Epstein-Barr virus, a form of herpesvirus) and HIV/AIDS. Many bacterial infections, such as tuberculosis or streptococcal infections, can also prompt lymph node enlargement as part of the immune response.
- Leukaemia and lymphoma: These cancers represent serious conditions where lymphadenopathy can signify disease progression. Leukaemia, characterized by the uncontrolled proliferation of white blood cells, can lead to widespread lymph node enlargement. Lymphomas, which include both Hodgkin and non-Hodgkin lymphoma, are cancers of the lymphoid tissue marked by affected lymph nodes throughout the body.
- Chronic inflammatory diseases: Patients suffering from chronic conditions such as rheumatoid arthritis or systemic lupus erythematosus may experience generalized lymphadenopathy as a consequence of the ongoing inflammatory processes. The immune response mounted against the underlying autoimmune condition can lead to an enlargement of lymph nodes.

Localized lymphadenopathy causes can arise from specific conditions, including:

- Cancer metastases: One of the grave consequences of cancer is its ability to metastasize—spread from its original site to other areas of the body. Lymph nodes often serve as the first site of metastasis for cancers of the lung, breast, kidney, and head and neck regions. As adjacent tissues infiltrate the lymph nodes, they become enlarged, which can often be palpated during clinical examination.
- Lymphoma: Hodgkin's disease, a type of lymphoma, is characterized by the presence of Reed-Sternberg cells and typically presents with localized lymphadenopathy, especially in the cervical and supraclavicular regions.
- Local infections: Suppurative infections, such as an abscess or localized cellulitis, generally lead to the enlargement of nearby lymph nodes as they respond to the infection. Inflammatory changes in the area prompt lymph nodes to swell as the immune system mobilizes to combat the infection.

Learning Point

Clinical examination of lymph nodes typically conducted a detailed assessment to evaluate lymphadenopathy during physical examinations. This assessment is crucial for determining the underlying cause of node enlargement and guiding further diagnostic measures. Below are the steps and considerations for effectively evaluating lymph nodes:

- Inspection and palpation: You initiate the examination by visually inspecting the lymph nodes for abnormal swelling. Larger nodes may be visible; however, many may require palpation for detection. The examination should focus on specific regions such as the head and neck, axillary region, and groin.
- Assessment of parameters: During palpation, clinicians should assess several characteristics of the lymph nodes:
- Size: Measure the diameter of palpable nodes and note if they are enlarged compared to baseline findings.
- Consistency: Evaluate whether the nodes feel firm, rubbery, or hard. Normal nodes should feel soft and mobile.
- Tenderness: Assess tenderness during palpation; tender nodes often indicate acute infection or inflammation.
- Mobility: Determine if the nodes are fixed to surrounding tissues may suggest malignancy, or mobile, which is often seen in reactive conditions.

Specific lymph node areas:

- Cervical nodes: Begin with lymph nodes in the head and neck region, which include preauricular, posterior auricular, submandibular, and supraclavicular nodes.
- Axillary nodes: These nodes, located in the armpit region, should be assessed, especially in patients with breast issues.
- Inguinal nodes: Evaluate the groin area for enlargement, which could relate to local infections or malignancies.

In cases of lymphadenopathy, additional diagnostic tests may be necessary to ascertain the underlying cause. Depending on the clinical presentation and physical findings, you may consider:

- Blood tests: Complete blood counts (CBC), basic metabolic panels, and specific markers for infections (such as HIV or specific antibodies) enable a better understanding of the patient's immunologic and hematologic status.
- Imaging studies: Ultrasound, computed tomography (CT) scans, or magnetic resonance imaging (MRI) can provide visual assessments of lymph nodes and surrounding structures, helping to reveal structural abnormalities, involvement with malignancies, or the presence of unclear masses.

- Biopsy: If the clinical picture suggests malignancy or if nodes remain unexplained despite non-invasive evaluations, a biopsy may be necessary to obtain tissue for pathological examination. Procedures may include fine needle aspiration (FNA) or excisional biopsy, depending on the node's size and localization.

3.7   Assessing Body Temperature

Core body temperature provides invaluable insight into a patient's health status. Understanding the mechanisms of temperature regulation, recognizing signs of fever and hyperpyrexia, and conducting a thorough clinical examination are imperative for effective patient management. By diligently assessing body temperature and its associated symptoms, healthcare professionals can address potential health concerns early, improving patient outcomes and experiences. It is crucial for clinicians to remain vigilant in these assessments, considering the complexities and implications of alterations in body temperature as they relate to broader health conditions.

The regulation of core body temperature is tightly controlled by homeostatic mechanisms that ensure optimal functioning of the body's systems. The body maintains a narrow temperature range, vital for enzymatic and metabolic processes, and any deviation from this norm can have significant health implications.

The body generates heat primarily through metabolic processes occurring in the deep organs, including the liver, muscles, and brain. To maintain optimal body temperature, excess heat produced must be expelled efficiently. One of the primary modes of heat loss involves the dilatation of blood vessels within the extensive network of subcutaneous tissues. This process, known as vasodilation, enables warm blood from the deeper tissues to flow closer to the surface of the skin, facilitating heat transfer to the environment. This heat exchange is essential, especially in hot conditions or during physical exertion.

Furthermore, the body's ability to lose excess heat is enhanced by the process of sweating. As sweat evaporates from the surface of the skin, it absorbs heat, thereby cooling the body. The hypothalamus, a key regulatory centre in the brain, integrates these responses to maintain a stable core temperature. It processes input from peripheral thermoreceptors and initiates appropriate physiological changes, such as vasodilation or increased sweating, to counteract fluctuations in temperature. It is also important to note that the body's temperature is not static; it exhibits daily variations influenced by various factors, including circadian rhythms, physical activity, and hormonal changes. Typically, core body temperature fluctuates slightly, peaking in the late afternoon and evening before decreasing during sleep. This natural variation underscores the body's remarkable ability to adapt to internal and external changes.

An abnormally high body temperature is termed fever, which is typically defined as a controlled rise in temperature as part of the body's immune response to infection or illness. Fever often presents with accompanying symptoms including shivering and chills, referred to as rigors. These sensations occur as the body tries to generate more heat to reach a new set-point temperature established by the hypothalamus in response to inflammatory signals. Fever can serve as a useful diagnostic sign, indicating that the body is fighting off an underlying infection or other illness.

When body temperature escalates to extreme levels, it is termed hyperpyrexia, which is defined as a body temperature of 40 °C (104 °F) or higher. Hyperpyrexia is often considered a medical emergency because prolonged elevated temperatures can cause cellular dysfunction and potentially lead to organ damage or death if untreated.

Learning Point

Symptoms associated with hyperpyrexia can vary widely but typically include:

- Increased or irregular heart rate
- Muscle spasms
- Rapid breathing
- Seizures
- Confusion or other changes in mental state
- Loss of consciousness
- Coma

In addition to its acute impacts, fever can also serve as an indicator in chronic illnesses. For instance, patients with cancer may frequently present with fever as a symptom, often indicating disease progression or metastasis. Though fever is rarely an early symptom of cancer, it may manifest in cases of hematologic malignancies such as leukaemia or lymphoma, highlighting the multifaceted role of immune responses in various diseases.

In clinical practice, the assessment of body temperature is an integral part of a comprehensive examination. Typically, clinical assessments begin with a general examination that includes evaluating posture, gait, and any subtle changes in the patient's condition. Following this initial assessment, healthcare providers examine several systems to gain a holistic understanding of the patient's health status. One of the first steps in clinical examination involves assessing the patient's body temperature. This task is usually accomplished using various tools, such as digital thermometers, infrared thermometers, or even tympanic thermometers, each providing a means to accurately measure core body temperature. Recognizing variances in temperature can often facilitate early diagnosis and intervention in various medical conditions.

In addition to temperature, the general examination includes an evaluation of:

- State of hydration: Assessing signs of dehydration, including skin turgor, mucous membrane moisture, and overall physical appearance.
- Nutritional status: Evaluating factors such as body mass index (BMI), muscle mass, skin condition, and overall vitality.

- Neurological assessment: Evaluating mental status and neurological reflexes can help determine the impact of elevated temperature on cognitive function and overall health.
- Respiratory and cardiac examination: A comprehensive examination may also include auscultation of breath sounds and heart rhythm, allowing for the assessment of the respiratory and cardiovascular system's response to fever.

If fever or hyperpyrexia is detected, you also evaluate potential underlying causes through a thorough history and additional diagnostic testing. This may include:

- Blood tests: Complete blood count (CBC), inflammatory markers (e.g. C-reactive protein), and specific pathogen tests (e.g. blood cultures) can aid in identifying infectious agents or inflammation.
- Imaging studies: X-rays, CT scans, or MRI can visualize any abscesses, tumours, or pathological processes contributing to febrile conditions.
- Pulmonary function tests: If respiratory involvement is suspected, these tests can help evaluate lung function and gas exchange capabilities.

Core body temperature is very tightly controlled by homeostasis. Most excess heat generated in the body is lost by dilatation of the extensive network of vessels in the subcutaneous tissues. This allows heat to be transferred from the deep organs, and the process is helped by sweat, which evaporates. The hypothalamus integrates all of these responses. There is also a daily variation in body temperature.

3.8 Part 2: Focused Learning

Learning Activity 1

In the table below, match the definition and cause(s) to the appropriate gait:

Gait	Definition	Causes
1. Spastic	(a) Stooped posture, difficulty in initiating movement, small shuffling steps	(i) Proximal muscle disorder (thyrotoxicosis)
2. Foot-drop	(b) Slow walking, stiff legs, may be dragging, weakness, and stiffness of one leg if unilateral	(ii) Cerebellar disease (tumour)
3. Ataxic	(c) Flexes leg at hip more than usual to prevent toes catching, stamping as foot hits ground	(iii) Cerebrovascular disorder (stroke)
4. Waddling	(d) Inability to tilt pelvis when swinging each leg through to take the next step, exaggerated lateral trunk movements	(iv) Peripheral neuropathy (weakness, sensory loss)
5. Parkinsonian	(e) Unsteady when standing and adopts a broad base, unsteady when walking, lurches from side-to-side	(v) Parkinson's disease

Answer
1. *Spastic*
   (b) Slow walking, stiff legs, may be dragging, weakness, and stiffness of one leg if unilateral
   (iii) Cerebrovascular disorder (stroke)
2. *Foot-drop*
   (c) Flexes leg at hip more than usual to prevent toes catching, stamping as foot hits ground
   (iv) Peripheral neuropathy (weakness, sensory loss)
3. *Ataxic*
   (e) Unsteady when standing and adopts a broad base, unsteady when walking, lurches from side-to-side
   (ii) Cerebellar disease (tumour)
4. *Waddling*
   (d) Inability to tilt pelvis when swinging each leg through to take the next step, exaggerated lateral trunk movements
   (i) Proximal muscle disorder (thyrotoxicosis)
5. *Parkinsonian*
   (a) Stooped posture, difficulty in initiating movement, small shuffling steps
   (v) Parkinson's disease

Learning Activity 2

Find some common facial and general body features associated with hyperthyroidism (overactive thyroid) and hypothyroidism (underactive thyroid):

Hyperthyroidism	Hypothyroidism

Answer

Hyperthyroidism:

Unintentional weight loss, even when your appetite and food intake stay the same or increase
Rapid heartbeat (tachycardia)—commonly more than 100 beats a minute
Irregular heartbeat (arrhythmia)
Pounding of your heart (palpitations)
Increased appetite
Nervousness, anxiety, and irritability
Tremor—usually a fine trembling in your hands and fingers
Sweating
Changes in menstrual patterns
Increased sensitivity to heat
Changes in bowel patterns, especially more frequent bowel movements
An enlarged thyroid gland (goitre), which may appear as a swelling at the base of your neck
Fatigue, muscle weakness
Difficulty sleeping
Skin thinning
Fine, brittle hair

Hypothyroidism:

Fatigue
Increased sensitivity to cold
Constipation
Dry skin
Weight gain
Puffy face
Hoarseness
Muscle weakness
Elevated blood cholesterol level
Muscle aches, tenderness, and stiffness
Pain, stiffness, or swelling in your joints
Heavier than normal or irregular menstrual periods
Thinning hair
Slowed heart rate
Depression
Impaired memory
Enlarged thyroid gland (goitre)

Learning Activity 3
List the main general physical features of Cushing's syndrome.

Answer
- *Weight gain in face (moon face)*
- *Weight gain on the back of neck (buffalo hump)*
- *Skin changes with easy bruising in the extremities and development of purplish stretch marks (striae) particularly over the abdomen or axillary region*
- *Red, round face (plethora)*
- *Central obesity with weight gain centred over the chest and abdomen with thin arms and legs*
- *Excessive hair growth (hirsutism) on face, neck, chest, abdomen, and thighs*
- *Generalized weakness and fatigue*
- *Blurry vision*
- *Vertigo*
- *Muscle weakness*
- *Menstrual disorders in women (amenorrhea)*
- *Decreased fertility and/or sex drive (libido)*
- *Hypertension*
- *Poor wound healing*

Learning Activity 4

What is meant by clubbing of the fingers and toes and what is its significance?

Answer
- *Clubbed fingers is a symptom of disease, often of the heart or lungs which cause chronically low blood levels of oxygen. Clubbing may result from chronic low blood-oxygen levels.*
- *Lung disease:*
    Lung cancer, lung abscess, empyema, bronchiectasis, cystic fibrosis
- *Heart disease (any disease featuring chronic hypoxia):*
    Congenital cyanotic heart disease
    Subacute bacterial endocarditis
- *Gastrointestinal:*
    Malabsorption
    Crohn's disease and ulcerative colitis
    Cirrhosis

Learning Activity 5

List the features that might lead you to diagnose dehydration associated with:

- The tongue
- The eyes
- The skin
- The pulse
- The blood pressures

Answer
List the features that might lead you to diagnose dehydration associated with:
The tongue: Dry mucosa
The eyes: Lost glistening and shiny appearance
The skin: In which situation could the skin signs be unreliable?
Skin turgor is lost, unreliable in elderly patients.
The pulse: Increase to compensate for intravascular volume loss.
The blood pressures: Droop

Learning Activity 6
Use your knowledge of basic physiology to explain how the capillary hydrostatic pressure, the plasma oncotic (colloidal osmotic) pressure, and the integrity of the capillary wall interact to control normal movement of fluid across the capillary wall.

Answer
In the capillaries hydrostatic pressure increases filtration by pushing fluid and solute out of the capillaries, while capillary oncotic pressure (also known as colloid osmotic pressure) pulls fluid into the capillaries and/or prevents fluid from leaving.
Pressure differences govern fluid movement across semi-permeable membranes and two of these forces are hydrostatic/hydraulic pressure and osmotic pressure. The third factor is the permeability of the capillary membranes. There will be an escape of water and solute into the interstitial space resulting in interstitial oedema whenever the hydrostatic pressure is much higher than the osmotic pressure inside the intravascular space. Oedema also occurs when there is capillary leakage due to impaired membrane integrity such as in burns or anaphylaxis.
Generalized oedema commonly results from heart disease, liver disease, and kidney disease. Explain failure or disease of these organs can lead to disruption of the three factors.
Congestive heart failure: Oedema is the result of the activation of a series of humoral mechanisms that promote sodium and water reabsorption by the kidneys and expansion of the extracellular fluid. Congestive heart failure also increases venous pressure which backs pressure in venous capillary and promotes fluid extravasation and oedema formation.
Liver disease: Cirrhosis slows the normal flow of blood through the liver, thus increasing pressure in the vein that brings blood to the liver from the intestines and spleen. The increased pressure in the portal vein can cause fluid to accumulate in the legs (oedema) and in the abdomen (ascites). Also, in liver failure the synthesis of proteins such as albumin may lead to plasma colloid osmotic pressure decreases. This happens becaues there is less fluid reabsorbed at venular ends of capillaries by osmosis.
Kidney disease: Oedema is the result of primary salt retention and GFR reduction due to glomerulopathy. The glomerular damage leads to urinary protein loss which may lead to plasma colloid osmotic pressure decreases. Furthermore, less fluid reabsorbed at venular ends of capillaries by osmosis.

Learning Activity 7
List the common sites where oedema can be detected. What other associated features might you see in some areas where oedema fluid has accumulated?

Answer
List the common sites where oedema can be detected.
In ambulant patients: Space behind the medial malleolus (ankles oedema).
In the recumbent patient: sacrum and lower back (sacrum oedema).

Learning Activity 8
The sitting height should be about 50% of the standing height—name a common disorder associated with a reduced sitting height.

Answer
In osteoporosis, the collapse of vertebrae causes shortening of the sitting height.

Learning Activity 9
List the features on general examination that would confirm weight loss and wasting.

Answer
Unusual prominence of the cheekbones, head of humerus, major joints, the rib cage,
    and bony landmarks of the pelvis.

Learning Activity 10
What feature in the hands is associated hypoalbuminaemia? What is the consequence of hypoalbuminaemia and how can this be clinically detected?

Answer
Hypoalbuminaemia causes white nails (Leukonychia)
Consequence of hypoalbuminaemia: Fluid retention that causes swelling, especially of the feet or hands.
How can this be clinically detected: Ankles oedema and/or sacrum oedema.

Learning Activity 11
What is jaundice due to? Where is it best detected on the body?

Answer
Jaundice is a condition in which the skin, sclerae, and mucous membranes turn yellow because of a high level of bilirubin, a yellow-orange bile pigment. Jaundice has many causes, including hepatitis, gallstones, and tumours.
Hyperbilirubinemia is the main cause of jaundice. Bilirubin, which is responsible for the yellow colour of jaundice, is a normal part of the pigment released from the breakdown of "used" red blood cells.
The best places to detect jaundice are sclerae (for white patients) and abdominal wall (for darker skin tones).

Learning Activity 12

Pallor is a major feature of anaemia. Which sites are the best for detecting pallor?

Answer

Pallor is paleness of the skin

Mild pallor is when pallor is detected in the conjunctiva and/or mucous membrane.

Moderate pallor when there is pallor of conjunctiva and/or mucous membrane but also pallor of the skin.

Severe pallor when pallor of conjunctiva and/or mucous membrane is involved in addition to pallor of the skin and palmar pallor.

Learning Activity 13

Cyanosis can be peripheral and central. Name the sites where peripheral and central cyanosis can be detected. State the mechanisms of peripheral and central cyanosis.

Answer

*Central cyanosis occurs when the level of deoxygenated haemoglobin in the arteries is below 5 g/dL with oxygen saturation below 85%. The bluish hue is generally seen over the entire body surface and visible mucosa, e.g. **tongue**, lips, cheek, extremities.*

*Peripheral cyanosis occurs when there is increased oxygen uptake in peripheral tissues; it is not associated with arterial desaturation. Peripheral cyanosis often involves only the extremities, e.g. lips, finger, toe, ear but **not tongue**.*

Learning Activity 14

List the differences on palpation between enlarged nodes due to infection and enlarged nodes due to malignant infiltration.

Answer

Causes	*Infection*	*Malignant infiltration*
Size	*Regularly enlarge*	*Irregularly enlarge*
Consistency	*Soft, firm*	*Rubbery, hard*
Tenderness	*Yes*	*No*
Mobility	*Moveable*	*Fixed*

Bibliography

1. Bickley, L. (2012). *Bates' guide to physical examination and history taking.* Lippincott Williams & Wilkins.
2. Douglas, G., Nicol, F., & Robertson, C. (Eds.). (2013). *Macleod's clinical examination E-book.* Elsevier Health Sciences.
3. Jarvis, C. (2023). *Physical examination and health assessment-Canadian E-book: Physical examination and health assessment-Canadian E-book.* Elsevier Health Sciences.

4. Lena, A., Ebner, N., & Anker, M. S. (2019). Cardiac cachexia. *European Heart Journal Supplements, 21*(Suppl L), L24–L27.
5. McCance, K. L., & Huether, S. E. (2014). *Pathophysiology: The biologic basis for disease in adults and children.* Elsevier Health Sciences.
6. Ruthven, A. K. B. (2016). *Essential examination, 3rd edition: Step-by-step guides to clinical examination scenarios with practical tips and key facts for OSCEs.* Scion Publishing Limited.

Useful Websites

7. https://medtube.net/

Assessing and Diagnosing Disorders of the Cardiovascular System (CVS)

4

Learning Objectives

In this part of the chapter, we revisit basic anatomy and physiology of the cardiovascular system and identify the clinical signs and symptoms diagnostic of heart disease and disorders.

> **Learning Objectives**
> By the end of this chapter, you will be able to:
>
> *Understand the basic pathophysiology of heart disease.*
> *Explain the physiological changes and anatomical features present in heart disease.*
> *Link symptoms and signs of basic pathology to heart disease.*
> *Identify general and specific signs and symptoms relevant to the diagnosis of heart disease and their significance in differential diagnosis.*
> *Undertake a step-by-step physical examination on a cardiac patient.*
> *Understand key concepts in cardiac conditions.*

Common Medical Terms

The list of medical terms below is cited for easy reference and the reader is expected to understand these medical terms before they proceed to read this chapter.

Cachexia
Carotid pulse
Conjunctival pallor
Corneal arcus

© The Author(s), under exclusive license to Springer Nature
Switzerland AG 2026
C. Leliopoulou, L. Holman, *Physical Examination and Diagnostic Skills for Nurses and Allied Health Professionals*,
https://doi.org/10.1007/978-3-032-26539-5_4

Clubbing
Cyanosis
First heart sound
Heaves
Jugular venous pressure (JVP)
Koilonychia
Mediastinal shift
Oedema
Pallor
Splinter haemorrhages
Sweatiness
Thrills
Tendon xanthomata
Xanthelasma

4.1　Part I: The Heart as a Pump—The Cardiac Cycle and the Factors Influencing Cardiac Output

The heart is a hollow muscular organ shaped with its base uppermost and the apex inclined to the left; it projects downwards (inferiorly) and forwards (anteriorly). The heart sits between the lungs in the *mediastinum*, extending from the sternum to the vertebral column. The heart beats over 100,000 times per day to pump 7000 l of blood per day over 60,000 miles of blood vessels.

The *left border* is formed almost entirely by the inferior vena cava, with the superior vena cava forming part of the *upper end of the border*. The *upper (superior) border*, where the great vessels enter and leave the heart, is formed by right atrium and tricuspid valve. The *right border* is formed by the right ventricle. The *inferior border* is formed by the pulmonary valve and slightly by the pulmonary trunk.

> **Learning Point**
> The human circulatory system consists of:
>
> - The heart: pumps the blood around the body.
> - Blood vessels: carry the blood around the body.
>   - Arteries move blood away from the heart and towards other organs.
>   - Veins transfer blood towards the heart and away from other organs.
>   - Capillaries pass blood through organs lining arteries and veins.
> - Blood: the transport medium

Lungs are linked to a circulatory system that carries oxygen and nutrients to the body. Blood is pumped to load oxygen and gas exchange takes place at alveoli level. The blood is pumped from the heart to the lungs and back to the heart and then to the rest of the body. There are two parts in this circulatory system: the *pulmonary circulation* and the *systemic circulation*. The pulmonary circulation involves deoxygenated blood that leaves the heart through the pulmonary arteries and is circulated through the lungs, where gas exchange takes place and becomes oxygenated. The oxygenated blood returns to the heart through the pulmonary veins.

The heart is covered by two layers of pericardium, the outer layer called parietal pericardium and the inner layer called visceral pericardium or epicardium. Between these two serious layers there is a serious fluid which lubricates and prevents friction as the heart contracts.

The *pericardial fluid* secreted by the pericardial membranes, and it is located between the two layers of pericardium. This fluid acts as a lubricant to reduce friction when the heart beats. The pericardium has two layers: the inner layer (visceral pericardium) and the outer layer (parietal pericardium). From outermost to innermost, the layers of the heart wall are the epicardium, myocardium, and endocardium. The wall of left ventricle is much thicker, because six to seven times as much force must be exerted to push blood around the systemic circuit. Unlike skeletal muscle, cardiac muscle fibres do not rely on nerve activity to tell them when to start a contraction, instead pacemaker cells (cardiac muscle) establish a regular rate of contraction.

The heart measures around 10 cm from base to apex and weights around 300 g. The base is level with the second costal cartilage and the apex can be located just to the midclavicular line in the fifth intercostal space.

The endocardium is an endothelial tissue which line the chambers of the heart and covers the valves. It also forms the lining of the vessels entering and leaving the heart. This smooth and glistering tissue allows blood flow without turbulence which would damage the vessel walls. The middle layer of the heart walls consists of highly specialized muscular tissue, the myocardium. It has striations, is involuntary and has an internal control system or pacemaker. Cardiac muscle has one or two nuclei and many mitochondrial which reflect high levels of metabolic activity and intercalated discs join the cells together. That allows ions exchange freely across the muscle cell walls allowing the waves of contraction to pass easily across the myocardium.

The general physiology of the heart

In simple terms:
   A. The heart is a pump.
   B. Heart muscle cells (the myocardium) require oxygen.
   C. Regular rate and rhythm are maintained by a system that conducts electricity.
   D. It pumps blood through a system of blood vessels that have a limited volume capacity.

Learning Point

- The heart has four chambers: right atrium, right ventricle, left atrium, and left ventricle.
- Blood returns to the heart via the inferior vena cava from the trunk and limbs and via the superior vena cava from the head and neck.
- This blood enters the right atrium and passes through the valve called tricuspid valve to the right ventricle.
- The blood is then ejected through the pulmonary valve into the pulmonary trunk, which divides into two main branches.
- These transport the blood to the lungs. From here, the blood is taken via the pulmonary veins to the left atrium. The blood passes from here through the valve called mitral valve to the left ventricle and is then ejected through the aortic valve into the aorta for distribution to the rest of the body.

The wall of the heart is supplied with blood by the coronary circulation. The major arteries serving the myocardium are the left and right coronary arteries. Both originate from the aorta. The left coronary artery which branches into the left anterior descending artery and the circumflex artery, supplies blood to the left side of the heart. The right coronary artery supplies blood mainly to the right side of the heart. Once oxygen has been delivered to the tissue, blood is collected by a large vein, called the *coronary sinus*, which drains into the right atrium.

The cardiac cycle describes the events occurring during one heartbeat. It lasts around 0.8 s when the heart rate is 70/min. It is divided into diastole and systole and refers to the ventricular activity. Although we will describe events in stages this is a continuous process. During a normal heart beat the two atria contract while the two ventricles relax. Then, when the ventricles contract, the atria relax. The phase of contraction is known as *systole* and the phase of relaxation is referred to as *diastole*. A cardiac cycle (heartbeat) comprises a systole and diastole of both atria and a systole and diastole of both ventricles.

	The stages of the cardiac cycle can be roughly divided into three stages:
Stage 1:	*Filling phase*—The ventricles fill during diastole and atrial systole. The heart is completely relaxed, and pressures are low. Blood enters from the circulation and flows through the atria and into the ventricles. The AV valves (tricuspid valve and mitral valves) are open, and the semilunar valves are closed
Stage 2:	*Systole phase*—The ventricles start to contract, pushing blood into the aorta and the pulmonary trunk. This is also known as systole. The atria are relaxed, and the pressure rises in the ventricles until the AV valve close.
Stage 3:	*Diastole phase*—The ventricles start to relax, ventricular pressure falls and back pressure in the great vessels causes the semilunar valves (pulmonary valves and aortic valves) to close. The ventricles are now ready to refill in the next filling phase.

4.2   **Cardiac Output and Heart Sounds**

Blood pressure in the arterial system varies with the cardiac cycle reaching a systolic peak and a diastolic trough. The difference between the systolic and diastolic pressures is called the pulse pressure. The blood pressure is affected by the following factors:

The left ventricular output per beat Stroke volume
The ability of the aorta and the large arteries to distend
The arteriolar peripheral resistance under the autonomic nervous system control
The blood volume
The viscosity (thickness) of the blood
Changes in any of these factors will alter the blood pressure.

Blood pressure (BP) is the pressure exerted by the blood on the wall of the vessel and in general refers to the pressure in arteries. The BP will be raised when:

The heart rate and the force of contraction are increased.
The resistance to blood flow is increased following vasoconstriction.

Since the heart pumps in a pulsating manner, the arterial pressure fluctuates between 120 mm (systolic) and 80 mm (diastolic) of mercury. The difference between the systolic and diastolic blood pressure is called the pulse pressure and is about 40–50 mm of mercury. In simple terms, the pulse pressure is the amount of pressure required to feel a pulse and it is a rough index of how stiff the arteries are. A consistently high pulse pressure increases the risk of cardiovascular disease and a risk of atrial fibrillation. Factors that can increase the pulse pressure include atherosclerosis, thyrotoxicosis, anaemia, and fever.

The systolic pressure varies by up to 10 mmHg between the right and left brachial arteries. Standing usually causes a slight reduction in systolic (<20 mm) and a slight increase in diastolic (<10 mm) pressure. In individuals who have postural hypotension there is a large fall in both systolic and diastolic pressure on standing-causes usually include drugs hypovolaemia, prolonged bed rest, and abnormalities of the autonomic nervous system.

The amount of blood ejected from the left or right ventricles into the aorta or pulmonary trunk per minute is called the *cardiac output*. It depends upon the heart rate (HR) and stroke volume (SV), the amount of blood pumped out with each ventricular contraction at rest.

The *stroke volume* is the amount of blood ejected by a ventricle during each contraction which is about 70 ml. The heart rate is normally 60–80 beats/min but can be altered by several factors. The cardiovascular centre situated in the medulla and pons controls the rate and force of the contraction. In the medulla and the pons there is also the vasomotor centre which controls blood vessels and blood pressure.

The cardiac output is dependent on the heart rate and the stroke volume.

$$\text{Cardiac output} = \text{heart rate} \times \text{stroke volume}.$$

For example, if heart rate is 75 beats per minute and the stroke volume is 70 ml then the cardiac output equals 75 min × 70 ml = 5250 ml/min.

Learning Point

A typical cardiac cycle in the left atrium and left ventricle (a similar sequence of events occurs on the right side of the heart, but the pressure changes are lower).

Here the heart chamber pressures change in aortic, ventricular, and atrial pressures with corresponding valve actions and heart sounds ("Lub" and "Dub").

A clear diagram of heart chamber pressures during the cardiac cycle with labelled aortic pressure (red), ventricular pressure (green), and atrial pressure (yellow). The graph should show phases with AV valves and semilunar valves opening and closing, as well as the "Lub" and "Dub" heart sounds corresponding to the first and second heart sounds respectively. The image should include a clear x-axis for time and y-axis for pressure (mmHg), and should visually represent the waveforms of pressure changes during systole and diastole.

The heart sounds are sound of the valves closing and opening. The first sound (Lub) is the tricuspid and mitral valves closing and the second sound (Dup) is heard as the pulmonary and aortic valves close. The heart sound can be listened through a stethoscope on the chest wall. The first heart sound (S1) is due to tricuspid valve and mitral valve closure. The second heart sound (S2) is due to pulmonary and aortic valves closure.

Learning Point

The anatomical position of each heart sound on auscultation.

Each letter stands for a specific heart auscultation point:

1. Aortic area—located at the right 2nd intercostal space.
2. Pulmonic area—located at the left 2nd intercostal space.
3. Erb's point—located at the left 3rd intercostal space.
4. Tricuspid area—located at the lower left sternal border (4th intercostal space).
5. Mitral area—located at the left 5th intercostal space, medial to the midclavicular line.

Damage to the valves from diseases such as rheumatic fever or endocarditis may cause the valves to have problem to close properly and leak and secondly the valves become narrow and stiff called *stenosis*. This valvular damage may produce abnormal sounds or *murmurs* caused by turbulence as blood leaks back into the heart or is forced through the narrowed valve. These conditions can lead to increased cardiac work, loss of efficiency, and heart failure. The mitral and aortic valves are most often affected by rheumatic fever or endocarditis.

4.3   The Electrical Conduction System of the Heart

The autonomic nervous system, sympathetic and parasympathetic nervous systems, control the heart. The sympathetic fibres arise from the pressure centre, while the parasympathetic fibres arise in the depressor centre. The sinus node (SA) can continuously generate electrical impulses, thereby setting the normal rhythm and rate in a healthy heart. Hence, the SA node is referred to as the natural pacemaker of the heart. The atrioventricular (AV) node can generate 40–60 action potentials (electrical impulses) per minute, if the AV node no longer receives electrical impulses from the SA node, the AV node will become the pacemaker for the heart, so the heart continues to beat without the SA node.

Heart muscle can contract without stimulation from the nervous system. This coordinated contraction of the heart depends upon a conduction system formed from specialized non-contractile muscle cells. An impulse can spread from atria to ventricles in an orderly manner.

Learning Point
This intrinsic conduction system consists of:

- A sinoatrial (SA) node
- An atrioventricular (AV) node
- An atrioventricular bundle or bundle of His
- The bundle branches and Purkinje fibres

The cells of the SA node are autorhythmic. These set the heart rate and for this reason is known as the pacemaker. The SA node (acts as the pacemaker of the heart) has the highest frequency of discharge (110 impulses per min) therefore they dominate the other cells.

The pulse from the SA node spreads through both atria causing depolarization and contraction. The next area to receive the impulse is the AV node at the bottom of the right atrium then it is passed down the AV bundle and right and left bundles to the apex of each ventricle. It travels fast through the Purkinje fibres to the ventricular muscle cells which contract simultaneously to produce a coordinated ventricular systole.

> **Learning Point**
> - The parasympathetic vagus nerve acts as a break on heart rate and the sympathetic nerves with adrenaline accelerate the heart rate.
> - Parasympathetic nerves release acetylcholine (heart less excitable & HR decreases).
> - Sympathetic nerves release noradrenaline (i.e. adrenaline) HR increases.

The pulse from the SA node spreads through both atria causing depolarization and contraction. The next area to receive the impulse is the AV node <u>at the bottom of the right atrium</u> then it is passed down the AV bundle and right and left bundles to the apex of each ventricle. It travels fast through the Purkinje fibres to the ventricular muscle cells which contract simultaneously to produce a coordinated ventricular systole.

> **Learning Point**
> The normal heart produces a typical waveform, sinus rhythm which consists of five deflection waves known as PQRS complex which represents a complete cardiac cycle and T. The small P wave represents the atrial depolarization while the QRS complex represents ventricular depolarization. The T wave represents ventricular repolarization. The PR interval is the time taken for impulse conduction from the SA node through the atria to the AV node and onto the ventricles. The ST segment represents a period of inactivity and ventricular depolarization.

The wall of the heart is supplied with blood by the coronary circulation. The major arteries serving the myocardium are the left and right coronary arteries. Both originate from the aorta. The left coronary artery which branches into the left anterior descending artery and the circumflex artery, supplies blood to the left side of the heart. The right coronary artery supplies blood mainly to the right side of the heart. Once oxygen has been delivered to the tissue, blood is collected by a large vein, called the coronary sinus which drains into the right atrium.

> **Learning Point**
> The anatomical structures of the coronary arteries around the heart.
> The myocardium receives its blood supply from the right and left coronary arteries. The left coronary artery forms the circumflex and anterior interventricular arteries and the right coronary artery the marginal and posterior interventricular arteries.

The body at rest the heart receives about 250 mls of blood every minute. Deoxygenated blood leaves the myocardium via cardiac veins and some of these veins form the coronary sinus which return most of the blood to the right atrium. The remainder is drained directly into the right atrium via cardiac veins.

Venous blood, low in oxygen and rich in carbon dioxide returns to the heart via superior and inferior venae cave and the coronary sinus. The blood enters the right atrium and passes through the tricuspid valve into the right ventricles. Blood is pumped from the ventricles through the tricuspid and mitral valve into the pulmonary which transports blood to the lungs in the pulmonary circulation. The close contact between the capillaries and alveoli enables gaseous exchange to occur and carbon dioxide from the blood moves into the alveoli and oxygen moves into the blood (diffusion).

The blood received in oxygen and low in carbon dioxide returns to the left atrium via four pulmonary veins, two from each lung and pass through the bicuspid valve into the left ventricle. Contraction of the ventricles moves the blood through the semilunar valve into the aorta and to all parts of the body. The flow of blood depends *on the pressure to move, and resistance encountered.*

Learning Point
The greater the resistance the smaller the flow (*hypertension*). Resistance depends on the size of the blood vessels and interactions between constituents of the blood (*viscosity*). Turbulence flow happens if the vessel is large (aorta), the viscosity and density is low (anaemia), and blood is moving very fast (as it does in the arteries).

4.4 Transport of Blood—The Arterial, Venous, and Capillary Circulation

Blood flow refers to the amount of blood passing through a vessel in a specified time. It depends on the blood pressure and the resistance (opposition) to the flow as blood travels through the vessels. The factors which produce resistance are **vessel diameter, blood viscosity, and vessel length**. Factors influencing blood pressure: *Cardiac output, peripheral resistance, and blood volume.*

Venous return of blood is influenced by the speed (velocity) of the blood leaving the heart and the action of the skeletal muscles in "milking" the blood back to the heart. The cardiovascular examination usually starts with the assessment of the pulse (radial artery) and the measurement of the blood pressure which is carried out along with the other vital signs at the beginning of the general examination. This is then followed by the examination of the major arterial pulses in the upper and lower limbs, the jugular venous pulse, and finally the heart itself.

In examining the arterial pulse you need to determine:
The rate
The rhythm
The volume (amplitude) and contour (shape)

Learning Point
- Most of the resistance occurs in the peripheral vessels and is known as the peripheral resistance (PR)
- The nervous system control is through the vasomotor centre (VMC) which is part of the cardiovascular centre in the brain.
- The level of activity in the VMC depends on the amount of inhibition by the baroreceptors (sensory receptors) responding to pressure changes in the carotid sinus and aortic arch.
- Low pressure reduces baroreceptors inhibition of the VMC which send more impulses to the vessels which constrict. High BP results in complete inhibition of the VMC and vasodilation.

Blood pressure (BP) is the pressure exerted by the blood on the wall of the vessel and, in general, refers to the pressure in arteries. The blood pressure will be raised when:

1. The heart rate and the force of contraction are increased.
2. The resistance to blood flow is increased following vasoconstriction.

Since the heart pumps in a pulsating manner, the arterial pressure fluctuates between 120 mm (systolic) and 80 mm (diastolic) of mercury. The difference between the systolic and diastolic blood pressure is called the *pulse pressure* and is about 40–50 mm of mercury.

Hypertension is when the BP is consistently above the normal level 140/90 mmHg, and it is a major cause of organ damage: stroke, kidney disease, increased atherosclerosis retinopathy, CHP, LVH, PVD.

Hypertension is broadly classified into primary (essential) hypertension and secondary hypertension. The cause of the primary hypertension is not known but evidence shows that there is a strong correlation with heredity and lifestyle. Important risk factors include high salt diet, obesity, lack of exercise, excess cholesterol, high alcohol intake, and high blood cholesterol levels. Secondary hypertension is caused by existing medical condition mainly kidney and hormonal disease, i.e. kidney disease, endocrine-pheochromocytoma, liver disease, aortic co-arctation, and pregnancy. Primary hypertension is further classified into labile hypertension, essential hypertension, and malignant hypertension.

Essential hypertension (90–95%) cause is not known.

Labile hypertension or borderline BP fluctuates between normal and hypertensive range.

Malignant hypertension, severe hypertension, ocular changes (i.e. papilledema), LVH, and prognosis are poor.

Learning Point
Venous return of blood is influenced by the speed (velocity) of the blood leaving the heart and the action of the skeletal muscles in "milking" the blood back to the heart. This is an important factor towards blood pressure regulation.

The muscle pump	
Muscle relaxed,	Muscle contracted,
Valves closed	Valve above muscle opens

Factors contributing to blood pressure are known to be:
Peripheral resistance
Cardiac output
Blood volume
Venous return
Blood viscosity affecting peripheral resistance
Elasticity of large arteries

4.5   The Symptoms and Signs of Cardiovascular Disease (CVS)

Heart disease causes five main symptoms:

- Chest pain
- Breathlessness
- Ankle swelling (oedema)
- Palpitations
- Dizziness and blackouts

Before assessing the heart, blood pressure, and peripheral pulses, you may also look for the following general features related to CVS disorders:

Clubbing
Cyanosis: Peripheral cyanosis is inadequate circulation due to excess oxygen removed from the blood. Detect by looking at the peripheries, i.e. lips, feet, fingers, ears. It indicates poor and/or inadequate circulation in the small vessels. For example, cold hands in cold weather (vasoconstriction), patients with low cardiac output, Raynaud's disease (vasoconstriction and excessive oxygen is removed from the blood). Central cyanosis: heart or lung problems leading to poor blood oxygenation in lungs. Detect by looking at the lips, under the tongue, but whole patient may be cyanosed. There is poor oxygenation of the blood when it passes through the lungs as seen in lung diseases. Also, when the blood bypasses the lungs completely as in

right to left shunt seen in congenital heart diseases. Common causes: LVF, pulmonary fibrosis, air flow obstruction.

Pallor

Cardiac cachexia is generalized body wasting condition—fatigue, muscle, fat, and bone wasting. Consequences of long-term conditions such as CHF indicate poor prognosis. Neurohormonal and metabolic waste disorder. Prognosis is usually poor when cachexia is evident.

Oedema

Cardiovascular disease involves disorders of the heart and/or arteries and veins and *there are key symptoms and signs which may be associated with CVS or heart disease as follows*:

> **Learning Point**
> - *Chest pain* can be a significant symptom for CVS disease. Many cardiac patients present with angina pectoris (the Latin pectus means chest) due to ischaemia (insufficient blood flow to the heart) and is typically presented as pressure or discomfort in the anterior chest. Coronary artery disease usually causes angina. Characteristics of pains: substernal, tight chest pain which may radiate to neck, jaw, arms usually left and it is usually aggravated by exertion and relieved by rest. The patient may be breathless, and pain is described as crushing, squeezing, and constricting.
> - Rarely, angina may be due to aortic stenosis, hypertrophic cardiomyopathy or due to spasm of the coronary arteries. Myocardial infarction or unstable angina causes nausea and a feeling of impending doom, severe pain, persistent, associated with rare but characteristic tearing sensation between the shoulder blades and back. Pain is severe and persistent and sometimes associated with pain of MI.
> - A rarer cause of cardiovascular chest pain is a dissecting aneurysm, in which there is a tearing of the muscle layer of the thoracic aorta leading to bulging of the wall. Patients complain of a severe "tearing" pain. Other non-cardiac causes of chest pain are those arising from the oesophagus, pleura, and chest wall.
>   *Differential diagnosis*: Musculoskeletal pain; GIT pain; Dissecting aortic aneurysm; pleuritic pain; Herpes zoster (shingles); Pericarditis (inflammation of the pericardium due to viral or bacterial infection; post-MI uraemia). *Differential by pain* described as constant soreness behind sternum, pain often worsens on inspiration and related to movements, for example, turning over in bed, pneumothorax. Pain at rest—differential diagnosis: MI, unstable angina, dissecting aortic aneurysm, oesophageal pain, pleuritic pain, musculoskeletal, herpes zoster (Shingles), pericarditis.

- ***Dyspnoea*** is awareness of increased respiratory effort that is perceived as unpleasant or inappropriate or an uncomfortable awareness of one's own breathing. Dyspnoea is associated with chest pain in CVS disease and can spread to arms, back, neck, or jaw. Respiratory disorders such as pulmonary oedema, asthma, bronchitis, pneumonia, pneumothorax, lung cancer, pulmonary embolism, anaemia, stroke, MI, valvular disease and arrhythmia and COPD can cause breathlessness but cardiac disorders, for example, congestive heart failure, arrhythmias also cause dyspnoea. In mild heart failure dyspnoea may only become apparent on exertion. In severe failure, however, breathlessness may be evident at rest and the patient cannot lie flat. Left ventricular failure and congestive cardiac failure are associated with cardiac dyspnoea. ***Orthopnoea*** means that the patient has shortness of breath when lying flat and ***paroxysmal nocturnal dyspnoea*** noted when the patient wakes at night and has to sit up gasping for breath.
- There is increased fluid volume in lungs leading to impaired gas exchange. In case of anaemia the reduced Hb/RBC reduces oxygen content of blood.
- Other causes may be obesity, anaemia, anxiety, high altitude with lower oxygen levels, allergic reaction, and anaphylaxis.
- ***Ankle swelling (oedema)*** is the accumulation of excess fluid in the tissues around the ankles. They are first affected due to gravity and develop when an imbalance occurs between the osmotic and hydrostatic pressures. Often **sacral oedema** is found on the lower back in heart failure patients. Differential diagnosis: increase in venous pressure in heart failure reduced plasma osmotic pressure due to loss of protein in liver or renal failure. Increase in permeability of capillary walls to proteins (leaky capillary due to inflammatory reactions). Blockage of lymphatic vessels due to malignant disease or parasitic diseases.
- **Palpitations** are an abnormal awareness of the heartbeat. Palpitations or arrhythmias may be due to an abnormal rate or an irregular rhythm due to a disorder of electrical conduction, overactive thyroid, anaemia, certain drugs, anxiety, very forceful heart contraction, e.g. an overactive thyroid, anaemia, drugs, and excessive vasodilatation, e.g. after a heavy meal. They are described as flattering or racing heartbeat.
- **Dizziness and blackouts** due to aortic stenosis can cause low oxygen levels in the brains and cause dizziness. The aortic valve regulates blood flow from the left ventricle to the aorta and the valve becomes rigid and narrow.
- **Cardiac syncope** is a sudden loss of consciousness followed by quick recovery. Abnormal heart rhythms may also be responsible.
- **Orthopnoea** is breathlessness when lying flat and it is caused in heart failure/lVF, CCF. Stimulation of nerve endings due to an increase in pulmonary capillary pressure caused by redistribution of fluid from periphery when the patient lies flat.

- **<u>Paroxysmal nocturnal dyspnoea</u>** means that the patient is being woken at night by breathlessness and causes them to sit upright or go to a window gasping for breath (severely breathless). Sometimes the patient produces a cough with a frothy pink/white sputum. Paroxysmal nocturnal dyspnoea usually is related to congestive heart failure and a similar mechanism to orthopnoea causes paroxysmal nocturnal dyspnoea but the patient may be extremely breathless and waken gasping for air and the patient often has a cough and produces a frothy sputum which may be pink or blood stained.
- **<u>Fatigue</u>** is an overwhelming feeling of lacking energy and in CVS disease there is also exercise intolerance particularly in heart failure patients due to weakened pumping ability of the heart. Fatigue is also associated with a heart attack either before or after a heart attack.
- **<u>Central cyanosis</u>** (blueness and purplish of the skin) occurs when the level of deoxygenated haemoglobin in the arteries is below 5 g/dL with oxygen saturation below 85%. The bluish/purplish discolouration is generally seen over the entire body surface, and it is more visible in mucosa, e.g. tongue, lips, cheek, extremities.
- **<u>Cough</u>** or **<u>wheezing</u>** is noted in congestive heart failure patients who may cough out pink, frothy sputum due to pulmonary oedema. Left ventricular failure reduces forward flow into the aorta and systemic circulation and causes an increase in lung pressure with fluid tracking into the interstitial space disrupting alveolar membrane junctions, and fluid and blood cells flood into the alveoli and leads to pulmonary oedema. This concentration of fluid and blood cells in the alveoli creates cough and the production of frothy sputum.

4.6   The Role of the Pulse

The radial pulse is commonly used to assess the following:

- Heart rate
- Rhythm
- Volume (amplitude)
- Contour intra-arterial recording of pressures versus time gives the shape of the pulse wave.

As the left atrium contracts (atrial systole) pressure increases and pushes blood into the open mitral valve (ventricles 70% full by passive filling due to higher pressures in major veins than ventricles) Atrial contraction "tops up" 30% End of the atrial systole ventricles mac amount to blood (End Diastolic volume (EDV) is approximately 130 ml at rest).

Left ventricular pressure increases (V systole) as atrial systole ends. Left ventricular pressure becomes higher than atrial pressure, which causes closure of the mitral valve (1st heart sound-Lubb). Ventricles contracting (isovolumetric contraction is the constant volume as ventricular pressure and tension increases and all valves closed, but pressure not high enough to force open the atrial valve). Left ventricular pressure continues to rise and exceeds that in aortic trunk this forces AV open. Blood flows into aortic trunk (ventricular ejection). Ventricular pressure reduces. Note that stroke volume is when each ventricles ejects 80 mls which is 60% of EDV which is the ejection fraction. EF is variable in response to physiological demand. At the end of ventricle systole pressure in LV falls rapidly.

Aorta: ventricular systole ends, LV pressure falls rapidly. Blood in aorta now flows back to LV this movement closes aortic valve. Pressure in aorta is reduced as back flows begins. After aortic valve closes pressure rises again due to recoil of the elastic wall. This produces a temporary rise called the dicrotic notch (wave form from produced due to transient increase in aortic pressure).

<u>Capillaries</u> are microscopic vessels connecting arterioles to small veins (venules). The main function of the capillaries is to permit exchange of nutrients and wastes between the blood and the tissue cells. They are composed only of a single layer of endothelium and basement membrane.

In the capillaries, hydrostatic pressure increases filtration by pushing fluid and solute out of the capillaries, while capillary oncotic pressure (also known as colloid osmotic pressure) pulls fluid into the capillaries and/or prevents fluid from leaving.

Pressure differences govern fluid movement across semi-permeable membranes and two of these forces are hydrostatic/hydraulic pressure and osmotic pressure. The third factor is the permeability of the capillary membranes. There will be an escape of water and solute into the interstitial space resulting in interstitial oedema whenever the hydrostatic pressure is much higher than the osmotic pressure inside the intravascular space. Oedema also occurs when there is capillary leakage due to impaired membrane integrity such as in burns or anaphylaxis or any other condition.

The cardiovascular physical examination usually starts with the assessment of the pulse (most commonly using the radial artery) and the measurement of the blood pressure, which are usually carried out along with the other vital signs (pattern and rate of breathing and assessment of temperature) at the beginning of the general examination. This is followed by examination of the major arterial pulses in the upper and lower limbs, the jugular venous pulse, and, finally, the heart itself.

In examining the arterial pulse, you need to determine the rate, the rhythm, and the volume and contour. Abnormalities of pulse rate and rhythm are called *arrhythmias.*

Tachycardia is the heart rate that exceeds the normal resting rate (60–100 beats per minute); for adults, a heart rate of more than 100 beats per minute is considered tachycardia. Bradycardia is a heart rate slower than 60 beats per minute. Bradycardia can occur when transmission of impulses between the atria and ventricles is either partially or completely stopped. This is called atrioventricular (AV) block and is divided into: first-degree block, in which all atrial impulses can get through but usually with some delay; second-degree block, also called partial AV block, in which some atrial depolarizations can get through to the ventricle, but others do not; third-degree block, also called complete AV block, in which no atrial impulses can get through. Heart activity is maintained by spontaneous ventricular impulses, called escape rhythms.

The pulse rhythm is assessed by feeling the radial pulse but may need to be confirmed on auscultation.

Two basic questions need to be asked:

- Is the rhythm *regularly irregular*—in other words, do extra beats occur in a basic regular rhythm?
- Is the rhythm *irregularly irregular*—i.e. is it totally irregular?

The Pulse Volume and Contour

The carotid pulse is the most accurate indicator of aortic pulse volume and contour because of its proximity to the heart. The *volume* or *amplitude* correlates with the pulse pressure. The peak represents the maximal systolic pressure, and the trough relates to diastolic pressure. The difference between the two is the pulse pressure usually about 40–50 mm mercury. The *contour (shape)* relates to the speed of the upstroke, the duration of the peak, and the speed of the down stroke. The normal pulse shows a smooth and rapid upstroke, a rounded smooth peak, and a slower, less abrupt downstroke.

The brachial arterial pulse is examined to assess the volume and contour of the peripheral vessels; examination of the carotid pulse provides the most accurate representation of changes in the central aortic pulse. A small weak pulse may indicate low blood pressure, heart disease, or a blood vessel blockage. The most common cause for small weak pulses is *shock*. This causes a small weak pulse, rapid heartbeat, shallow breathing, and unconsciousness.

A bounding pulse is a strong throbbing felt pulse. It is due to a forceful heartbeat which means the stroke volume is likely large, creating a wide pulse pressure. Bounding pulses are present in febrile states, hyperthyroidism, during exercise, anxiety, severe anaemia, or complete heart block and with aortic regurgitation.

Learning Point

Regular irregular arrhythmias:

- Atrial flutter is a common supraventricular arrhythmia characterized by rapid, regular atrial rate at a rate around 300 beats/min and a regular ventricular rate corresponding to one-half or one-quarter of the atrial rate (150 or 75 beats/minute).
- Paroxysmal supraventricular tachycardia (SVTs) is a very fast heart rhythm (150–200 beats/min). Most SVTs are due to one or more extra electrical pathways between the atria and the ventricles.
- Ventricular tachycardia is a very fast heart rhythm (more than 120 beats/min) that begins in the ventricles.

Pulsus alternans is the alternation of one strong and one weak pulse beat without a change in the cycle length. It is most associated with left ventricular dysfunction. Therefore, patients with heart failure, cardiomyopathy, or coronary artery disease are at greatest risk for developing pulsus alternans.

Paradoxical pulse is a fall of systolic blood pressure of more than 10 mmHg during inspiration. It is usually due to a heart or lung condition, such as asthma, it can also be the result of heavy blood loss.

Collapsing pulse is a pulse that is bounding and forceful, with a rapid upstroke and descent. It is typically associated with aortic regurgitation.

Learning Point
Irregularly irregular rhythms

- <u>Premature atrial ectopic beat</u> is an extra heartbeat caused by a signal to the atria from an abnormal electrical focus. It is also called an atrial premature beat or a premature atrial contraction. The main symptom is a perception of a skipped heartbeat.
- <u>Atrial fibrillation</u> is an irregular and often rapid heart rate that occurs when the atria experience chaotic electrical signals (400~600 beats/min). The result is a fast and irregular heart rhythm. The heart rate in atrial fibrillation may range from 100 to 200 beats a minute. Atrial fibrillation is the most common irregular heartbeat.
- <u>Premature ventricular ectopic beat is</u> extra heartbeats that begin in ventricles. The main symptom is a perception of a skipped heartbeat.
- <u>Ventricular fibrillation</u> is considered the most serious cardiac rhythm disturbance. Disordered electrical activity causes ventricles to quiver or fibrillate (150~500 beats/min), instead of contracting normally. This prohibits the heart from pumping blood, causing collapse and cardiac arrest.

Look for a past history of myocardial infarction, angina, or stroke. Enquire about a childhood history of rheumatic fever since this commonly affects the heart valves. Also do ask about drugs that a patient may have been on including any complementary therapies such as herbal medication.

4.7   Part 2: Case Studies

Competent case history taking is the key to make accurate diagnosis. It is important to identify those cases where the problem. For example, pain may appear to arise from the joint, but is in fact referred pain, left shoulder pain which might in fact be referred pain from neck, diaphragm, or heart.

Musculoskeletal symptoms lasting more than 6 weeks are generally described as chronic. The way in which symptoms evolve can be import guide in making a diagnosis. Was the onset sudden or gradual? Chronic disease may start insidiously and may have a variable course with remissions. Was the onset associated with trauma or infection?

The main symptoms of musculoskeletal conditions are pain, stiffness, and joint swelling.

Pain needs to record the location, onset, character, radiation, aggravation, and relieving factors. The pain may feel radiating from the joint or even from an adjacent joint, for example, pain from the knee may be felt in the knee but can sometimes be felt in the hip or ankle. Also, the tennis elbow, pain will usually be felt on the outside of elbow joint. Pain due to pressure on nerves often has numbness and tingling but the character of musculoskeletal pain can be very variable. Non-inflammatory pain is more directly related to use, and pain caused by inflammation is often present at rest as well as on use. Ask whether the pain is constant (probably inflammatory) or intermittent (probably mechanical). The activity or positions make the mechanical joints disorder worse, and rest relieves the pain. Bone pain may be localized or diffuse but muscle pains are difficult to localize and are usually continuous and deep. Another major symptom of muscle disorder is weakness which may be generalized or localized and may be associated with wasting. Tendon or bursa pains are usually localized, often accompanied by signs of inflammation.

Stiffness and joint swelling are common to many joint problems, both may have been noticed by the patient and volunteered during history taking. If the patient has noticed, licit for how long they have been present, prolonged morning stiffness or short-lasting (less than 30 min), whether they are associated with pain.

Learning Point
History of presenting complaint:

- Timing of symptoms: onset, frequency, duration, pattern
- Mode of onset
- Initiating, aggravating, and relieving factors
- Quality, intensity, and severity of symptoms
- Associated manifestations
- Life events preceding and/or at onset
- Previous episodes of similar symptoms
- Diagnosis and/or treatment by other healthcare practitioners

Also consider:

- Occupation
- Hobbies
- Exercise
- Lifestyle
- Ethnicity

Each individual case study consists of a summary of the patient's clinical presentation starting with a list of diagnostic features and any other clinical details that may be important for a differential diagnosis. Becoming competent at interpreting signs and symptoms depends on seeing as many examples as possible and discussing them with a senior colleague. You may wish to use this chapter as a guide to build a comprehensive collection of your own. We have endeavoured to include commonly encountered case studies as well as less common findings which are of clinical importance. Here we include case studies which feature clinical sign sand symptoms that a competent practitioner should be able to recognize and diagnose.

Using the enhanced Cambridge-Calgary (Kurtz et al. 2003) consultation model, the practitioner should collect data on the patient's presenting complaint and taking a patient-centred approach should assess and diagnose the problem. This consultation model enables healthcare practitioners to communicate the patient's problem and plan for a safe and effective management plan. The Calgary-Cambridge model also focuses on the patient's perspective on the problem and builds on the rapport with patients.

The dividing line between history taking and clinical examination is an artificial one since the examination begins from the moment the patient walks into the room. The practitioner uses their observational skills to inspect and assess the general appearance of the patient, uses verbal and non-verbal skills to assess the patient's physical health but also engage with the patient, observe their tone of speech, mood, and orientation for time, place, and person. Throughout the physical examination, we need to be aware of the patient's body language and use our senses of hearing, sight, and touch to communicate and listen to the patient.

Make sure that you apply the principles of the Cambridge-Calgary consultation model and note key findings before you proceed with the physical examination of the patient to maximize patient-centred care and utilize quaternary prevention.

Case Study 1

Gerald, a 54-year-old teacher, was admitted to hospital, complaining of severe central chest pain radiating to the back which had come on suddenly. At the onset of the pain, he took an antacid which had no effect on the pain, apart from making him belch. The pain persisted for about 1 h and became associated with increasing breathlessness, together with a cough, productive of a large amount of pink-stained sputum.

About 10 years ago, he had developed asthma. Since bronchodilators had been ineffective, his GP prescribed Gerald prednisone, which he was still taking. He had since gained 2 stone (12.8 kg) in weight and his blood pressure averages of 180/125.

On examination, he was overweight with obesity around the trunk. Gerald who was distressed, pale, and clammy (a cold sweat), was unable to lie flat. His pulse was 120 per minute and regular and the blood pressure was now 120/90 mmHg, but the GP could not feel pulses bilaterally below the femoral artery.

Before, you examine the patient you may want to reflect on the following question:

1. What are the plausible causes and differential diagnoses for the chest pain, breathlessness, and pink-stained sputum?
2. What is the significance of the weight increase and raised blood pressure noted in his history?
3. What is the significance of the distress, pallor, clamminess, inability to lie flat and the pulse and current blood pressure reading?
4. Why could the practitioner not feel the pulses below the femoral artery?

Case Study 2

Muhammad is a 56-year-old man; he has type 2 diabetes and smokes about 20 cigarettes a day. He lives with his wife. Muhammad was admitted to Emergency Department 2 days ago following an episode of chest pain and cardiac arrhythmias. He was diagnosed with an inferior STEMI (ST elevation myocardial infarction).

He was treated with percutaneous coronary intervention (PCI). He also prescribed atropine for his bradycardia and GTN for his chest pain, but his chest pain becomes worse on inspiration and coughing. Muhammad is sitting forward in the bed leaning on the table.

Muhammad has a BMI of 36, and his BP is 130/90 mmHg, Pulse: 70, SaO_2: 96%, Respirations: 22, temperature: 38.6 °C. On auscultation the doctor found a pericardial rub and he was sent for an echocardiogram which shows a small pericardial effusion.

1. What are the likely causes and differential diagnosis of chest pain, bradycardia, and pyrexia? What is the likeliest diagnosis?
2. Brief discussion of the possible pathophysiology of the presenting complaint.
3. Based on the results of the history, choose and describe the clinical exams you will perform in order to localize the lesion responsible for the clinical presentation of this patient.
4. What is the significance of the pericardial rub in this patient?

Case Study 3

George is a 65-year-old man with a history of hypertension, treated with a thiazide diuretic, a low-sodium diet, and a weight control programme. Recently, George was diagnosed with type 2 diabetes and he has been managing his diabetes with an oral hypoglycaemic agent, exercise, and diet control. George also suffers from mild to moderate anxiety, but he has not been diagnosed with depression. He also suffers from headaches and dizziness; he recently got diagnosed with first-degree heart block.

1. What are the likely causes and differential diagnosis of headaches and dizziness? What is the likeliest diagnosis?
2. Brief discussion of the possible pathophysiology of the presenting complaint.

3. Based on the results of the history, choose and describe the clinical exams you
   will perform in order to localize the lesion responsible for the clinical presentation of this patient.
4. What is the significance of the blood pressure reading in this patient?

Case Study 4

Claire is a 71-year-old retired school cook who has been complaining of severe
fatigue and indigestion in the last couple of days. Her son took her to the Emergency
Department, and she was given oxygen, and an intravenous line was inserted.
Bloods were taken for serum enzymes and electrolytes and a tentative diagnosis if
myocardial infarction was made. Claire is a type 2 diabetic and she also suffers from
osteoarthritis. Her BMI is 30.6 kg/m^2 and on admission her HbA1C was 75. Her BP
is 90/60 mmHg, and her pulse is 90 beats per minute, weak, and irregular.

1. What are the likely causes and differential diagnosis of the weak and irregular
   pulse and fatigue? What is the likeliest diagnosis?
2. Brief discussion of the possible pathophysiology of the presenting complaint.
3. What is the significance of the blood pressure reading in this patient?

Case Study 5

Alistair is a 43-year-old man who has complained of palpitations for the last month.
He had first noticed these when climbing the stairs of the house. He became aware
of his heart beating rapidly. There was also an associated pain and mild shortness of
breath which would last for about 5 min. The pain was felt across the sternum. He
smokes about 30 cigarettes a day and tends to drink more than he should when
stressed. He is not on any medication but sometimes takes anti-diarrhoea remedies
for occasional bouts of diarrhoea.

   He also noted some swelling of his ankles, particularly in the evening, and shifting dullness was noted on abdominal examination.

   On examination, his pulse was 104 per minute and regular and the blood pressure
was 155/95 mmHg.

1. What are the likely causes and differential diagnosis of the palpitations, chest
   pain, mild shortness of breath? What is the likeliest diagnosis?
2. Brief discussion of the possible pathophysiology of the presenting complaint.
3. What is the significance of the pulse reading in this patient?

Case Study 6

Nita is a 40-year-old woman who has been unwell for 6 months. She complained of
being irritable and had lost about 6 kg in weight. When she visits you at your practice, she also complains of shortness of breath on exertion and some swelling of the
ankles. On examination you find her to be thin and tense, with a temperature of
38.5 °C. The pulse is 140/min. and totally irregular. There is pitting oedema of the
ankles and feet and the JVP is raised to the angle of the jaw. The heart apex cannot

be felt and the heart sounds are soft. In the chest, there are crackles over both lung fields and the signs of a left-sided pleural effusion.

1. What other questions would you want to ask in the history to help you with the diagnosis?
2. What features would you look for on general (not systemic) examination that would help you in the differential diagnosis. In each case, state your reasons for looking for the particular feature (or groups of features)
3. Comment on the significance of Nita's JVP finding on examination.
4. Discuss the causes and differential diagnosis of Nita's symptoms, signs, and features of cardiac failure. Why might the heart sounds be soft and the apex not felt?
5. If the apex beat had been shifted to the anterior axillary line, what would this signify and what would be the mechanism for this?

4.8   Part 3: Physical Examination Technique

In this section discuss step by step the physical examination we need to undertake for the above patient. Before we start make sure that we follow the below:

- Wash hands.
- Introduce yourself.
- Position patient at 45° supine.
- Expose area for examination.

Inspection
By standing at the end of bed and we observe for and note:

General appearance (facial appearance and skin features), shortness of breath, cyanosis central, malar flush, features of congenital disorders associated with heart problems, for example, Downs trisomy 21 extra chromosome (endocardial cushion defect), Turner's syndrome, cyanosis, pallor, sweatiness, and cachexia.

> **Learning Point**
> *Cyanosis* is a bluish colour of the skin and mucus membranes. It may be caused by Raynaud's disease, cardiac problems and hypothermia and the skim on fingertips, toes, palms and feet appears bluish or greenish, or ashen. Darker skin tones may appear more ashen.
> *Pallor* is a pale colour of the skin and in darker skin tones this may not be noted easily. Underlying cause of pallor is usually anaemia or poor perfusion with a cardiac cause.
> *Sweatiness* is associated with heart attack and heart failure due to an overactive sympathetic nervous system (hyperhidrosis)
> *Cachexia* is the loss of muscle mass due to gut malabsorption, also known as "body wasting". Cachexia can make worse heart failure-associated anaemia.

We look and feel their hands and note:

- Feel temperature and check capillary refill time.
- Peripheral cyanosis (blue hands due to peripheral vascular disease).
- Raynaud's syndrome, heart failure shock, and central cyanosis.

Tendon xanthomata (cholesterol deposits in tendons, they appears as enlarged subcutaneous nodules found over the knuckles and Achilles tendon).

Observe their face and examine their eyes:

A *Corneal arcus* is a white ring around the cornea that is commonly a normal finding in elderly people. However, when it is present in younger people and is associated with fat deposits in the skin around the eyes (xanthelasmata), it indicates excess lipids in the blood—an associated risk factor in heart disease. HDL >/ 1 mmol/l in people with CVD or at high risk, LDL cholesterol <2.0 mmol/l

Xanthelasma, a yellow growth at the corners of the eyelids and they are cholesterol deposits build up under the skin. They are a sign of heart disease.

Conjunctival pallor is a sign of anaemia and it is an unhealthy paleness. It is observed in the anterior palpebral conjunctiva or conjunctival rim

---

Examine the mouth for:

- Central cyanosis causes blue lips and tongue and when severe can also cause blue hands but usually warm.
- Poor dentation.

We observe and feel the neck:

Carotid pulse is felt on either side of the front of the neck just below the angle of the jaw and carries blood from the heart to the brain.

The *JVP* reflects the pressure in the right atrium and the waveform of the pulsation can aid in diagnosing several important conditions. There are no valves between the jugular veins and the right atrium, which means that the height of the column of blood in the neck veins directly reflects the pressure in the right atrium. In physical examination, we observe the external jugular vein because it is easier to see than the internal jugular vein when it is distended. The external jugular vein runs from the mid-point of the clavicle obliquely across the sternomastoid muscle.

The deeper internal jugular vein passes from the sternoclavicular joint upwards and beneath the external jugular vein towards the angle of the jaw.

JVP helps diagnose right-sided heart failure and in differentiating a cardiovascular cause of acute shortness of breath (right ventricular failure, pulmonary embolism) from an intrinsic pulmonary cause (asthma, chronic obstructive pulmonary disease).

All systemic veins collect blood from the tissues and return it to the right atrium. The venous return from the gut is collected by the portal venous system which carries the blood first to the liver. The venous system has a much lower pressure than the arterial system. Blood from the chest abdomen and limbs drains passively into right atrium via the inferior vena cava. This alone is inadequate and contraction of the upper and lower limbs is required to actively propel blood back to the heart.

Valves are present in the lower limb veins to prevent blood from flowing in the wrong direction. Venous drainage from the head and neck drains via the superior vena cava and is gravity-assisted when the individual is upright.

We note differences between the JVP and carotid pulses as shown in the table below. The JVP reflects the pressure in the right atrium and the waveform of the pulsation can aid in diagnosing a number of important conditions. There are no valves between the jugular veins and the right atrium which means that the height of the column of blood in the neck veins directly reflects the pressure in the right atrium. The external jugular vein is easier to see than the internal jugular vein when it is distended. The external jugular vein runs from the mid-point of the clavicle obliquely across the sternomastoid muscle. The deeper internal jugular vein passes from the sternoclavicular joint upwards and beneath the external jugular vein towards the angle of the jaw. The JVP is best measured using the internal jugular vein.

Jugular venous pulse	Carotid pulse
Increases when pressure applied over liver	The pulsation can be felt
More than one peak	Breathing has no effect on the pulse
The pulsation cannot be felt	Does not alter when neck position changed
Pressure increased by deep inspiration	No change when pressure applied over liver
Alters when neck position changed	Single peak

Interpretation of the JVP

If we palpate the JVP waveforms on the patient's neck it will consist of a, v, and c wave in one cardiac cycle. So, this picture illustrates these waveforms:

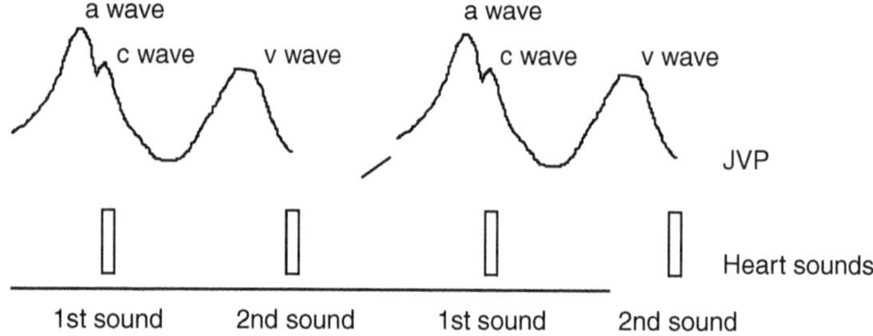

We are concerned with the "a" and "v" waves, since the "c" wave is transmitted from the carotid pulse. The cardiac cycle on the right side consists of contraction (systole) of the right atrium, during which the right ventricle is in diastole and fills with blood, followed by ventricular contraction during which the right atrium is in diastole and fills with blood. Ventricular contraction forces the tricuspid valves to close and the pulmonary valve to open. Bearing this in mind:

What do you think the "a" wave is associated with?
What do you think the "v" wave is associated with?

What is the major pathological reason for a general increase in the JVP?
Which wave is very prominent if there is right ventricular hypertrophy? Can you think of two likely reasons for this?
Which wave is very prominent if the tricuspid valve is damaged and is allowing blood to leak back to the right atrium?

The "a" wave produced by atrial systole precedes tricuspid valve closure.
The "v" wave produced by atrium filling passively during ventricular systole.
The major pathological reason for a general increase in the JVP is:
Congestive or right-sided heart failure
Pulmonary embolism
Superior vena cava obstruction
Tricuspid valve closure
Constrictive pericarditis
Right ventricular infarction

The physical assessment of JVP involves putting the patient in the correct position, sitting at 45° angle, neck muscle relaxed, visualize or use torch if necessary and look out for double pulsation to be observed. JVP is visible but not raised.

When the pressure of the blood in the right atrium is very high it may cause hepatic congestion. That is because back pressure leads to RAP increase followed by increase in pressure in the super vena cava artery leading to high pressure in the hepatic veins. Likely causes of this is CCF, obstructive pulmonary disease, and on examination you find enlarged tender liver and spleen, ascites, and jaundice. The patient usually complains of feeling fatigue, having indigestion and abdominal discomfort.

On the other hand, when the pressure in the left atrium is very high the pressure in the left atrial pressure increases and pulmonary capillaries engorge and stiffen the lungs causing fluid leak into alveoli. On auscultation, crackling sounds can be heard. Raised pulmonary venous pressure may lead to pulmonary oedema. This happens because the increased hydrostatic pressure in the pulmonary veins leads to the accumulation of fluid in the alveoli of the lungs and there is fluid accumulation in the basal areas of the lungs causing the basal alveoli to collapse on expiration usually due to LVF. Patient may complain of acute shortness of breath, exercise-related dyspnoea, orthopnoea, paroxysmal nocturnal dyspnoea, cool skin, and cyanosis. On auscultation, bilateral crackle sounds were found due to the opening of collapsed alveoli on inspiration.

Furthermore, we examine their nails for any of the signs below:

Koilonychia, or spoon nails, is related to iron deficiency anaemia and poor blood flow weakens and depresses the underlying connective tissue giving the nails this peculiar shape and form. Other causes are celiac disease and GI bleeding malignancy and heart disease.

Finger *clubbing* of the fingernails is also associated with CVS disease. The normal angle between the fingernail and nail bed is 160° and the base is firm to palpation. In clubbing, the angle increases and if press the nail base and the nail appear to "float" in severe clubbing, the fingers may have a drumstick appearance. Although clubbing is a common finding in many illnesses. In the cardiovascular system is caused by two main conditions: Congenital cyanotic heart disease and subacute bacterial endocarditis.

Splinter haemorrhages are linear discoloration described as "splinters under the nail" and are associated with endocarditis (infection of the heart valves). Other causes are vasculitis or clots in the small capillaries.

We feel their wrist:

- Radial pulse (absent radial pulse can be caused by congenital heart failure, arterial embolism, or atheroma)
- Collapsing pulse

Inspect their arms:

- Scars
- Visible heave

In normal individuals, nothing is usually visible on inspection of the heart. If pulsations are noted, they could be considered abnormal. Sometimes we see the slight pulsation of the *apical impulse* with some normal, slim individuals. The position of the apical impulse should be noted. Percussion is of little value since it is very difficult to percuss the outline of the heart due to its position behind the sternum and the presence of lung partly in front of it.

We use palpation to:

- Locate the apex beat, count, and assess character.

In the fourth to fifth left intercostal space, on the mid-clavicular line (patient lying supine at 45°). There are three common pathological situations which can displace the *apex beat*:

(a) *Mediastinal shift*: Collapsed or fibrotic lung, large pleural effusion, pneumothorax.
(b) *Left ventricular hypertrophy*: Hypertension, aortic stenosis or incompetence, mitral incompetence.
(c) *Right ventricular hypertrophy*: Pulmonary stenosis, chronic lung disease, multiple pulmonary emboli, right to left shunt (congenital heart disease).

Pulmonary hypertension and pulmonary stenosis are the likely reasons for right ventricular hypertrophy. The wave that is very prominent if the tricuspid valve is damaged and is allowing blood to leak back to the right atrium is the v wave.

Heaves and thrills

A heave is a palpable lifting sensation under the sternum and anterior chest wall to the left of the sternum usually in right ventricular hypertrophy.

Thrills feel like a vibration or buzzing on the skin of the precordium underneath your hand. Thrills are palpable murmurs, the examine hand will detect a vibration. These are always accompanied by an easy heard murmurs on auscultation.

In normal individuals, nothing is usually visible on inspection of the heart. If pulsations are noted they must be considered abnormal. Percussion is of little value since it is very difficult to percuss the outline of the heart due to its position behind the sternum and the presence of lung partly in front of it. The most important part for palpation is the detection of the cardiac apex (5th intercostal space and mid-clavicular line). Palpable heart or cardiac impulse is the lowest and most lateral point at which the heart impulse can be felt or heard. Use the sternal angle (angle of Louis) as a landmark for the 2nd IC then count down. Make sure that you examine the trachea and then apex. Start palpating in the axilla and move anteriorly until the apex is felt. If not then can miss an apex that is significantly displaced. A forceful apex beat suggests increased cardiac output. For example, a forceful apex beat can be felt after exercise or if the person has a fever. Thrusting heave-LVH/RVH MR.AR if it is diffused then it is LVF cardiomyopathy if tapping the MS.

Common pathological situation which can displace the apex beat are abnormalities of the heart, lungs, and rib cage, such as collapsed lungs, which can move the mediastinum and heart to the right.

Pneumothorax, pleural effusion, collapsed lungs and thoracic scoliosis can move the mediastinum to right or left as well as abnormalities of the hearts such as LVH, cardiomyopathy, RVH. The apex is usually just palpable however it may be heaving or thrusting in nature on inspection if there is hypertrophy of the ventricles or dilation of the ventricles. Sometimes the apex beat is not palpable. You may ask the patient to turn to the left or ask them to lean forward, which can facilitate location of the apex beat.

The heart may become hypertrophic or dilated because of cardiac failure and its inability to produce sufficient CO to meet the needs of the body. The myocardium responds to physiological and pathological stimulus as well as hormonal and neural stimuli including compensatory mechanisms such as the sympathetic NS renin-angiotensin system. Impaired cardiac function reduced CO leading to failure of ventricles to empty, and retain venous blood. Compensatory mechanizes activated and increase pressure workloads, leading to increased muscle mass (ventricular hypertrophy) or dilation of ventricles. Dilation of the ventricles may occur in some conditions such as dilated cardiomyopathy.

We auscultate using the stethoscope to listen for normal 1st and 2nd heart sounds, any 3rd or/and 4th heart sound and murmurs. Thrills are palpable murmurs, and they feel like a vibration. These occur at specific point in cardia cycle resulting from turbulent blood flow within the heart and great vessels. Causes of murmurs are valve stenosis, incompetence, abnormally large amount of blood flow past a normal valve. There are two types of murmurs: systole and diastole. Murmurs are usually associated with heart pathology and they may be heard in some common physiological and pathological situations as a secondary phenomenon such as pregnancy, anaemia, aortic coarctation fever, hypertension, and thyrotoxicosis.

Learning Point

Use stethoscope to listen for normal, 1st and 2nd heart sounds, any 3rd or/and 4th heart sound, and murmurs.

Place the digraph of the stethoscope on the

- Apex (mitral)
- Tricuspid
- Pulmonary (2nd left intercostal space)

Common physiological situation causing a loud 1st sound may be exercise but a loud 1st sound (Lap) can be caused by mitral stenosis or hyperthyroidism.

Softer 1st sounds can also be produced in healthy individual because of poor conduction of sounds through chest walls or calcified mitral valve or poor LV contraction.

The 2nd sound has two components, aortic and pulmonary. Normally split sound not heard as very close together but in inspiration there is more blood returning back to the pulmonary circulation thus there is a slight pulmonary valve delay in closing. This occurs because the aortic valve closes before the pulmonary valve when the individual inspires, the RV takes a little longer to eject the increased venous return. Or on inspiration increase BV to RV. Reduce BF to LV. Increasing the BV in RV causes PV to stay open longer as RV takes a little longer to eject increased venous return. Conversely, AV closes marginally earlier due to reduced LV volume. Splitting of 2nd sound occurs in children or younger people during inspiration (2nd ICS sternal border)

Aortic (2nd right intercostal space)

The diaphragm is used most widely and is best for hearing higher-pitched sounds such as the second heart sound and most murmurs.

The bell is used for lower pitched sounds, such as the 3rd and 4th heart sounds. The first heart sound is due to the closure of the mitral and tricuspid values. Some common physiological and pathological situations which cause a loud first sound are high cardiac output (e.g. exercise, fever, anaemia), low cardiac output (e.g. rest and heart failure), first-degree heart block, and mitral regurgitation can cause a softer first heart sound.

Second heart sounds are due to the closure of aortic and pulmonary valves. Inspiration causes second heart sound physiological splitting into aortic, followed by pulmometry components because increased venous return to the right-side heart.

In children or young adults, the second heart sound splits into two components during inspiration. This is due to small changes in the stroke volume of left and right ventricles during the normal respiratory cycle, the heart delays pulmonary valve closure. Systemic hypertension due to increased aortic pressure is associated with a loud aortic component.

Aortic valve stenosis is the part of the heart that is likely to be diseased if the aortic component is very soft. Pulmonary hypertension due to increase in pressure associated with a loud pulmonary component. The 3rd and 4th heart sounds are low frequency sounds occur early and late in diastole respectively. They are caused by abrupt tension of the ventricular walls, following rapid diastolic filling.

The 3rd heart sound is likely to be heard in dilated cardiomyopathy after acute myocardial infarction. Murmurs are the sounds occurring at specific points in the cardia cycle and resulting from turbulent blood flow within the heart and great vessels. They may indicate valve disease.

Murmurs are usually associated with heart pathology. However, they may be heard in some common physiological and pathological situations as a secondary phenomenon, i.e. where the heart is normal.

Such as innocent murmurs of this type are common in children. In adults, they usually reflect hyperkinetic circulation, such as anaemia, fever, pregnancy, and thyrotoxicosis, which lead to turbulent flow in the aortic or pulmonary outflow tracts.

The first heart sound (S1) represents closure of the atrioventricular (mitral and tricuspid) valves as the ventricular pressures exceed atrial pressures at the beginning of systole. S1 is normally a single sound because mitral and tricuspid valve closure occurs almost simultaneously.

The second heart sound (S2) represents closure of the semilunar (aortic and pulmonary) valves. S2 is normally split because the aortic valve (A2) closes before the pulmonary valve (P2). The closing pressure (the diastolic arterial pressure) on the left is 80 mmHg as compared to only 10 mmHg on the right.

This higher closing pressure leads to earlier closure of the aortic valve.

The venous return to the right ventricle (RV) increases during inspiration due to negative intrathoracic pressure and P2 is even more delayed, so it is normal for the split of the second heart sound to widen during inspiration and to narrow during expiration.

The 3rd heart sound happens due to rapid filling of the left ventricle as blood thuds against the left ventricle while the 4th heart sound is due to contraction of the atria against a taut ventricle.

We listen to their back for:

Auscultate lung bases for crepitations (this is an important sign of heart failure deterioration)

Palpate for sacral oedema (heart failure)

We examine their ankles for:

Peripheral oedema

Peripheral oedema is due to a raised hydrostatic pressure. Fluid first collects around the ankles because of gravity in the ambulant patient and is always symmetrical, unlike the oedema due to venous obstruction. Once the patient is bedridden, the fluid also accumulates around the sacrum and buttocks.

The major local and general causes of ankle swelling. In each case, indicate whether the swelling is likely to be unilateral or bilateral happen in:

- Heart failure
- Venous obstruction in pelvis or abdomen
- Immobility
- Low plasma albumin
- Venous insufficiency (varicose veins)
- Venous thrombosis
- Regional lymphatic obstruction

Heart failure deprives the liver from the blood it needs to work this build up puts extra pressure on the portal vein and induce liver disease. The very high pressure of the blood in the right atrium may lead to the following clinical features:

- Hepatic congestion (liver enlargement)
- Right-side heart failure
- Obstructive pulmonary disease
- Fatigue
- Abdominal discomfort
- Loss of appetite
- Jaundice
- Ascites
- Splenic enlargement

When the pressure in the left atrium is very high then the following clinical features may be noted:

- Engorgement & stiffening of lung (pulmonary oedema)
- Left-side heart failure
- Exercise-related dyspnoea
- Orthopnoea (breathlessness when lying flat) due to heart failure/LVF, CCF
- Paroxysmal nocturnal dyspnoea
- Breathlessness
- Tachycardia

Finally, we conclude by:

- Washing our hands
- Reviewing the observation chart
- Recording the examination and peripheral pulse

4.9   Part 4: Focused Learning

Learning Activity 1

The main causes of cardiac chest pain are shown in the table below. Use the keywords below to build up the main characteristics of each pain:

Angina	Myocardial infarction	Pericardial involvement

Keywords and phrases:

1. Worse on movement but not physical exertion	2. Constricting feeling
3. Worse on physical exertion but not movement	4. Retrosternal (behind the sternum)
5. Worse on breathing in	6. Crushing (vice-like) feeling
7. Lasts at least 30 min but more often hours	8. Seldom lasts more than 15 min
9. Brought on by physical or emotional exertion	10. Comes on suddenly usually without warning
11. Radiates (spreads) to neck, jaw, and down left arm	12. Radiates to tip of left shoulder
13. Affected by posture	14. Relieved by rest

Answer:

Angina	Myocardial infarction	Pericardial involvement
2. Constricting feeling *3. Worse on physical exertion but not movement* *4. Retrosternal (behind the sternum)* *6. Crushing (vice-like) feeling* *8. Seldom lasts more than 15 min* *9. Brought on by physical or emotional exertion* *10. Comes on suddenly usually without warning* *11. Radiates (spreads) to neck, jaw, and down left arm* *14. Relieved by rest*	*2. Constricting feeling* *3. Worse on physical exertion but not movement* *4. Retrosternal (behind the sternum)* *6. Crushing (vice-like) feeling* *7. Lasts at least 30 min but more often hours* *10. Comes on suddenly usually without warning* *11. Radiates (spreads) to neck, jaw, and down left arm*	*1. Worse on movement but not physical exertion* *4. Retrosternal (behind the sternum)* *5. Worse on breathing in* *12. Radiates to tip of left shoulder* *13. Affected by posture*

Learning Activity 2

(a) Can you think of some important causes of breathlessness (cardiac and non-cardiac)?

Answer:

Respiratory disorders: Asthma, bronchitis, pneumonia, pneumothorax, lung cancer, pulmonary embolism, COPD …

Cardiac disorders: Congestive heart failure, arrhythmia …

Other: Obesity, anaemia, anxiety, high altitude with lower oxygen levels, allergic reaction, anaphylaxis…

(b) Patients with orthopnoea or paroxysmal nocturnal dyspnoea usually have congestive heart failure and often have a cough accompanied by frothy sputum which may be pink, or blood stained. What is the underlying mechanism for this?

Answer:

Congestive heart failure is an imbalance in pump function in which the heart fails to maintain the circulation of blood adequately. Left ventricular failure will reduce forward flow into the aorta and systemic circulation which causes an increase in lung pressure. Increased lung pressure, fluid can track into the interstitial space disruption of alveolar membrane junctions, fluid and blood cells floods into the alveoli and leads to pulmonary oedema. When the liquid and blood cells accumulate in the alveoli, thus creating cough accompanied by frothy sputum.

(c) What questions would you ask a patient who presents with breathlessness?

Answer:

How much can you do before getting breathless?

How many pillows do you sleep on?

Do you ever wake up gasping for breath?
If so, do you have to sit up or get out of bed?
Do you cough or wheeze when you are short of breath?

Learning Activity 3

Palpitations

This is best defined as an abnormal awareness of the heartbeat. Palpitations may be due to:

- An abnormal rate or an irregular rhythm due to a disorder of electrical conduction, overactive thyroid, anaemia, certain drugs, anxiety
- Very forceful heart contraction, e.g. an overactive thyroid, anaemia, drugs
- Excessive vasodilatation, e.g. after a heavy meal

What questions would you ask a patient who presents with palpitations?

Answer:

Please describe your heartbeat during an attack, regular or irregular?
Is there anything that sets it off?
Can you do anything to stop it?
Is there anything that seems to make it better or worse?
Do you take any medicine now?

Learning Activity 4

(a) Describe the appearance of finger clubbing:

Answer:

The normal angle between the fingernail and nail bed is 160° and the base is firm to palpation. In clubbing, the angle increases and if press the nail base the nail appears to "flot", in severe clubbing, the fingers may have a drumstick appearance.

(b) Clubbing is a common finding in many illnesses. In the cardiovascular system list two main causes:

Answer:

Congenital cyanotic heart disease
Subacute bacterial endocarditis

Learning Activity 5

(a) The pain of myocardial infarction is severe. What is the expression on the patient's face likely to be and what important skin findings will be noted on examination.

Answer:

Lowering the brow, pressing the lips, parting the lips, and turning the head left.

(b) What posture is the patient likely to adopt if there is pericardial pain?

Answer:

Sitting up and leaning forward tends to ease the pain.

Learning Activity 6

Where should one look for peripheral and central cyanosis and what are their mechanisms?

Answer:

Central cyanosis occurs when the level of deoxygenated haemoglobin in the arteries is below 5 g/dL with oxygen saturation below 85%. The bluish hue is generally seen over the entire body surface and visible mucosa, e.g. tongue, lips, cheek, extremities.

Peripheral cyanosis occurs when there is increased oxygen uptake in peripheral tissues; it is not associated with arterial desaturation. Peripheral cyanosis often involves only the extremities, e.g. lips, finger, toe, ear but not tongue.

Differential cyanosis, in which the upper extremities are pink and the lower extremities are cyanotic, is associated with conditions such as co-arctation of the aorta and interrupted aortic arch when there is right-to-left shunting through a patent ductus arteriosus.

Learning Activity 7

Complete the following and define the terms that follow:

(a) The pulse rate is commonly assessed by feeling the radial pulse. The normal rate varies between 60 and 80 beats per minute. Although cardiac muscle has its own inherent ability to contract, the control of the rate is exercised by the *autonomic nervous system*. The _______1_______ division slows the rate down and the ______2_____ speeds it up. Consequently, a _______3____ in _______4____ division activity or a ______5_____ in _____6____ division activity will increase the heart rate.

Keywords and phrases:

Sympathetic   Parasympathetic   Increase   Decrease

Answer:

1. *Parasympathetic*
2. *Sympathetic*
3. *Increase*
4. *Sympathetic*
5. *Decrease*
6. *Parasympathetic*

(b) Define the following terms and list some common causes:

(i) Tachycardia

Answer:

A heart rate that exceeds the normal resting rate, for adults, a heart rate of more than 100 beats per minute is considered tachycardia.

(ii) Bradycardia

Answer:

Bradycardia is defined as a heart rate slower than 60 beats per minute.

Learning Activity 8

What is atrial flutter?

Answer:

Atrial flutter is a relatively common supraventricular arrhythmia characterized by rapid, regular atrial rate at a characteristic rate around 300 beats/min and a regular ventricular rate corresponding to one-half or one-quarter of the atrial rate (150 or 75 beats/minute).

What is paroxysmal supraventricular tachycardia?

Answer:

Paroxysmal supraventricular tachycardia (SVTs) is a very fast heart rhythm (150–200 beats/min). Most SVTs are due to one or more extra electrical pathways between the atria and the ventricles.

What is ventricular tachycardia?

Answer:

Ventricular tachycardia is a very fast heart rhythm (more than 120 beats/min) that begins in the ventricles.

Learning Activity 9

Complete the table using the keywords and phrases provided:

Jugular venous pulse	Carotid pulse

Keywords and phrases:

The pulsation can be felt	The pulsation cannot be felt
Breathing has no effect on the pulse	Pressure increased by deep inspiration
Does not alter when neck position changed	Alters when neck position changed
Increases when pressure applied over liver	No change when pressure applied over liver
More than one peak	Single peak

Answer:

Jugular venous pulse	Carotid pulse
Increases when pressure applied over liver	*The pulsation can be felt*
More than one peak	*Breathing has no effect on the pulse*
The pulsation cannot be felt	*Does not alter when neck position changed*
Pressure increased by deep inspiration	*No change when pressure applied over liver*
Alters when neck position changed	*Single peak*

Learning Activity 10
Interpretation of the JVP
Study the following diagram of the JVP pulsations and answer the questions that follow:

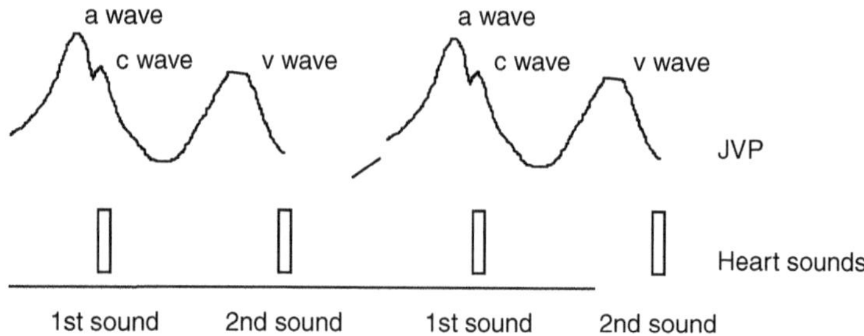

(a) What do you think the "a" wave is associated with?
Answer:
The "a" wave produced by atrial systole precedes tricuspid valve closure.

(b) What do you think the "v" wave is associated with?
Answer:
The "v" wave produced by atrium filling passively during ventricular systole.

(c) What is the major pathological reason for a general increase in the JVP?
Answer:
Congestive or right-side heart failure
Pulmonary embolism
Superior vena cava obstruction
Tricuspid valve closure
Constrictive pericarditis
Right ventricular infarction

(d) Which JPV wave is very prominent if there is right ventricular hypertrophy? Can you think of two likely reasons for this?
Answer:
"a" waves due to pulmonary hypertension and pulmonary stenosis.

(e) Which JPV wave is very prominent if the tricuspid valve is damaged and is allowing blood to leak back to the right atrium?
Answer:
"v" wave

Learning Activity 11
List the major local and general causes of ankle swelling. In each case, indicate whether the swelling is likely to be unilateral or bilateral.
Answer:
Heart failure (bilateral)

Venous obstruction in pelvis or abdomen (bilateral)
Immobility (bilateral)
Low plasma albumin (bilateral)
Venous insufficiency (varicose veins) (unilateral)
Venous thrombosis (unilateral)
Regional lymphatic obstruction (unilateral)

Learning Activity 12

(a) What happens to the liver when the pressure of the blood in the right atrium is
     very high? What is the cause of this raised pressure? What will the patient com-
     plain of and what will you find on examining the abdomen?
     Answer:
     (i) *Hepatic congestion (liver enlargement)*
     (ii) *Right-side heart failure or obstructive pulmonary disease*
     (iii) *Fatigue, abdominal discomfort, loss of appetite*
     (iv) *Jaundice, ascites, splenic enlargement*

(b) What happens to the lungs when the pressure in the left atrium is very high?
     What is the cause of this raised pressure? What is the patient likely to complain
     of and what will you hear at the lung bases through the stethoscope?
     Answer:
     (i) *Engorgement & stiffening of lung (Pulmonary oedema)*
     (ii) *Left side heart failure.*
     (iii) *Exercise-related dyspnoea, orthopnoea, and paroxysmal nocturnal
     dyspnoea*
     (iv) *Breathlessness, tachycardia, inspiratory crackles*

Learning Activity 13

(a) Where is the apex beat normally felt?
     Answer:
     *In the fifth or sixth left intercostal space, on the mid-clavicular line (Patient
     lying supine at 45°).*

(b) List three common pathological situations which can displace the apex beat:
     Answer:
     (i) *Mediastinal shift: Collapsed or fibrotic lung, large pleural effusion,
     pneumothorax.*
     (ii) *Left ventricular hypertrophy: Hypertension, aortic stenosis or incompe-
     tence, mitral incompetence.*
     (iii) *Right ventricular hypertrophy: Pulmonary stenosis, Chronic lung disease,
     multiple pulmonary emboli, right to left shunt (congenital heart disease)*

(c) The apex beat is usually just palpable. However, it may be heaving or thrusting
     in nature (you may also see this on inspection). What is the pathological mecha-
     nism for this, and which part of the heart is involved?
     Answer:
     Left ventricular hypertrophy or dilatation.

(d) Sometimes the apex beat is not palpable. Can you think of any physiological and pathological mechanisms for this?
Answer:
Obesity, emphysema, left pleural effusion, myocardial infarction, pericardial effusion.

(e) Sometimes a heave close to the left sternal border (parasternal heave) can be felt with the flat part of the hand. What is the pathological mechanism for this, and which part of the heart is involved?
Answer:
Right ventricular hypertrophy or dilatation.

(f) What are thrills and which anatomical structures of the heart are they associated with?
Answer:
Thrills are palpable murmurs, the examine hand will detect a vibration. These are always accompanied by an easy heard murmurs on auscultation.

Learning Activity 14
<u>Auscultation</u>

The diaphragm is used most widely and is best for hearing higher-pitched sounds such as the second heart sound and most murmurs. The bell is used for lower pitched sounds, such as the 3rd and 4th heart sounds. You need not concern yourself with the bell.

You should again refer to your knowledge of the cardiac cycle for the following questions:

(a) What is the mechanism for the 1st heart sound?
Answer:
The first heart sound is due to the closure of the mitral and tricuspid values.

(b) Name some common physiological and pathological situations which cause a loud first sound:
Answer:
High cardiac output, exercise, fever, anaemia.

(c) Name some common physiological and pathological situations which cause a softer first heart sound:
Answer:
Low cardiac output (rest, heart failure), first-degree heart block, mitral regurgitation.

(d) What is the mechanism for the second heart sound?
Answer:
Second heart sound is due to the closure of aortic and pulmonary valves.

(e) The second sound often has two components, aortic and pulmonary. Which comes first and why is this?

Answer:

Inspiration causes second heart sound physiological splitting into aortic followed by pulmometry components because increased venous return to the right-side heart.

(f) In which type of normal individuals are you likely to hear a split-second sound?
Answer:
In children or young adults, the second heart sound splits into two components during inspiration. This is due to small changes in the stroke volume of left and right ventricles during the normal respiratory cycle, the heart delays pulmonary valve closure.

(g) Name a very common cardiovascular disease associated with a loud aortic component. What do you think the mechanism might be?
Answer:
Systemic hypertension due to increase the aortic pressure.

(h) Name the part of the heart that is likely to be diseased if the aortic component is very soft:
Answer:
Aortic valve stenosis

(i) Name a cardiorespiratory disorder associated with a loud pulmonary component. What do you think the mechanism might be?
Answer:
Pulmonary hypertension due to increase in pressure.

(j) Briefly state the physiological mechanisms for the 3rd and 4th heart sounds.
Answer:
These low frequency sounds occur early and late in diastole respectively. They are caused by abrupt tension of the ventricular walls, following rapid diastolic filling.

(k) In which common cardiac disorder is a third heart sound likely to be heard?
Answer:
It can be heart in dilated cardiomyopathy after acute myocardial infarction.

(l) What are murmurs and with which anatomical parts of the heart are they associated?
Answer:
Murmurs are the sounds occurring at specific points in the cardiac cycle and resulting from turbulent blood flow within the heart and great vessels. They may indicate valve disease.

(m) Murmurs are usually associated with heart pathology. However, they may be heard in some common physiological and pathological situations as a secondary phenomenon, i.e. where the heart is normal. Can you name some of these?
Answer:
Innocent murmurs of this type are common in children.

In adults, they usually reflect hyperkinetic circulation, such as anaemia, fever, pregnancy, and thyrotoxicosis, which lead to turbulent flow in the aortic or pulmonary outflow tracts.

Learning Activity 15

(a) Complete the following using the keywords and phrases that follow:

The heart is part of the *mediastinum*, the mass of tissue between the *lungs*, extending from the sternum to the vertebral column. The pointed end is called the *apex* and projects downwards (inferiorly) and forwards (anteriorly). The *left border* is formed almost entirely by the _______ a _______, with the _______ b _______ forming part of the upper end of the border. The *upper (superior) border*, where the great vessels enter and leave the heart, is formed by _______ c _______ and _______ d _______. The *right border* is formed by the _______ e _______. The *inferior border* is formed by the _______ f _______ and slightly by the _______ g _______.

Answer:
Inferior vena cava
Superior vena cava
Right atrium
Tricuspid valve
Right ventricle
Pulmonary valve
Pulmonary trunk

(b) Where does pericardial fluid originate from? Where is it located? What is its function?

Answer:

The pericardial fluid secreted by the pericardial membranes. It is located between the two layers of pericardium, acts as a lubricant to reduce friction when the heart beats.

(c) One of the layers that comprises the wall of the heart is the myocardium. What are the names of the other two layers?

Answer:

From outermost to innermost, the layers of the heart wall are the epicardium, myocardium, and endocardium.

(i) How does the wall of the left ventricle differ from that of the right and what is the reason for this?

Answer:

The wall of left ventricle is much thicker, because six to seven times as much force must be exerted to push blood around the systemic circuit.

(ii) What is unique about the structural arrangement of cardiac muscle?

Answer:

Unlike skeletal muscle, cardiac muscle fibres do not rely on nerve activity to tell them when to start a contraction, instead it specialized cardiac muscle fibres-pace marker cells, establish a regular rate of contraction.

(d) Complete the following using the keywords and phrases that follow:

Blood returns to the heart via the _______a_______ from the trunk and limbs and via the _______b_______ from the head and neck. This blood enters the _______c_______ and passes through the _______d_______ valve to the _______e_______. The blood is then ejected through the _______f_______ valve into the _______g_______, which divides into two main branches. These transport the blood to the _______h_______. From here, the blood is taken via the _______i_______ to the _______j_______. The blood passes from here through the _______k_______ valve to the _______l_______ and is then ejected through the _______m_______ valve into the _______n_______ for distribution to the rest of the body.

Keywords and phrases:

Left atrium	Tricuspid valve
Aortic valve	Pulmonary valve
Superior vena cava	Lungs
Inferior vena cava	Left ventricle
Aorta	Pulmonary trunk
Pulmonary veins	Right ventricle
Mitral (bicuspid valve)	Right atrium

Answer:
Inferior vena cava
Superior vena cava
Right atrium
Tricuspid valve
Right ventricle
Pulmonary valve
Pulmonary trunk
Lungs
Pulmonary veins
Left atrium.
Mitral (bicuspid valve)
Left ventricle.
Aortic valve
Aorta

Case Study 1

Gerald, a 54-year-old teacher, was admitted to hospital, complaining of severe central chest pain radiating to the back which had come on suddenly. At the onset of the pain, he took an antacid which had no effect on the pain, apart from making him belch. The pain persisted for about 1 h and became associated with increasing breathlessness, together with a cough, productive of a large amount of pink-stained sputum.

About 10 years ago, he developed asthma. Since bronchodilators had been ineffective, his GP prescribed Gerald prednisone, which he was still taking. He had since gained 2 stone (12.8 kg) in weight and his blood pressure averages of 180/125.

On examination, he was overweight with obesity around the trunk. Gerald who was distressed, pale, and clammy (a cold sweat), was unable to lie flat. His pulse was 120 per minute and regular and the blood pressure was now 120/90 mmHg, but the GP could not feel pulses bilaterally below the femoral artery.

Before you examine the patient you may want to reflect on the following question:

1. What are the plausible causes and differential diagnoses for the chest pain, breathlessness, and pink-stained sputum?

   Answer 1:

   The chest pain could be due to cardiovascular, lung or upper gastrointestine track (GIT) causes. He had a history of asthma, and his chest pain could link to that—he may well have sustained muscular damage from bouts of coughing. However, the chest pain is far too severe and there is no evidence of the pain being worse on movement, which excludes asthma and muscle strain. The pink-stained sputum also does not fit with asthma.

   He could have had a spontaneous pneumothorax which can occur with severe asthma. However, he would have been in severe respiratory distress and there would have been evidence of this on physical examination.

   The pain is unlikely to be due to an upper GIT problem since antacids did not help.

   The predicted cause is a myocardial infarct which has resulted in breathlessness due to left ventricular failure. His copious pink, frothy sputum may confirm his diagnosis. An inferior myocardial infarct could cause pain to radiate to the back, the duration of the pain also suggests a myocardial infarction.

2. What is the significance of the weight increase and raised blood pressure noted in his history?

   Answer 2:

   The weight increase could be due to over-reacting in view of his cardiac state and the type of work that he does. However, it is much more likely to be because of long-term steroids. Steroids are the commonest cause of Cushing's syndrome, which is associated with obesity around the trunk. High blood pressure is a common finding in Cushing's disease and is due to increased salt and water retention.

   Other plausible causes of increased weight in a patient of this age are hypothyroidism and late-onset diabetes mellitus, but there is no evidence in the history for either of these disorders nor in the physical examination.

3. What is the significance of the distress, pallor, clamminess, inability to lie flat and the pulse and current blood pressure reading?

   Answer 3:

   The distress, pallor, clamminess, pulse, and current blood pressure reading plus the inability to lie flat are consistent with left ventricular failure. The pallor and clamminess are the effects of poor peripheral perfusion of the tissues,

*the fall in blood pressure from the previous high reading is also consistent
with decreased ventricular output. The pulse is rapid, which means that the
heart is compensating for decreased myocardial contractility by decreasing
its rate.*

*The inability to lie flat is due to orthopnoea may be a result of pulmonary
oedema. You can look out for the pink-stained sputum associated with pulmonary oedema.*

4. Why could the practitioner not feel the pulses below the femoral artery?
Answer 4:

*You were not able to feel the pulses because of decreased blood supply to the
limbs. As a result of poor left ventricular output. There is a possibility of an
abdominal aortic aneurism to rule out since there were no other findings on
examination (no abdominal pain or pulsatile mass). Also, it is unlikely that
you would feel the femoral pulses if there was an aneurism.*

Case Study 2

Muhammad is a 56-year-old man; he has type 2 diabetes and smokes about 20 ciga-
rettes a day. He lives with his wife. Muhammad was admitted to Emergency
Department 2 days ago following an episode of chest pain and cardiac arrhythmias.
He was diagnosed with an inferior STEMI (ST elevation myocardial infarction).

He was treated with percutaneous coronary intervention (PCI). He also prescribed atropine for his bradycardia and GTN for his chest pain, but his chest pain
becomes worse on inspiration and coughing. Muhammad is sitting forward in the
bed leaning on the table.

Muhammad has a BMI of 36, and his BP is 130/90 mmHg, Pulse: 70, SaO_2:
96%, Respirations: 22, temperature: 38.6 °C. On auscultation, the doctor found a
pericardial rub and he was sent for an echocardiogram which shows a small pericardial effusion.

1. What are the likely causes and differential diagnosis of chest pain, bradycardia,
   and pyrexia? What is the likeliest diagnosis?

   *Pericardial effusion is not common after a heart attack. A pericardial rub is dif-
   ferent from a heart murmur. This is likely to be acute pericarditis or pleuritic
   pain due to musculoskeletal or nerve-related pathology.*

2. Brief discussion of the possible pathophysiology of the presenting complaint.

   *There is visceral and parietal pleural rubbing over each other, or it could be
   due to inflammation of the tissues lining the lungs and chest cavity. Another
   possible cause might be the heart attack or angina or pneumonia (this patient
   has pyrexia).*

3. Based on the results of the history, choose and describe the clinical exams you
   will perform in order to localize the lesion responsible for the clinical presentation of this patient.

   *Auscultation and palpation of the heart and lungs to discern other possible
   causes of chest pain such as pneumonia.*

4. What is the significance of the pericardial rub in this patient?
    This may be significant in the differential diagnosis of pleuritis.

Case Study 3

George is a 65-year-old man with a history of hypertension, treated with a thiazide diuretic, a low-sodium diet, and a weight control programme. Recently, George was diagnosed with type 2 diabetes and he has been managing his diabetes with an oral hypoglycaemic agent, exercise, and diet control. George also suffers from mild to moderate anxiety, but he has not been diagnosed with depression. He also suffers from headaches and dizziness; he recently got diagnosed with first-degree heart block.

1. What are the likely causes and differential diagnosis of headaches and dizziness? What is the likeliest diagnosis?
    Headaches can be caused by high blood pressure but it is also a symptom of second-degree heart block (Mobitz type 1 and Mobitz type 2)
2. Brief discussion of the possible pathophysiology of the presenting complaint.
    First-degree heart block does not cause symptoms.
    Second-degree heart block can cause dizziness, nausea, and skipped beats. There are two types: Mobitz type 1 is less serious and usually does not require treatment, while Mobitz type 2 is more serious and may require a pacemaker.
    Third-degree heart block: Also known as complete heart block, this can cause heart palpitations and cardiac arrest.
3. Based on the results of the history, choose, and describe the clinical exams you will perform in order to localize the lesion responsible for the clinical presentation of this patient.
    The full physical examination is recommended for this patient to ensure that a correct diagnosis and treatment offered to the patient who is clearly quite anxious and upset with his new diagnosis.
4. What is the significance of the blood pressure reading in this patient?
    Chronic high blood pressure can cause long-term heart failure and if hypertension has not been controlled well with medication can cause arrhythmias.

Case Study 4

Claire is a 71-year-old retired school cook who has been complaining of severe fatigue and indigestion in the last two days. Her son took her to the Emergency Department, and she was given oxygen, and an intravenous line was inserted. Bloods were taken for serum enzymes and electrolytes and a tentative diagnosis if myocardial infarction was made. Claire is a type 2 diabetic and she also suffers from osteoarthritis. Her BMI is 30.6 kg/m^2 and on admission her HbA1C was 75. Her BP is 90/60 mmHg, and her pulse is 90 beats per minute, weak, and irregular.

1. What are the likely causes and differential diagnosis of the weak and irregular pulse and fatigue? What is the likeliest diagnosis?

   It may be a complication of diabetes such as ketoacidosis, but further blood samples are needed to work this out. This could be a silent MI or cardiogenic shock post MI so further investigations are required to exclude these.

2. Brief discussion of the possible pathophysiology of the presenting complaint.

   Severe fatigue can be implicated in many different conditions, but it is not uncommon post MI and this patient reported to have hypotension due to diminished cardiac output and ischemia. This usually increases cardiac afterload and there is ineffective stroke volume and insufficient circulation.

3. What is the significance of the blood pressure reading in this patient?

   This may indicate that the patient is getting worse and urgent review is needed to start them on medication and fluid management.

Case Study 5

A 43-year-old man who has complained of palpitations for the last month. He had first noticed these when climbing the stairs of the house. He became aware of his heart beating rapidly. There was also an associated pain and mild shortness of breath which would last for about 5 min. The pain was felt across the sternum. He smokes about 30 cigarettes a day and tends to drink more than he should when stressed. He is not on any medication but sometimes takes anti-diarrhoea remedies for occasional bouts of diarrhoea.

He also noted some swelling of his ankles, particularly in the evening, shifting dullness was noted on abdominal examination.

On examination, his pulse was 104 per minute and regular and the blood pressure was 155/95 mmHg.

1. What are the likely causes and differential diagnosis of the palpitations, chest pain, mild shortness of breath? What is the likeliest diagnosis?

   There is some indication of right-sided heart failure but further investigation is needed to exclude this diagnosis.

2. Brief discussion of the possible pathophysiology of the presenting complaint.

   The right ventricle is not contracting properly which leads to fluid overload. Swelling in the neck veins, ankles, and legs, and accumulation of fluid in the abdomen are also noted.

3. What is the significance of the pulse reading in this patient?

   HR is significant in heart failure because it may indicate better or worse outcomes for the patient.

Case Study 6

Nita is a 40-year-old woman who had been unwell for 6 months. She complained of being irritable and had lost about 6 kg in weight. When she visits you at your practice, she also complains of shortness of breath on exertion and some swelling of the ankles. On examination you find her to be thin and tense, with a temperature of

38.5 °C. The pulse is 140/min. and totally irregular. There is pitting oedema of the ankles and feet and the JVP is raised to the angle of the jaw. The heart apex cannot be felt and the heart sounds are soft. In the chest, there are crackles over both lung fields and the signs of a left-sided pleural effusion.

1. What other questions would you want to ask in the history to help you with the diagnosis?

   When did they notice the swelling? How long ago? Did they also feel short of breath? Have they had a temperature in the past 2 days? How is their appetite?

2. What features would you look for on general (not systemic) examination that would help you in the differential diagnosis. In each case, state your reasons for looking for the particular feature (or groups of features)

   Signs of anaemia or jaundice to exclude general illness. Breathlessness, how often and for how long?

3. Comment on the significance of Nita's JVP finding on examination

   In patients with heart failure, weight gain may indicate hypervolemia, while weight loss may indicate cardiac cachexia (unintentional, non-oedematous weight loss of >5% within the last 12 months). History and additional findings from the physical examination such as jugular veins, lung, and extremity examinations are required to determine whether weight changes are related to changes in volume status and/or amount of muscle or fat.

4. Discuss the causes and differential diagnosis of Nita's symptoms, signs, and features of cardiac failure. Why might the heart sounds be soft and the apex not felt?

   Due to enlarged heart, on examination heart sound may be soft and the apex not felt but it could be aortic stenosis or valvular regurgitation or left bundle branch block or it could be due to pericardial effusion (fluid in the heart) or pleural effusion (fluid in the pleura).

5. If the apex beat had been shifted to the anterior axillary line, what would this signify and what would be the mechanism for this?

   It could be a number of things such as cardiomyopathy or cardiomegaly right tension pneumothorax or left ventricular hypertrophy. Palpitation of the apex and auscultation should help determine the cause.

   The apex is produced by the left ventricle systole so the direction of the shift can indicate the type of heart condition. In this case it is suggestive of left ventricular hypertrophy.

Bibliography

1. Bickley, L. (2012). *Bates' guide to physical examination and history taking.* Lippincott Williams & Wilkins.
2. Jarvis, C. (2023). *Physical examination and health assessment-Canadian e-book.* Elsevier Health Sciences.

3. Kurtz, S., Silverman, J., Benson, J. & Draper, J. (2003). Marrying content and process in clinical method teaching: enhancing the Calgary–Cambridge guides. *Academic Medicine, 78*(8), 802–809.
4. Lena, A., Ebner, N., & Anker, M. S. (2019). Cardiac cachexia. *European Heart Journal Supplements: Journal of the European Society of Cardiology, 21*(Suppl L), L24–L27.
5. McCance, K. L., & Huether, S. E. (2014). *Pathophysiology: The biologic basis for disease in adults and children*. Elsevier Health Sciences.
6. Wieling, W., Kaufmann, H., Claydon, V. E., et al. (2022). Diagnosis and treatment of orthostatic hypotension. *Lancet Neurology, 21*(8), 735–746. https://doi.org/10.1016/S1474-4422(22)00169-7

Assessing and Diagnosing Disorders of the Respiratory System (RS)

5

Learning Objectives

In this part of the chapter, we revisit basic anatomy and physiology of the respiratory system and identify the clinical signs and symptoms diagnostic of respiratory disease and disorders.

Learning Objectives

By the end of this chapter, you will be able to:

Understand the basic pathophysiology of respiratory disease.
Explain the physiological changes and anatomical features present in respiratory disease.
Link symptoms and signs of basic pathology to respiratory disease.
Identify general and specific signs and symptoms relevant to the diagnosis of respiratory disease and their significance in differential diagnosis.
Undertake a step-by-step physical examination on a cardiac patient.
Understand key concepts in respiratory conditions.

Common Medical Terms

The list of medical terms below is cited for easy reference and the reader is expected to understand these medical terms before they proceed to read this chapter.

Cough
Clubbing
Breathlessness
Dyspnoea
Cyanosis

© The Author(s), under exclusive license to Springer Nature
Switzerland AG 2026
C. Leliopoulou, L. Holman, *Physical Examination and Diagnostic Skills for
Nurses and Allied Health Professionals*,
https://doi.org/10.1007/978-3-032-26539-5_5

Haemoptysis
Lymphadenopathy
Sputum
Stridor
Wheeze

5.1   Part 1: The Lungs and the Function of Breathing

Breathing provides a good example of polarity. There is a relationship between *breathing in* and *tension* and *breathing out* and *relaxation* respectively. Since breathing is an exchange process, it embraces the polarities of accepting and giving. Breath continually connects us with all life forms, and we are all bound by breath, whether we like it or not. Consequently, breathing is the basis of contact and relationship.

Lungs are one of the major structures of the respiratory system and they are separated into *lobes* by *fissures* which are oblique on both sides, the left lung consists of *two lobes*: the *superior* and *inferior* lobes, the right lung consists of *three lobes*: the *superior*, *middle*, and *inferior* lobes.

On the right lung we have the upper, middle, and lower lobes and on the left the upper and lower. The respiratory system supplies *oxygen to tissues* via the blood from inspired air and removes carbon dioxide from the blood into expired air but there are other important functions of the respiratory system such as to regulate the acid-base balance, the pulmonary defence mechanism, and speech.

Learning Point
The anatomy of the respiratory system involves:
   The nasal cavities:

- Nose
- Pharynx
- Larynx

   The thoracic cages and supporting structures:

- Trachea
- Right and left lung
- Bronchi
- Bronchioles
- Pleural membrane
- Alveoli
- Diaphragm
- Pulmonary vessels
- Intercoastal muscles

Lungs are one of the major structures of the respiratory system and they are separated into lobes by fissures which are oblique on both sides, the left lung consists of **two lobes**: the superior and inferior lobes, the right lung consists of **three lobes**: the superior, middle, and inferior lobes. On the right lung, we have the upper, middle, and lower lobes and on the left the upper and lower.

Learning Point
When we exam the lungs it is important to exam the front, sides, and back of the chest so we can pick up pathology in the upper, middle, and lower lobes.

Anterior: The lower border of the lung at rest extends down to the 6th rib in the mid-clavicular line.
Lateral: The lower border of the lung extends to the 8th rib in the mid-axillary line.
Posterior: The lower border of the lung is marked by the 10th rib.

Learning Point
The physiology of the respiratory system involves:

- Lung function
- Mechanism of breathing
- Compliance
- Perfusion
- Gas exchange

Respiration is concerned with gas exchange between the atmosphere and the alveoli of the lung.

Air enters the lungs when the pressure inside the lungs is less than that of the atmosphere and leaves the lungs when the pressure in the lungs is greater than the atmospheric pressure. Effective gas exchange depends on:

- Ventilation
- Diffusion of gases
- Pulmonary capillary blood flow
- The carriage of gases by the blood

Two other important physiological functions of the lungs are ventilation and perfusion, which they must be matched for efficient gas exchange to take place. Understanding ventilation and perfusion can enable the learner to understand the lung disease processes and that these two functions are going hand in hand because ventilation is the movement of air in and out of the lungs while perfusion is the supply of deoxygenated blood to the lungs to be oxygenated and sent around the rest of the body. This is measured by the V/Q ratio which should be approximately equal to 1 and when this ratio V/Q > 1 so ventilation with reduced perfusion is found in haemorrhage, shock, and pulmonary embolism. When the ratio V/Q < 1 perfusion with reduced ventilation is found in asthma and COPD and lung collapse and consolidation. The ability of the lungs to expand known as *lung compliance* is key to ventilation.

Bronchi connect the windpipe with the lungs, there are the lobar bronchi in the left lung, and three exist in the right lung. The lobar bronchi, in turn, give rise to segmental or tertiary bronchi. The tertiary bronchi supply the bronchopulmonary segments. Bronchioles are the terminal divisions of the bronchi; they have no cartilage and they are thin walled with a total surface area of 40-80 m2 and there are also wall thinned cavities surrounded by dense network of capillaries that allow exchange of oxygen and carbon dioxide. This large surface area provided by the alveoli is extremely important for efficient gas exchange and prevents hypoxia and hypercapnia.

In conditions such as emphysema the surface area is greatly reduced and therefore efficient gas exchange is no longer possible. Each alveolus is very closely associated with a network of capillaries containing deoxygenated blood from the pulmonary artery. The capillary and alveolar walls are very thin allowing rapid exchange of gas by passive diffusion along concentration gradients. Carbon dioxide moves into the alveolus as the concentration is much lower in the alveolus than in the blood and oxygen moves out of the alveolus because the continuous flow of blood through the capillaries prevents saturation of the blood with oxygen and allows maximal transfer across the membrane. They also contain *surfactant* which aids in the *compliance of the lung* but also contains macrophages which are part of the lung defence. *Surfactant* exists in the fluid lining in the inner surface of the alveoli and is a *mixture of substances* secreted by the cells of the alveolar epithelium. It is important in *the lung expansion because it reduces the surface tension in the lung.*

One other important aspect of the physiology of the lungs is the mechanism of breathing that involves active (inspiration) and passive (expiration) breathing. *Inspiration* or active breathing happens when the external intercostal muscles contract and the rib cage moves *upwards* and *outwards* while the diaphragm contracts or moves down. This is followed by an increase in the intrathoracic volume which creates a negative pressure within the thorax. The lungs are held to the thoracic wall by the pleural membranes and so expand outwards. This in turn creates negative pressure in the lung and air rushes in. In *expiration* the diaphragm relaxes and moves upwards and the lungs collapse under the influence of their own elastic force and pressure within the lung increases to higher than atmospheric pressure air rushes out.

Compliance, the ability of the lungs and thorax to expand, is determined by the elastic retractive force that is an inherent property of the lungs and the lung volume that is how inflated it is. *Pulmonary surfactant* greatly reduces surface tension in the alveoli increasing compliance and allowing the lung to inflate much more easily, thereby eliminating the work of breathing. Examples of high compliance are observed in emphysema and low compliance in lung fibrosis.

Respiration is concerned with gas exchange between an organism and its environment, i.e. between the atmosphere and the alveoli of the lung. Air enters the lungs when the pressure inside the lungs is less than that of the atmosphere and leaves the lungs when pressure in the lungs is greater than the atmospheric pressure. Effective gas exchange depends on:

- Ventilation
- Diffusion of gases
- Pulmonary capillary blood flow
- The carriage of gases by the blood

It is important that the nurse understands the difference between respiration, breathing, and ventilation. Respiration is the oxidation reaction that releases energy from foods such as glucose. Breathing on the other hand is the mechanism that moves air into and out of the lungs allowing gas exchange to happen. Ventilation means moving air in and out of the lungs which requires a difference in air pressure (the air moves from high to low pressure) and therefore, ventilation depends on the airtight cavity of the thorax as we breath the volume of air in our thoracic cage changes and the pressure inside changes with it which causes the air to move in or out of the lungs. Now there are two structures which are important for ventilation to happen. During inhalation or breathing in the outer intercostal muscles contract pulling our ribs up while the muscles of the diagraph contract pulling the diagraph down into a more flattened shape. These movements increase the volume of air in the chest and cause a drop in pressure in the thorax, so air enters the lungs again. Reduction in ventilation will lead to an accumulation of carbon dioxide (aka hypercapnia).

Another important consideration is the amount of blood ejected from the left or right ventricles into the aorta or pulmonary trunk per minute called the cardiac output. The cardiac output is directly proportional to the stroke volume—the amount of blood ejected by a ventricle during each contraction which is about 70 ml. The heart rate—which is about 75 beats per minute. The cardiac output is closely related to pulmonary capillary blood flow and the pulmonary blood flow depends on the volume and distribution of right ventricular output. Capillaries wrap up organs and their sole purpose is to bring blood close to every cell in an organ, therefore their walls are only one cell thick in order to allow substances and materials such as oxygen, glucose, amino acids and water get exchanged and diffused.

During the filling phase—the ventricles fill during diastole and atrial systole.

In isovolumetric contraction—the ventricles contract, building up pressure ready to pump blood into the aorta/pulmonary trunk.

In the outflow phase—the ventricles continue to contract, pushing blood into the aorta and the pulmonary trunk. This is also known as systole.

Followed by isovolumetric relaxation—the ventricles relax, ready to re-fill with blood in the next filling phase.

Hypoxia is diagnosed when respiration cannot meet the metabolic needs of the body either because the lungs cannot extract enough oxygen from the atmospheric air (aka hypoxaemia) or because the cardiovascular system cannot transport oxygen to meet the needs of the body effectively. This type of respiratory failure is also known as respiratory failure type 1. When a patient is diagnosed to be hypoxaemic (aka low oxygen levels) and hypercapnic (aka high levels of carbon dioxide) this patient is diagnosed to have respiratory failure type 2 or respiratory acidosis. This type of respiratory failure or acidosis can only be managed if ventilation (aka patient's depth of breathing) is improved.

Some other factors the nurse needs to bear in mind when diagnosing a patient with breathing difficulties are malignant hypertension (when diastolic is above 120 mmHg) and isolated systolic hypertension (an increase in cardiac output or peripheral vascular resistance (aka hardening of the arteries and rigidity of the veins) can cause a systolic blood pressure of over 140 mmHg and a diastolic of less than 90 mmHg). Both types of hypertension can cause cardiac failures and therefore they needed to be noted on patients' medical history. Blood pressure is the result of the cardiac output and the peripheral vascular resistance found in the body and therefore a critical determinant in health and illness.

5.2   The General Pathophysiology of Lung Disease

The volume of air breathed in and out and the respiratory rate vary from person to person according to age, sex, build, and activity and at rest a normal person will inspire and expire about 500 ml of air with each breath (tidal volume) but in general lung volumes depend on the physiology of the lung. However, these functional categories often show overlap and they do not account for localized disorders such as tumours or infections (pneumonia).

> **Learning Point**
> Lung function can be disturbed in four ways:
>   (a) Obstruction to airflow; the term chronic obstructive airways disease is commonly used. All these diseases show the common abnormalities of:
>   • Limitation to expiration
>   • Similarity in some symptoms and signs
>   • Frequent existence together of these disorders
>   (b) Restriction of lung expansion
>   (c) Abnormalities of gas diffusion
>   (d) Changes in pulmonary blood flow

Different parts of the nervous system provide information to the respiratory centres and chemoreceptors monitor the amounts of oxygen and carbon dioxide in the blood, because the ventilation responds to establish the concentration of these two gases in the blood. Lung capacity can also be affected by the person's position, the strength of respiratory muscle, and the distensibility of lungs and chest cage. When we breath the lungs expand, and some effort is put forward to achieve this, but this depends on the compliance of the lung. Compliance can be reduced with age or disease, i.e. pulmonary oedema.

Vital capacity (VC) is the maximum amount of air a person can expel from the lungs after a maximum inhalation. It is equal to the sum of inspiratory reserve volume, tidal volume, and expiratory reserve volume and the vital capacity for a healthy adult is between 3 and 5 L.

Spirometry measures FEV1 = Forced expiratory volume over 1 s and FVC = forced vital capacity to assess what kind of lung disease the patient may suffer from. These values can be used to calculate the ratio of FEV1/FVC and a healthy individual should be >0.7.

Learning Point

Consider the following:

Total lung capacity (TLC) is the maximum volume to which the lungs can be expanded with the greatest possible inspiration effort. The average lung capacity is about 6 L.

Tidal volume is the amount of air that can be inhaled or exhaled during one respiratory cycle—about 500 ml. This depicts the functions of the respiratory centres, respiratory muscles, and the mechanics of the lung and chest wall.

Inspiratory reserve volume is the extra amount of air that can still be inhaled forcefully after the end of a normal tidal inspiration—about 3000 ml.

Expiratory reserve volume is the volume of air that can still be exhaled forcefully after the end of normal tidal expiration—about 1100 ml. This expiratory reserve volume is reduced with obesity, ascites, or after upper abdominal surgery.

Residual volume is the volume of air remaining in the lungs after maximal exhalation. Normal adult value is averaged at 1200 ml (20–25 ml/kg). It is indirectly measured from summation of FRC and ERV and cannot be measured by spirometry. In obstructive lung diseases with features of incomplete emptying of the lungs and air trapping, residual volume may be significantly high.

Inspiratory capacity is the maximum volume of air that can be inhaled following a resting state about 3500 ml. It is calculated from the sum of inspiratory reserve volume and tidal volume. IC = IRV + TV.

Functional residual capacity is the amount of air remaining in the lungs at the end of a normal exhalation. It is calculated by adding together residual and expiratory reserve volumes. The normal value is about 1800–2200 ml. FRC = RV + ERV.

FRC does not rely on effort and highlights the resting position when inner and outer elastic recoils are balanced. FRC is reduced in restrictive disorders. The ratio of FRC to TLC is an index of hyperinflation. In COPD, FRC is up to 80% of TLC.

Obstructive lung disease such as asthma and COPD, presents with a normal FVC, but FEV1 is reduced to <80% normal/predicted and FEV1/FVC is reduced to <0.7. Restrictive lung disease such as lung fibrosis, severe scoliosis present with reduced FVC and normal or reduced FEV1 and FEV1/FVC normal at >0.7. These are useful investigations in the management of patients with respiratory disease or respiratory weakness secondary to neurological impairment. They aid diagnosis, help monitor response to treatment, and can guide decisions regarding further treatment and intervention. Spirometry can measure all the lung volumes except residual volume.

This is particularly recommended when investigating patients with symptoms that suggest pulmonary disease (e.g. cough, wheeze, breathlessness, crackles, or abnormal chest x-ray). When monitoring patients with known pulmonary disease for progression and response to treatment (e.g. interstitial fibrosis, COPD, asthma, or pulmonary vascular disease). Also, patients with diseases that may have a respiratory complication (e.g. connective tissue disorders or neuromuscular diseases) and as part of preoperative evaluation prior to lung resection, abdominal surgery or cardiothoracic surgery these tests are recommended. Also in patients at risk of lung diseases (e.g. exposure to pulmonary toxins such as radiation, medication, or environmental or occupational exposure) or as part of surveillance following lung transplantation to assess for acute rejection, infection, or obliterative bronchiolitis.

5.3   General Symptoms and Signs of Lung Diseases

During history taking and physical examination, it is important to note what symptoms are troubling the patient recently and which symptom has brought them to us. It is important to note the patient's own words when describing their symptom(s) and establish the duration of the symptom, when it started and when have they had this before in the past? Was it gradual or intermittent or was it sudden? Varying durations can give clues to different underlying causes and help establish the facts around duration of the symptom. For example, breathlessness is a serious symptom but needs to be differentiated from dyspnoea. Pulmonary embolism and pneumothorax usually present with a sudden onset of dyspnoea while pneumonia and COPD may take hours or days to develop. Anaemia and pleural effusion or lung fibrosis can develop over weeks and years. A sudden onset of dyspnoea is critical when seeking to differentiate diagnosis.

Cough

Cough is the most common respiratory symptom, and it is initiated when irritant receptors on the mucous membrane of the respiratory tract are stimulated. Cough which persists for more than 6 weeks should always be taken seriously.

Drugs, head injury, and anaesthesia can suppress the cough reflex leading to retention of secretions and infection. Cough can be classified into:

Productive
Non-productive (dry)

Learning Point

It is also important to establish the character of the cough when asking question in the history regarding cough.

- Is it dry or purulent or barking?
- When does it happen?
- Daytime? Nocturnal?
- Are there any exacerbating or alleviating factors?
- If it is productive what colour is the sputum?
  - Green/yellow may indicate infection, such as in lung abscess or bronchiectasis, acute bacterial bronchitis sputum is purulent (pus containing) and in a large volume
  - Bright red in pulmonary infarction or tuberculosis
  - Pink and frothy sputum is associated with pulmonary oedema
  - White, clear, mucoid found in chronic bronchitis
  - Rust coloured in pneumonia
  - Sticky mucous plugs in asthma, cystic fibrosis
- Another major consideration is how much is produced?
- Are we talking about teaspoonful or less?
  - Sputum is produced every day normally about 100 ml of sputum, which is carried upwards by ciliary action and swallowed
  - Sputum should always be inspected

Breathlessness

Dyspnoea or breathlessness is shortness of breath, and most causes are easily diagnosed on history and examination. The time period over which breathlessness develops is of great significance. If the patient complains of immediate breathlessness, then this may suggest pneumothorax, or acute pulmonary oedema due to heart arrythmias, pulmonary embolism, or a foreign body.

If the breathlessness lasts for hours then you may be need to consider asthma, left heart failure, pneumonia, or laryngeal oedema. When this symptom lasts for days then we are looking for pneumonia or left heart failure. If the patient complains of breathlessness for weeks, then the diagnosis may be around pleural effusion, anaemia, or respiratory muscle weakness. But for long-standing breathlessness, the nurse should be looking to diagnose bronchial cancer, lung fibrosis, thyrotoxicosis, or muscle weakness. On this note, some patients may complain of breathless for years due to muscle weakness, chronic obstructive airways disease, lung fibrosis, or chest wall disorders.

At this point, it is important that we also understand the terms *dyspnoea* and *orthopnoea* because both symptoms can point out towards a respiratory diagnosis. *Dyspnoea* is usually detected when the patient takes up some exercise or walked a long distance on flat level before the patient experiences dyspnoea. Some important assessment questions should be around how many steps can you climb before you get short of breath? Is there a diurnal variation of the symptom? Does it vary from day to day?

Orthopnoea, on the other hand, is when the patient experiences difficulty or painful breathing when lying flat. So some important assessment questions should be around how many pillows do you sleep with at night? Why do you sleep with this number of pillows? But remember that not every patient with four pillows is breathless when lying flat. Most causes of breathlessness are easily diagnosed on history and examination.

Haemoptysis

Haemoptysis is another significant respiratory symptom, and it is coughing up blood. The nurse needs to establish how much sputum mixed with blood and the colour of it is important. *Epistaxis* is not true haemoptysis but when the patient coughs up blood this may indicate infective pneumonia or TB, bronchiectasis or benign and malignant lung tumours. One should always differentiate true haemoptysis from a lesion of the nose, nasopharynx, and vocal cords. A definite diagnosis is only achieved in 60–70% of cases and some of the causes include:

Learning Point
Some important causes of haemoptysis include:

- Acute or chronic bronchitis
- Bronchial carcinoma
- Foreign body (trauma)
- Left ventricular failure (pulmonary oedema)
- Pulmonary infarction
- Tuberculosis
- Bleeding disorders

Wheeze

Wheeze is a common finding in chronic obstructive airways disease and asthma. Both produce expiratory wheezing. Narrowing of the larynx, trachea, and main bronchi causes mainly inspiratory wheezing.

When wheezing occurs on one side, a local obstruction such as a tumour infiltrating a main bronchus should be suspected. Wheeze is a sign and symptom of airway obstruction and in auscultation is an added breath sound typically seen in asthma and COPD, but it helps to establish when this may happen and find out from the patient whether wheezing is related to exercise or any other type of activity. It is always helpful to know what may exacerbate and/or relieve wheezing.

Stridor

Stridor is an inspiratory noise as a result of upper airway obstruction, and it is usually caused by upper airway lesions (masses) or severe infection from pharynx to carina of trachea. Have you noticed that you make any extra sounds when you breathe? It may be useful to give an example of exactly what you mean.

Chest Pain

Chest pain, however, can have many different causes and some are related to cardiovascular disease. In general, diseases of the lung tissue are usually painless, since there are no pain receptors within the lungs. When chest pain related to lung disease occurs, it invariably means that the pleura, which contains pain receptors, is also involved. The common causes are best considered with regard to the type of pain and the duration:

Learning Point
Continuous chest pain is associated with any of the following:

- MI—crushing, central chest pain, radiates to jaw and arms
- Pneumothorax—sharp, stabbing, on one side
- Bronchial cancer—infiltration of mediastinal nodes—central chest pain
- Dissecting aneurysm—tearing, central chest or upper abdominal

Intermittent chest pain is associated with any of the following:

- Angina—constricting, central chest pain, related to exertion, radiates to jaw and arms
- Pleuritic—sharp, worse on inspiration or coughing, radiates to shoulder, lower chest wall, upper abdomen. Found in pleural inflammations (e.g. pneumonia, pulmonary infarction, connective tissue diseases) and tumour infiltrations.
- Spinal nerve root irritation—worse on moving
- Peptic ulcer, hiatus hernia—burning, related to eating

Chest pain is also associated with lung disease, and it needs to be assessed fully using either the mnemonic SOCRATES and it is important to exclude cardiac pain. Lung tissue does not have pain receptors therefore disease of the lung tissue is usually painless, but lung pleura does have pain receptors therefore chest pain related to the lung indicates pleural involvement.

Learning Point

The mnemonic SOCRATES is used to assess pain and evaluate the patient experience with respiratory discomfort and stands for:

S—Site
O—Onset
C—Character: dull/sharp/pleuritic
R—Radiation
Alleviating factors
T—Time
E—Exacerbating factors
S—Severity, sleep disturbance

Other relevant questions may help you differentiate pain are asking system question such as have you lost your appetite, or have you noticed any weight loss? Have you experienced any malaise or lethargy recently? Did you have any infectious contacts? Are you aware of sustaining any trauma? Do you smoke? How long? Have you got any pets? This may help exclude allergens and budgerigars in atypical pneumonias.

Learning Point

It is also sensible to assess the patient for any previous and ongoing medical problems and this can be undertaken by using the mnemonic M J T H R E A D S

- M: MI or other underlying cardiac disorders
- J: Jaundice
- T: TB
- R: Rheumatic fever
- E: Epilepsy
- A: Asthma—control? ITU admissions? Last attach? Intubations?
- D: Diabetes
- S: Stroke

You may need to establish whether the patient had any previous medical admission or any recent surgeries and explore the reasons why they had surgery. Look out for any incidents of pulmonary embolism. You may also look into taking a good history of previous childhood infections, such as TB but also establish the past medical history of any prolonged whooping cough or untreated cough which may cause bronchiectasis later in life. Assessing for allergies and regular medications is also important should we look for side effects or interactions of prescribed medication the patient may be on such as ACE-I. This group of drugs may be responsible for exacerbating cough. There is also a possibility that any past recovery especially with bronchodilators and steroids may need to be taken note or any over-the-counter drugs the patient may have had.

Some conditions may not obviously appear respiratory and therefore they may be ignored. A full history taking may help pick up clues and questions around any medical conditions within the family may help establish a fuller picture for our patients.

Learning Point

Systematic interrogation: the lungs are closely related to the heart. Weight loss is a major sign in bronchial carcinoma. Fever may imply infection, e.g. pneumonia and tuberculosis.

Family history questions particularly with regard to asthma or tuberculosis can be passed in families. Sexual habits need to be considered since lung disease is a manifestation of HIV disease.

- Where do they live?
- Who do they live with?
- Are they married? Do they have children?
- Do they have any pets?
- What do they do for living? Past occupation?
- Have they ever been exposed to asbestos?
- Have they travelled within the last 6 months?
- Does anyone in the family have asthma?
- Is there a family history of TB?

Social history questions on smoking, exposure to pets and hobbies that can lead to lung disease, e.g. cats, dogs, pigeons, occupation, e.g. miners, industrial workers

- Do they smoke?
- What do they smoke?
- How much do they smoke?
- How often do they smoke?
- When did they start smoking?
- Do they drink any alcohol?
- How much in a day or a week?
- How often during a day or a week?
- What do they drink?

Drug history questions particularly past treatment with bronchodilators and steroids

Ideas, Concerns, Expectations (ICE)

- What do you think it may be? Any ideas? Any concerns? Any expectations?
- When ending the session, we can sum up the history and symptoms back to the patient and inform the patient of the plan.

Fever

Fever is also a typical respiratory symptom, and the nurse needs to find out if this fever is current and if the patient had a fever previously. Any night sweats-drenching deb clothes/sheets? When does it happen? Possible causes can be infection and malignancies.

In lung diseases fever is a symptom associated with consolidation which is the patchy thickening of the lung seen in bronchopneumonia.

Clubbing

Clubbing is considered one of those clinical signs strongly associated with lung disease such as bronchial carcinoma, lung fibrosis, lung abscess, emphysema, bronchiectasis, and tuberculosis.

Some cardiac diseases can also cause clubbing such as congenital cyanotic heart disease, bacterial endocarditis, and atrial myxoma but also gastrointestinal tract disease, for example, inflammatory bowel disease such as Crohn's disease, ulcerative colitis, coeliac disease and GI lymphomas and cirrhosis found to be associated with clubbing. Familial predisposition to clubbing and hypertrophic osteoarthropathy can be some other causes for this pathological process.

> **Learning Point**
> Clubbing can be categorized in four stages:
>
> - Stage 1: increased sponginess of nail bed
> - Stage 2: loss of angle between nail bed and skin
> - Stage 3: increased longitudinal curvature of nail
> - Stage 4: bulbous appearance of distal phalanges (drumstick like)

Cyanosis

Central cyanosis is seen in lung disease and is a main symptom and sign. A typical sign of central cyanosis is the bluish colour of the tongue, caused by the reduced oxygenation of blood leaving the lungs. Other causes include high altitude, severe hypoventilation (due to head injury, drugs, or chest injury), congenital heart disease (shunting of venous blood from the right side to the left side of the heart), and chronic obstructive airways disease (decreased blood flow through diseased lungs).

Peripheral cyanosis is noted in the bluish colour of nail beds of fingers and toes, tips of ears, and nose caused by peripheral vasoconstriction (cold or vascular disease), sluggish blood flow (due to increased blood viscosity), or left ventricular failure.

Pulsus paradoxus

Pulsus paradoxus is another important respiratory sign and symptom found in patients with greater than normal fall in blood pressure and pulse volume during inspiration (e.g. in severe asthma).

Lymphadenopathy

Enlarged lymph nodes of the neck palpated indicate infection. Lymph from the lung drains from the hilum, up the paratracheal nodes to the supraclavicular and cervical nodes. Lung disease rarely involves the axillary nodes, since these receive lymph from the chest wall and breast. Examination of submental, submandibular, tonsillar, and cervical chain can be carried out by palpation from the front of the patient. Examination of the supraclavicular lymph nodes is best detected from behind.

5.4 Part 2: Case Studies

Each individual case study consists of a summary of the patient's clinical presentation starting with a list of diagnostic features and any other clinical details that may be important for a differential diagnosis. Becoming competent at interpreting signs and symptoms depends on seeing as many examples as possible and discussing them with a senior colleague. You may wish to use this chapter as a guide to build a comprehensive collection of your own. We have endeavoured to include commonly encountered case studies as well as less common findings which are of clinical importance. Here we include case studies which feature clinical sign sand symptoms that a competent practitioner should be able to recognize and diagnose.

Using the enhanced Cambridge-Calgary [3] consultation model, the practitioner should collect data on the patient's presenting complaint and taking a patient-centred approach should assess and diagnose the problem. This consultation model enables health care practitioners to communicate the patient's problem and plan for a safe and effective management plan. The Calgary-Cambridge model also focuses on the patient's perspective on the problem and builds on the rapport with patients.

The dividing line between history taking and clinical examination is an artificial one since the examination begins from the moment the patient walks into the room. The practitioner uses their observational skills to inspect and assess the general appearance of the patient, uses verbal and non-verbal skills to assess the patient's physical health but also engage with the patient, observe their tone of speech, mood, and orientation for time, place, and person. Throughout the physical examination, we need to be aware of the patient's body language and use our senses of hearing, sight, and touch to communicate and listen to the patient. Make sure that you apply the principles of the Cambridge-Calgary consultation model and note key findings before you proceed with the physical examination of the patient to maximize patient-centred care and utilize quaternary prevention.

Case Study 1

A 66-year-old man who has come to hospital with a 2-month history of cough, haemoptysis, malaise, and weight loss. He has smoked 25 cigarettes a day for the past 40 years. There is a history of chronic winter cough productive of some white sputum, but no other history of note. On examination, he is thin; examination of the lungs shows evidence of collapse in the upper zone of the left lung. There are also some generalized expiratory wheezes over both lung fields. The blood tests show that he has a raised serum calcium level.

1. What is the likely diagnosis for the current 2-month symptoms? What is the likely diagnosis for the chronic winter cough and what sign found on examination supports this diagnosis?
2. What are the underlying mechanisms for the cough, and haemoptysis, malaise, and weight loss?
3. State the pathological basis (mechanisms) for the following:
   - The cough and signs of consolidation:
   - The haemoptysis
4. What is the mechanism for the collapse of the left upper zone? What features would you find on examination that would confirm collapse?
5. Why is the plasma calcium raised?

Case Study 2

A previously healthy 56-year-old woman was admitted to hospital with 6-day history of fever and chills, she also complained of a cough productive of yellow-green sputum, tinged with rusty-coloured blood. On examination, the patient had a temperature of 38.9 °C, a pulse rate of 110 beats/min, and a respiratory rate of 25 breaths/min. Lung signs of consolidation are found localized to the middle lobe of the right lung. She is commenced on antibiotics, but her symptoms worsen, and she begins to produce large amounts of foul-smelling sputum indicating that she had developed a lung abscess. Following culture of the organism, her antibiotic treatment is changed, and she makes a slow recovery. Pneumonia is the likeliest diagnosis.

1. Outline the clinical features associated with bacterial (pneumococcal) pneumonia.
2. Discuss the mechanism for the consolidation of the middle lobe of the right lung.
3. What is lung abscess?
4. List the features that you would expect to find on examination of the respiratory system that would confirm consolidation?
5. Compare and contrast the terms aspiration pneumonia and inhalation pneumonia. State one cause for each

Case Study 3

A 65-year-old teacher was admitted to hospital complaining of severe breathlessness of 1 week and his symptom had come on rapidly over a period of 24 h. He had also experienced severe breathlessness at night and had to sleep propped up with pillows. Over the next days following the onset of his severe breathlessness, his legs and ankles had also become very swollen. He smokes 30 cigarettes a day and has got a 15-year history of a chronic cough productive of sputum and for the last past year he has noticed gradual swelling of both ankles, together with increasing shortness of breath on exertion. For the past 3 months prior to admission, he has had experienced haemoptysis, coughing up small amounts of fresh blood and he has also lost about 3 kg in weight.

On examination, he was very short of breath and cyanosed. The pulse was 130 beats per minute, regular with a very small volume, the blood pressure was 70/40 mmHg and the jugular venous pressure was grossly elevated. The heart sounds were faint, and the apex beat was not palpable. He was barrel chested, and the trachea was central. There was swelling of both legs right up to the groin. The lower one-third of the left lung showed the features of a pleural effusion and liver was enlarged, tender with a smooth edge and surface.

1. Comment on the 15-year history of chronic productive cough, the 1-year history of progressive ankle swelling and the barrel chest.
2. What is the likely significance of the weight loss and 3 months history of haemoptysis? Discuss the causes of haemoptysis that you should consider in this patient.
3. Discuss the possible causes and mechanisms for the blood pressure, pulse, faint heart sounds, absent apex beat, and rapid deterioration in the shortness of breath. What is the link with the raised JVP, swollen legs, and liver enlargement?
4. Briefly state the findings on examination of the lungs (inspection, palpation, percussion, and auscultation) that led to the diagnosis of pleural effusion. How might the presence of underlying chronic bronchitis and emphysema affect the classical features of a pleural effusion. What is the likely cause for the pleural effusion.

5.5   Part 3: Respiratory Examination

In this section discuss step by step the physical examination we need to undertake for the above patient. Before we start make sure that we follow the below:

- Wash hands.
- Introduce yourself.
- Position patient at 45° supine
- Expose area for examination.

Inspection

By standing at the end of bed and we observe for and note:

General appearance (facial appearance and skin features), shortness of breath, cyanosis central, fatigue, loss of appetite, and nausea are associated with lung problems, for example, sickle cell anaemia, thalassaemia, asthma, bronchitis, pneumonia, or COPD.

We look and feel their hands and note:

- Feel temperature and check capillary refill time.
- Peripheral cyanosis (blue hands due to peripheral vascular disease).
- Raynaud's syndrome, heart failure shock, and central cyanosis.

Observe their face and examine their eyes:

- Conjunctiva
- Lymph glands

Examine the mouth for:

- Central cyanosis causes blue lips and tongue and when severe can also cause blue hands but usually warm (peripheral cyanosis)
- Glossitis
- Angular stomatitis
- Clubbing

We feel their wrist:

- Radial pulse (absent radial pulse can be caused by congenital heart failure arterial embolism or atheroma)
- Collapsing pulse

Inspect their arms:

- Scars
- Visible heave
- Trunk/lower limbs
- Sacral oedema
- Ankle oedema
- Ascites

Examine the Lungs

Garibaldi and Elder [2] explain how physical examination ensures patient safety, relevant investigations and eliminate unnecessary tests, aids diagnosis, patient contact, clinical reasoning, prognosis and ongoing care and teaching through observation to others by demonstrating the four pillars of practice. Physical examination is the evaluation of objective anatomic findings with observation, palpation, percussion, and auscultations [5]. In doing so the practitioner may yield up to 20% necessary data for diagnosis and management. The examination of the lungs requires a systematic approach involving inspection (looking), palpation (feeling), percussion (tapping), and auscultation (listening) but it can help diagnose the problem but remember we always examine both the front and the back and compare one side with the other as we proceed.

On inspection should ***observe*** for any chest wall abnormalities such as:

Learning Point

Scoliosis is the lateral curvature of the spine largely congenital and in some cases neurological for example in poliomyelitis.

Kyphosis is an increased flexion of the spine and anterior curvature of the spine. It can be congenital, due to ankylosing spondylitis, spinal tuberculosis, or osteoporosis.

Pectus excavatum (funnel chest) is usually associated with underlying disease and the sternum is depressed. The causes are congenital, not secondary to lung disease. It may compress the heart and displace the apex, giving a serious impression of cardiac enlargement. Pectus carinatum (pigeon chest) is a congenital posterior displacement of lower aspect of sternum and this gives the chest a somewhat "hollowed-out" appearance. It can commonly cause the sternum and costal cartilages project outwards, and it is associated with severe childhood asthma. Abnormal chest movement and symmetry is decreased on one side could be due to lung fibrosis, pleural thickening, pleuritic pain, or musculoskeletal problems. Note that increased volume of chest on one side could be due to pneumothorax. Do not forget to look for other lesions and swellings on the chest wall.

Patterns of Breathing

Note the rate, depth, rhythm, effort, and symmetry of breathing. The symmetry of chest wall movement is considered in the section on palpation. Normal rate is 10–20 breaths per minute. Increased rate could be due to asthma, lung fibrosis, and pulmonary oedema or fever. Decreased rate could be due to CNS injury and CNS depressant drugs.

Learning Point

- *Tachypnoea* is increased rate of breathing due to asthma, lung fibrosis, pulmonary oedema, and fever. Decreased rate is due to CNS injury and CNS depressant drugs.
- *Cheyne-Stokes respiration* is often seen in terminal illness. Cheyne-Stokes is cyclical variation in depth and rate of breathing. Each cycle can last up to 2 min and involves a period of apnoea followed by light slow breathing then deep fast breathing before this declines again to another period of apnoea. The nurse and/or practitioner should also examine the patient for any of prolonged expiration caused by either chronic bronchitis or emphysema and the patient's face look like as if they were whistling when there

is severe difficulty with expiration because many of these patients breath out through pursed lips.

- *Kussmaul breathing* is deep sighing respiration and a type of breathing pattern associated with patients with metabolic acidosis (excess hydrogen ions in the blood). Renal failure, diabetic ketoacidosis, and aspirin overdose can cause this Kussmaul breathing because the metabolic acidosis stimulates the respiratory centre as it tries to excrete carbon dioxide.
- *Wheezes* are high-pitched whistling sound produced by airway walls oscillation between the open and nearly closed position. It occurs in both inspiratory and expiratory but is always louder in the expiration. Stridor is a loud, mainly inspiratory noise produced by laryngeal, tracheal, or major airway obstruction.

Note that patients with severe respiratory distress increase the effort of breathing and use of accessory muscle. Breathing difficulties can cause extreme distress. Some patients have great difficulty in lying flat known as orthopnoea. A healthy individual, when they lie flat, breath more with the diaphragm and less with the chest wall. In patients with airways obstruction, the diaphragm is often flat and inefficient draw ribs inwards. Thus, when they lie down, the diaphragm cannot provide the ventilation required. Patients with severe respiratory distress need to use their accessory muscles of respiration and audible noises such as wheezes or stridor may be heard.

Palpitation

In palpitation we need to identify tender areas, assess respiratory expansion, and assess tactile vocal fremitus (palpable vibrations when a patient repeats a sound).

The Trachea and Mediastinum

Trachea lies in midline of the neck and extends from cricoid cartilage (C6) superiorly to the trachea bifurcation at the level of sternal angle (T5). A smooth indentation on the trachea is commonly seen just above the bifurcation on the left side this is caused by the arch of the aorta. Its diameter is 15–20 mm and becomes intrathoracic at 6th cartilaginous ring. The intimate relationship between the arch of the aorta and the trachea and left bronchus is responsible for the physical sign known as "tracheal tug" and of characteristic of aneurysms of the aortic arch.

To locate the patient's trachea, we need to palpate with the fingertips between the sternocleidomastoid muscle at the suprasternal notch. Palpating the position of the trachea gives an indication of mediastinal displacement. Any deviation from the midline is considered abnormal. The position of the apex beat should always be checked when palpating the trachea. This is important because the trachea moves with the upper part of mediastinum, the apex beat moves with the lower part of mediastinum. Large effusion pushes the position of the apex beat but very large effusions are needed to displace the trachea.

Chest Wall Movements

The chest wall comprises ribs, dorsal spine, and muscles associated with respiration. The chest cavity contains, among other structures, the lungs, lined by two layers of pleura, which comprise air passages and air sacs.

Learning Point

Bearing this in mind:

- Chest wall expansion can be assessed by placing thumbs together and laying outstretched hands across anterior and posterior chest wall. On inspiration the thumbs will move apart.
- Bilateral reduction in chest wall movement is found in hyper-inflated chest (emphysema), reduced compliance (lung fibrosis), reduced rib cage movement (ankylosing spondylitis), weak inspiratory muscles (myasthenia gravis).
- Local or unilateral reduction in chest wall movement is found in pleural effusion, pleural thickening, lung collapse, consolidation (due to inflammatory exudate in alveoli from infections like pneumonia), and pneumothorax.

Tactile Vocal Fremitus

This is a crude test for assessing the transmission of sound to the chest wall and is normally palpable as a low frequency vibration. Reduced or absent fremitus is found in bronchial obstruction, chronic bronchitis, pleural thickening and effusion, pneumothorax, and a large infiltrating lung cancer. Increased fremitus is found over an area of lung consolidation (pneumonia). The value of this test and its interpretation are also considered in the section on vocal resonance (auscultation).

Percussion

Bilateral hyperresonant sound is associated with over-inflated lungs seen in emphysema and asthma. This is often not a reliable sign. Unilateral hyper-resonant sound is associated with pneumothorax. Percussion is an important technique and is used to determine whether underlying tissues are air filled, fluid filled or solid. The normal percussion note gives a resonant sound.

Dullness or dull note is found when the lung is filled with fluid or replaced by solid tissue. Causes may include pneumonia, pulmonary oedema, pleural effusion, lung fibrosis, and lung tumour.

Learning Point

Common causes for the following changes are:

Dullness

Bilateral Hyperresonance

Unilateral hyperresonance

Auscultation

The diaphragm of the stethoscope is preferred by many practitioners. However, the bell may give a more airtight fit in thin bony people and those with excessive chest hair. The diaphragm is said to be better for high-frequency sounds and the bell for low-frequency sounds.

Classification of the breath sounds:

Normal or vesicular breath sounds are those heard over the normal lung fields and are soft, low pitch have a rustling quality.

Bronchial breath sounds are heard in situations where the sound heard in the trachea and main bronchi are transmitted to the chest wall. Bronchial breath sounds have a higher frequency and are harsher than normal breath sounds. You can get an idea of their sound by placing the stethoscope over the trachea or larynx.

Additional breath sounds include:

- Wheezes are sounds which can be audible without a stethoscope in severe disease.
- Crackles.
- Pleural rub.

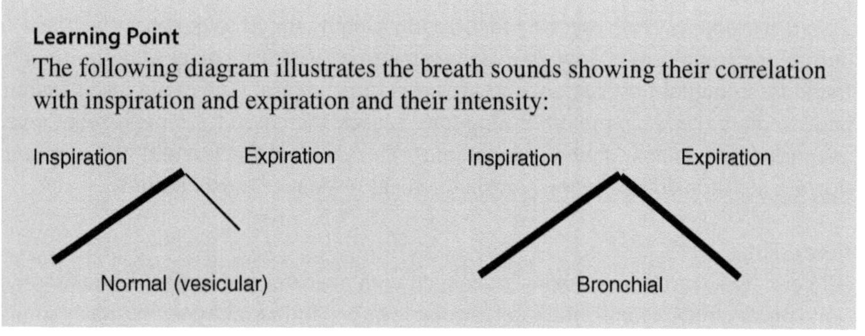

Learning Point
The following diagram illustrates the breath sounds showing their correlation with inspiration and expiration and their intensity:

The pathological processes may cause bilateral reduction in normal (vesicular) breath sounds, such as airway obstruction such as in asthma, emphysema, and tumour or anything interspersed between the lung and the chest wall, such as air, fluid or pleural thickening can cause unilateral reduction in breath sounds such as wheezes.

In pneumonia the lung substance is solid as in consolidation, but the air passage remains open which is a common lung condition associated with the localized transmission of bronchial breath sounds to the lung field. Wheezes are due to narrowing of the airways generalized wheezes are heard in asthma, chronic bronchitis/emphysema, and pulmonary oedema. Localized wheezes are heard in lung cancer (infiltrating a large bronchus), foreign body, and bronchial secretions.

Learning Point

Possible cause of unilateral and bilateral wheeze

Unilateral (localized) wheeze	Bilateral (generalized) wheeze
Foreign body	Asthma
Bronchial tumour	Chronic bronchitis
	Emphysema

Crackles are discrete, explosive sounds found in diseases involving small bronchioles and alveoli such as pneumonia, pulmonary oedema, chronic bronchitis/emphysema, and lung fibrosis.

Unilateral (localized) crackle	Bilateral (generalized) crackle
Bronchiectasis	Chronic bronchitis
Pneumonia	Pulmonary oedema

A pleural rub is a creaking sound heard when two layers of pleura rub together during breathing and is associated with pleural disease.

Vocal Sounds

Vocal resonance is a "fuzzy" sound heard through the stethoscope when individuals with normal lungs say "99" and is the equivalent of tactile vocal fremitus, refers to the vibration of the chest wall that results from sound vibrations created by speech "99" and when a person speaks, airflow from the lungs causes the vocal cords in the larynx to vibrate. These vibrations are vocal fremitus, which transmitted down the tracheobronchial tree and through the lung tissue to the chest. Increased fremitus is found over an area of lung consolidation (pneumonia) which is the pathological process in the lungs, associated with increased vocal fremitus and resonance. Reduced or absent fremitus is common in bronchial obstruction, chronic bronchitis, pleural thickening and effusion, pneumothorax, and a large infiltrating lung cancer.

Learning Point

Lung diseases usually lead to one or more of these pathological processes. These are known as consolidation found within lung tissue which may become solid, for example, in pneumonia. Fibrosis is another pathological process found when fibrous tissue replaces normal lung tissue. Collapse on the other hand happens when the lung is reduced in size and pleural effusion is the accumulation of fluid in the pleural cavity.

Learning Point

Pneumothorax is diagnosed by the presence of air in pleural space and tension pneumothorax is a medical emergency. During inspiration air is drawn into the pleural space which cannot escape during expiration.

There are two types of pneumothorax: *spontaneous* (especially in young thin men) and *pneumothorax secondary to trauma* or an existing lung disease. The clinical presentation of pneumothorax is sudden onset of pleuritic chest pain and progressively increasing shortness of breath. Please note that patients with asthma or COPD may present with sudden deterioration in their condition.

Clinical signs of pneumothorax include:
- Reduced chest expansion
- Percussion is hyperresonant
- Absent or reduced breath sounds
- Absent or reduced vocal resonance

The patient with tension pneumothorax shows respiratory distress:
- Increased respiratory rate noted on observation
- Tachycardia
- Pallor
- Hypotension
- Distended neck veins
- Deviation of the trachea and mediastinum away from the side of the pneumothorax

Physical examination for pneumothorax includes:
- Mediastinal shift: away from the lesion
- Chest wall movement: reduced
- Resonance/fremitus: reduced
- Percussion note: normal or hyperresonant
- Breath sounds: reduced vesicular

Pneumonia is an inflammation of the substance of the lung and it is usually bacterial in origin and there are four classifications:

Community-acquired pneumonia caused by either streptococcus or influenza or mycoplasma

Hospital-acquired pneumonia may be caused by gram-negative enterobacteria or staphylococcus aureus

Aspiration pneumonia

Immunocompromised pneumonia

Risk factors for pneumonia:
- Cigarette smoking
- Alcohol excess
- Cystic fibrosis
- Immunosuppression
- Bronchial obstruction

The clinical symptom of pneumonia includes:
- Fever
- Rigors
- Malaise
- Dyspnoea
- Cough with purulent sputum
- Haemoptysis
- Pleuritic chest pain
- Confusion

The clinical signs of pneumonia are:
- Fever
- Cyanosis
- Tachypnoea
- Tachycardia
- Hypotension

Physical examination for pneumonia includes:
Signs of consolidation (reduced chest expansion)
- Percussion note is dull
- Tactile vocal fremitus/vocal resonance increased
- Bronchial breathing present
- Pleural rub

Pulmonary embolus (PE) involves a circulating blood clot which has become lodged in the pulmonary circulation. These clots usually arise from a venous thrombosis in the pelvis or the legs. Pulmonary embolus can be small to massive. This may depend on the risk factors such as:
  Recent surgery
  Trauma/fractures
  Malignancy
  Previous pulmonary embolus
  Thrombophilia or antiphospholipid syndrome
  Prolonged bed rest
  Long-haul flights
The clinical presentation of pulmonary embolus includes:
  Acute shortness of breath
  Pleuritic chest pain
  Haemoptysis
  Tachypnoea
  Pleural rub on auscultation

Severe central chest pain (in massive PE)
Shock: hypotensive, tachycardia, tachypnoea, and raised JVP (in massive PE)
Central cyanosis
Syncope
Clinical features of massive PE:
  Sudden onset of breathlessness
  Chest pain
  Hypoxia
  Haemoptysis
  Tachycardia
  Pleural rub
  Chest X-ray: normal or small pleural effusion

Pulmonary oedema may be caused by conditions such as trauma to the lung, sepsis, drugs, and fluid overload. On many occasions there is usually underlying left ventricular failure, mitral stenosis, arrhythmias, or malignant hypertension. *Pulmonary oedema* is diagnosed when fluid is found in the lungs, and it is characterized by the following symptoms:
  Extreme breathlessness
  Orthopnoea
  Wheezing
  Production of pink frothy sputum
  Anxiety
  Profuse sweating
The clinical signs of the patient with pulmonary oedema are:
  Pale and sweaty
  Cough productive of frothy pink sputum
  Crackles and wheezes
  Tachycardia
  Tachypnoea
  Raised JVP
  Fine crackles and wheezing bilaterally

Lung collapse is caused by either compression or bronchial obstruction. Bronchial obstruction is caused by mucus, pus, secretions, clot, foreign body, and malignancy. Compression, however, can be caused by enlarged lymph nodes in malignancy or caused by pleural effusion and pneumothorax.
The patient usually complains of breathlessness and the severity of the breathlessness depends on the aetiology.
The clinical signs of lung collapse include:
  Reduction of chest wall movement
  Trachea and mediastinum shifted towards the affected side
  Percussion note is dull
  Breath sounds are absent or reduced
  Vocal resonance is absent or reduced

5.6   Summary of Pathological Processes in Respiratory Disease

Physical examination findings in ***Consolidation (solid)***:

- Mediastinal shift: No, Trachea central
- Chest wall movement: May be reduced on affected side
- Resonance/fremitus: Over area-increased
- Percussion note: Dull
- Breath sounds: Bronchial breathing sounds

Physical examination findings in ***Pneumothorax (Air)***:

- Mediastinal shift: Yes, Trachea may be deviated away from affected side
- Chest wall movement: May be reduced on affected side
- Resonance/fremitus: Reduced over affected area
- Percussion note: Hyperresonant
- Breath sounds: Reduced vesicular breath sounds over affected area

Physical examination findings in ***Pleural Effusion (fluid)***:

- Mediastinal shift: Yes, Trachea deviated away from affected side (if large)
- Chest wall movement: May be reduced on affected side
- Resonance/fremitus: Reduced over affected area
- Percussion note: Dull over affected area
- Breath sounds: Reduced vesicular breath sounds over affected area

5.7   Part 4: Focused Learning

Learning Activity 1

Using the figures for stroke volume and heart rate, calculate the cardiac output:

Answer:

$$Cardiac\ output = stroke\ volume \times heart\ rate$$

$$= 70ml \times 75beats\ /\min = 5250ml\ /\min = 5.25L\ /\min$$

Learning Activity 2

Answer the questions:

(a) Ventilation:

    (i) What is meant by the term, ventilation?

    Answer:

    The movement of air in and out of the lungs.

(ii) Name the structures in the chest wall and the property of the lung tissue that allow ventilation to be accomplished:

Answer:

Ventilation is accomplished by contraction and relaxation of the respiratory muscles and elastic recoil of the lungs.

(iii) What is meant by the term, *lung compliance*;

Answer:

Compliance refers to the ease with which the lungs and thoracic wall expand.

(iv) What is the function of *lung surfactant?*

Answer:

Lung surfactant lowers the surface tension in the alveoli, otherwise the alveolar tissue would resist expansion.

(v) Use the diagram and table to match the lung volumes and capacities with their definitions:

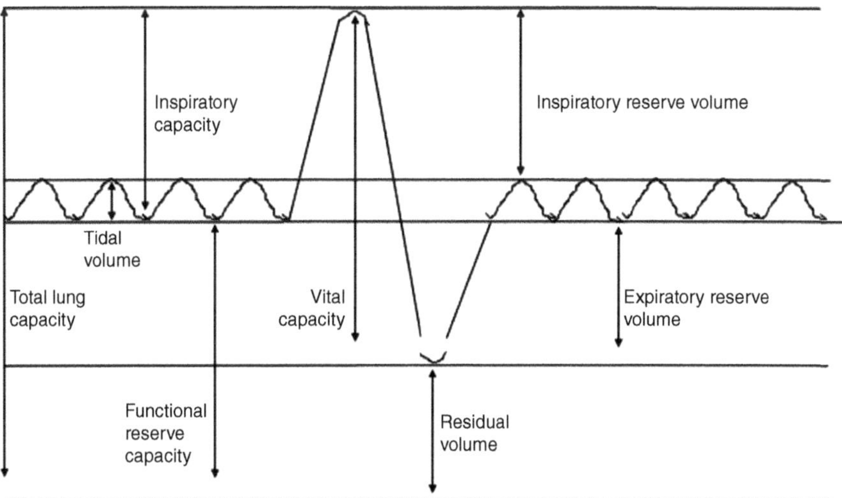

1. Total lung capacity	a. Volume of air breathed in and out with each normal breath—about 500 ml
2. Tidal volume	b. The volume of air that can still be exhaled forcefully after the end of normal tidal expiration—about 1100 ml
3. Inspiratory reserve volume	c. Volume still remaining in the lungs after the most forceful expiration—about 1200 ml
4. Expiratory reserve volume	d. Extra volume of air that can be inhaled forcefully after the end of normal tidal inspiration—about 3000 ml
5. Residual volume	e. The maximal volume to which the lungs can be expanded with the greatest possible inspiratory effort—about 5800 ml
6. Inspiratory capacity	f. Maximum amount of air that can be expelled after first filling the lungs maximally and then expiring maximally—about 4600 ml

7. Functional residual capacity	g. Amount of air that can be breathed beginning at normal expiratory level and then distending the lungs to maximal capacity—about 3500 ml
8. Vital capacity	h. The amount of air remaining in the lungs at the end of normal expiration about—2300 ml

Answer:
1. *Total lung capacity-e*
2. *Tidal volume-a*
3. *Inspiratory reserve volume-d*
4. *Expiratory reserve volume-b*
5. *Residual volume-c*
6. *Inspiratory capacity-g*
7. *Functional residual capacity-h*
8. *Vital capacity-f*

(b) Diffusion of gases: The passive exchange of gases between the alveoli and the blood. On which factors does normal gas diffusion depend?

Answer:
Normal gas diffusion depends on adequate ventilation and pulmonary blood flow, the capacity of gases to diffuse from the alveoli to the blood cells and sufficient quantities of red cells and haemoglobin.

(c) Pulmonary capillary blood flow. On which factors does an adequate pulmonary blood flow depend?

Answer:
The adequate pulmonary blood flow depends on the volume and distribution of right ventricular output.

(d) The transport of gases by the blood. State in which ways oxygen and carbon dioxide are transported in the blood.

Answer:
Oxygen is transported mainly in combination with haemoglobin, with a small amount being carried in solution in the plasma. Carbon dioxide is transported in combination with haemoglobin, in solution, and as bicarbonate ion.

Learning Activity 3
Complete the table below using the keywords provided:

Airways obstruction	Restricted expansion	Decreased gas diffusion	Blood flow changes

Keywords/phrases: Rib cage disease; bronchoconstriction; loss of elastic recoil; pleural disease; pulmonary capillary destruction; under-inflated chest; bronchial muscle hyperplasia; anaemia; pulmonary embolism; lung tissue fibrosis; reduced right ventricular output; bronchial secretions; respiratory muscle disorders; bronchial mucosal oedema; hyper-inflated chest

Answer:

Airways obstruction	Restricted expansion	Decreased gas diffusion	Blood flow changes
Bronchoconstriction; bronchial muscle hyperplasia; bronchial secretions; bronchial mucosal oedema; hyper-inflated chest	Rib cage disease; pleural disease; respiratory muscle disorders; lung tissue fibrosis	Loss of elastic recoil; under-inflated chest; anaemia	Pulmonary capillary destruction; pulmonary embolism; reduced right ventricular output

Learning Activity 4
Answer the questions related to the following symptoms:

Cough is the most common symptom. Cough is initiated when irritant receptors on the mucous membrane of the respiratory tract are stimulated. Cough which persists for more than 6 weeks should always be taken seriously. Drugs, head injury, and anaesthesia can suppress the cough reflex leading to retention of secretions and infection. Cough can be classified into:

- _Productive_
- _Non-productive (dry);_

(a) Complete the table below using the keywords provided:

Productive cough	Non-productive cough

Keywords and phrases:
Asthma; anxiety; foreign body in upper respiratory tract or bronchi; bronchial cancer; nervous habit; chronic bronchitis; pneumonia; fibrosis in interstitial tissue; lung abscess; pulmonary oedema; Irritations (fumes, dust); upper respiratory tract infection (e.g. influenza); bronchiectasis
Answer:

Productive cough	_Non-productive cough_
Asthma, chronic bronchitis, bronchial cancer, pneumonia, pulmonary oedema, lung abscess, bronchiectasis, foreign body	_Anxiety, foreign body in upper respiratory tract and bronchi, nervous habit, fibrosis in interstitial tissue (connective tissue between alveoli), irritations (fumes, dust), upper respiratory tract infection (e.g. influenza)_

(b) What questions should you ask in the history regarding cough?

Answer:
   Do you have a cough?
   How long has the cough been present?
   Day time or nigh time persistent?
   Is the cough dry or bring up productive?
   Any foreign body inhalation?

Sputum. Normally about 100 ml of sputum is produced every day, which is carried upwards by ciliary action and swallowed. Sputum should always be inspected.

(c) Match the following sputa with the appropriate conditions in the table below:

1. Chronic bronchitis	a. Purulent
2. Lung abscess	b. Sticky mucous plugs
3. Asthma,	c. Yellow/green
4. Bronchiectasis (dilatation of bronchi)	d. Large volume
5. Pulmonary infarction	e. Frothy, pink
6. Pneumonia	f. Bright red
7. Tuberculosis	g. Rust coloured
8. Cystic fibrosis	h. Clear, white, mucoid
9. Acute bacterial bronchitis	
10. Pulmonary oedema	

Answer:

   1. *Chronic bronchitis-h. Clear, white, mucoid*
   2. *Lung abscess- c. Yellow/green—i.e. purulent (pus containing); d. Large volume*
   3. *Asthma- b. Sticky mucous plugs*
   4. *Bronchiectasis- c. Yellow/green—i.e. purulent (pus containing); d. Large volume*
   5. *Pulmonary infarction- f. Bright red*
   6. *Pneumonia-g. rust coloured*
   7. *Tuberculosis-f. Bright red*
   8. *Cystic fibrosis- b. Sticky mucous plugs; d. Large volume*
   9. *Acute bacterial bronchitis- c. Yellow/green—i.e. purulent (pus containing)*
   10. *Pulmonary oedema- e. Frothy, pink*

(d) What questions would you ask in the history regarding sputum?

Answer:
What colour is the phlegm?
How often do you bring it up?
How much do you bring up?

Do you have trouble getting it up?

Haemoptysis; the coughing up of blood. One should always differentiate true haemoptysis from a lesion of the nose, nasopharynx, and vocal cords. A definite
  diagnosis is only achieved in 60–70% of cases. Causes include:

(e) List some important causes of haemoptysis

Answer:
Causes include:
Acute or chronic bronchitis
Bronchial carcinoma
Foreign body (trauma)
Left ventricular failure (pulmonary oedema)
Pulmonary infarction
Tuberculosis
Bleeding disorders
Breathlessness; most causes are easily diagnosed on history and examination. The
  time period over which breathlessness develops is of great significance:

(f) Place the disorders listed on page 7 in the appropriate column

Immediate (minutes)	Short (hours to days)	Long (weeks to years)

Disorders

Pulmonary embolism	Pneumonia	Pneumothorax
Pulmonary oedema	Asthma	Lung fibrosis
Anaemia	Pleural effusion	Chronic airways obstruction

Answer:
*Immediate; pneumothorax, acute pulmonary oedema due to heart arrythmias, pul-
  monary embolism, foreign body*
Hours; asthma, left heart failure, pneumonia, laryngeal oedema

Days; pneumonia, left heart failure
Weeks; pleural effusion, anaemia, respiratory muscle weakness
Months; bronchial cancer, lung fibrosis, thyrotoxicosis, muscle weakness
*Years; muscle weakness, chronic obstructive airways disease, lung fibrosis, chest
wall disorders*

(g) What questions would you ask in the history regarding shortness of breath?

Answer:
Timescale of onset/duration of the symptoms?
Is it constant or does it come and go?
How severe is the breathlessness?
What makes the breathing worse?
Does anything make it better?

Wheeze; a common finding in chronic obstructive airways disease and asthma. Both
produce expiratory wheezing. Narrowing of the larynx, trachea and main bronchi
causes mainly inspiratory wheezing. When wheezing occurs on one side, a local
obstruction such as a tumour infiltrating a main bronchus should be suspected.

Chest pain; there are many causes of chest pain and those related to cardiovascular
disease have already been considered. Diseases of the lung tissue are usually
painless, since there are no pain receptors within the lungs. When chest pain
related to lung disease occurs, it invariably means that the pleura, which contains
pain receptors, is involved. The common causes are best considered with regard
to the type of pain and the duration:

(h) Match the condition with the appropriate description and place tick in continuous or intermittent column:

Condition	Pain description	Continuous	Intermittent
1. Myocardial infarction	a. Sharp, stabbing, unilateral		
2. Pneumothorax	b. Central chest, progressively worsening, mediastinal infiltration		
3. Bronchial cancer	c. Crushing, central chest pain, radiates to jaw and arms		
4. Dissecting aneurysm	d. Sharp, worse on inspiration radiates to shoulder, lower chest		
5. Angina	e. Burning, related to eating		
6. Pleuritic pain	f. Tearing, central chest or upper abdomen		
7. Upper GIT disease	g. Worse on moving		
8. Spinal nerve root irritation	h. Constricting, central, radiates to jaw, arms, related to exertion		

Answer:
Continuous;
MI—crushing, central chest pain, radiates to jaw and arms
Pneumothorax—sharp, stabbing, on one side
Bronchial cancer—infiltration of mediastinal nodes—central chest pain
Dissecting aneurysm—tearing, central chest or upper abdominal

Intermittent;
Angina—constricting, central chest pain, related to exertion, radiates to jaw and arms
Pleuritic—sharp, worse on inspiration or coughing, radiates to shoulder, lower chest wall, upper abdomen. Found in pleural inflammations (e.g. pneumonia, pulmonary infarction, Connective tissue diseases) and tumour infiltrations.
Spinal nerve root irritation—worse on moving
Peptic ulcer, hiatus hernia—burning, related to eating

Learning Activity 5
Clubbing of the fingers:

The clinical features of clubbing have already been considered in the lessons on cardiovascular diagnosis:

(a) List the main respiratory, cardiovascular, and gastrointestinal causes of clubbing:

Answer:
The main causes are:
Respiratory diseases; bronchial carcinoma, lung fibrosis, lung abscess, bronchiec-tasis, tuberculosis
Cardiac; congenital heart disease, bacterial endocarditis
Gastrointestinal tract; inflammatory bowel disease, cirrhosis
Familial

Cyanosis:

The diagnosis of central and peripheral cyanosis was considered in the lessons on cardiovascular diagnosis.

(b) List the main causes of central and peripheral cyanosis

Answer:
Central cyanosis; bluish colour of the tongue, due to the reduced oxygenation of blood leaving the lungs causes include high altitude, severe hypoventilation (head injury, drugs, chest injury), congenital heart disease (shunting of venous blood from the right side to the left side of the heart), chronic obstructive airways disease (decreased blood flow through diseased lungs)
Peripheral cyanosis; bluish colour of nail beds of fingers and toes, tips of ears and nose. Causes include peripheral vasoconstriction (cold or vascular disease), sluggish blood flow (due to increased blood viscosity), left ventricular failure.

Pulsus paradoxus:
A greater than normal fall in blood pressure and hence, pulse volume, during inspiration, e.g. severe asthma.

Raised jugular venous pressure:
The interpretation of the JVP was considered in the lessons on cardiovascular diagnosis.

(c) In addition to right heart failure, which lung conditions may cause a raised JVP?

Answer:
Raised jugular venous pressure; found in right heart failure, pneumothorax, hyperinflated chest (e.g. severe asthma, tumour mass compressing the superior vena cava)

Peripheral oedema:
We have already noted that peripheral oedema is a common finding in right heart failure due to chronic obstructive airways disease (chronic bronchitis).

Enlarged lymph nodes (lymphadenopathy):
The important nodes to consider are those of the neck. Lymph from the lung drains from the hilum, up the paratracheal nodes to the supraclavicular and cervical nodes. Lung disease rarely involves the axillary nodes, since these receive lymph from the chest wall and breast.

Learning Activity 6
Explain the following:

(a) Consolidation.

Answer:
Lung tissue become solid.

(b) Fibrosis.

Answer:
Fibrous tissue replacement of normal lung tissue.

(c) Collapse.

Answer:
Lung is reduced in size.

(d) Pneumothorax.

Answer:
Collapse of lung due to air in the pleural space.

(e) Pleural effusion.

Answer:
Fluid in the pleural cavity.

Learning Activity 7
Use your books to define the following terms and to answer the associated questions:

(a) *Scoliosis*. Try to find some common causes of scoliosis.

Answer:
Lateral curvature of the spine.
Congenital, Neurological (poliomyelitis)

(b) *Kyphosis*. Try to think of some common reasons for kyphosis.

Answer:
Increased flexion of the spine
Congenital, Ankylosing spondylitis, Spinal tuberculosis, Osteoporosis

(c) *Pectus excavatum (funnel chest)*. Is this condition usually associated with underlying disease? What apparent effect could it have on the heart if it is severe?

Answer:
Sternum is depressed.
Congenital, not secondary to lung disease.
It may compress the heart and displace the apex, giving a serious impression of cardiac enlargement.

(d) *Pectus carinatum (pigeon chest)*. What common lung disease can cause pectus carinatum;

Answer:
Sternum and costal cartilages project outwards.
Severe childhood asthma.

Do not forget to look for other lesions and swellings on the chest wall.
<u>Patterns of breathing</u>
Note the rate, depth, rhythm, effort, and symmetry of breathing. The symmetry of chest wall movement is considered in the section on palpation.

Learning Activity 8
Answer the following questions related to rate, rhythm, depth, and effort:

(a) Rate.
    (i) What is the normal range for the rate of breathing?
    Answer:
    Normal rate is 10–20 breaths per minute.
    (ii) What is meant by the term tachypnoea.
    Answer:
    Increased rate of breathing.
    (iii) List some common causes of an increase and a decrease in breathing rate.
    Answer:
    Increased rate is due to asthma, lung fibrosis, pulmonary oedema, fever. Decreased rate is due to CNS injury and CNS depressant drugs.

(b) Rhythm:
    (i) Cheyne-Stokes respiration is often seen in terminal illness. Look up a good definition of it.
    Answer:
    Cheyne-Stokes is cyclical variation in depth and rate of breathing. Each cycle can last up to 2 min and involves a period of apnoea followed by light slow breathing then deep fast breathing before this declines again to another period of apnoea.
    (ii) Name two common causes of prolonged expiration. What does the patient's face look like when there is severe difficulty with expiration?
    Answer:
    Chronic bronchitis, Emphysema
    Many of these patients breath out through pursed lips as if they were whistling

(c) Depth:
    (i) What type of breathing pattern do patients with metabolic acidosis (excess hydrogen ions in the blood) have?
    Answer:
    Deep sighing respiration (Kussmaul breathing)
    (ii) What is the mechanism for this breathing pattern? Can you think of some serious diseases that cause it?
    Answer:
    Metabolic acidosis stimulates the reparatory centre as it tries to excrete carbon dioxide.
    Renal failure
    Diabetic Ketoacidosis
    Aspirin overdose

(d) Effort:

  (i) Breathing difficulties can cause extreme distress. Some patients have great difficulty in lying flat. What is this called and what are the likely mechanisms that could lead to it?

  Answer:

  Orthopnoea

  Normal subjects when they lie flat, breath more with the diaphragm and less with the chest wall. In patients with airways obstruction, the diaphragm is often flat and inefficient draw ribs inwards. Thus, when they lie down, the diaphragm cannot provide the ventilation required.

  (ii) Patients with severe respiratory distress need to use their accessory muscles of respiration and audible noises such as wheezes or stridor may be heard. Define these terms and, in each case, explain the underlying mechanism:

  Answer:

  Wheezes are high pitched whistling sound produced by airway walls oscillation between the open and nearly closed position. It occurs in both inspiratory and expiratory but is always louder in the expiration.

  Stridor is a loud, mainly inspiratory noise produced by laryngeal, tracheal, or major airway obstruction.

Learning Activity 9

(a) The position of the apex beat should always be checked when palpating the trachea. Why is this important?

Answer:

The trachea moves with the upper part of mediastinum, the apex beat moves with the lower part of mediastinum. Large effusion pushes the position of the apex beat but very large effusions are needed to displace the trachea.

(b) The table below lists common causes of mediastinal displacement. In each case, indicate whether the mediastinum is pulled towards the lesion or pushed away from it and try to briefly explain the mechanism in each case.

Lesion	Towards	Away
Pleural effusion		
Lung collapse		
Pneumothorax		
Unilateral fibrosis		

Answer:

Lesion	Towards	Away
Pleural effusion		*Away*
Lung collapse	*Towards*	
Pneumothorax		*Away*
Unilateral fibrosis	*Towards*	

Learning Activity 10
The chest wall comprises ribs, dorsal spine, and muscles associated with respiration. The chest cavity contains, among other structures, the lungs, lined by two layers of pleura, which comprise air passages and air sacs. Bearing this in mind:

(a) State four mechanisms that can lead to bilateral reduction in chest wall movement. Give a disease example for each.

Answer:
Bilateral reduction in chest wall movement is found in; hyper-inflated chest (emphysema), reduced compliance (lung fibrosis), reduced rib cage movement (ankylosing spondylitis), weak inspiratory muscles (myasthenia gravis)

(b) State four mechanisms that can lead to unilateral reduction in chest wall movements. Give a disease example for each.

Answer:
Local or unilateral reduction in chest wall movement is found in; pleural effusion, pleural thickening, lung collapse, consolidation (due to inflammatory exudate in alveoli from infections like pneumonia), pneumothorax.
Tactile vocal fremitus
This is a crude test for assessing the transmission of sound to the chest wall and is normally palpable as a low frequency vibration. The value of this test and its interpretation are considered in the section on vocal resonance (auscultation).
Percussion
Percussion is an important technique and is used to determine whether underlying tissues are air filled, fluid filled or solid. The normal percussion note gives a resonant sound.

Learning Activity 11
List common causes for the following changes:

(a) Dullness.

Answer:
Dull note; found when the lung is filled with fluid or replaced by solid tissue. Causes include; pneumonia, pulmonary oedema, pleural effusion, lung fibrosis and lung tumour.

(b) Bilateral hyperresonance.

Answer:
Bilateral hyperresonant sound is associated with over-inflated lungs seen in emphysema and asthma. This is often not a reliable sign.

(c) Unilateral hyperresonance.

Answer:
Unilateral hyperresonant sound is associated with pneumothorax.

Learning Activity 12
(a) What pathological processes cause bilateral reduction in normal (vesicular) breath sounds?

Answer:
Airway obstruction: asthma, emphysema, tumour.

(b) What pathological processes cause unilateral reduction in breath sounds? Give some disease examples.

Answer:
Anything interspersed between the lung and the chest wall, i.e. air, fluid or pleural thickening.

(c) Which lung conditions are commonly associated with the localized transmission of bronchial breath sounds to the lung field? What is the underlying mechanism for this?

Answer:
Pneumonia
Lung substance is solid as in consolidation, but the air passage remains open.

(d) What are wheezes and what is the underlying mechanism that gives rise to them?

Answer:
Wheezes are due to narrowing of the airways generalized wheezes are heard in asthma, chronic bronchitis/emphysema and pulmonary oedema. Localized wheezes are heard in lung cancer (infiltrating a large bronchus), foreign body, and bronchial secretions.

(e) Complete the following table with regard to wheezing:

Unilateral (localised) causes	Bilateral (generalised) causes

Answer:

Unilateral (localized) causes	Bilateral (generalized) causes
Foreign body	Asthma
Bronchial tumour	Chronic bronchitis
	Emphysema

(f) What are crackles and what is the underlying mechanism that gives rise to them?

Answer:

Crackles are discrete, explosive sounds found in diseases involving small bronchioles and alveoli such as pneumonia, pulmonary oedema, chronic bronchitis/ emphysema and lung fibrosis.

(g) Complete the following table with regard to crackles:

Unilateral (localised) causes	Bilateral (generalised) causes

Answer:

Unilateral (localized) causes	Bilateral (generalized) causes
Bronchiectasis	Chronic bronchitis
Pneumonia	Pulmonary oedema

(h) What causes pleural rubs and what do they sound like?

Answer:

A pleural rub is a creaking sound heard when two layers of pleura rub together during breathing and is associated with pleural disease.

Learning Activity 13

(a) Which pathological processes in the lungs are associated with increased vocal fremitus and resonance? Name a disease that can cause this pathological change.

Answer:

Increased fremitus is found over an area of lung consolidation (pneumonia)

(b) What pathological processes in the lungs are associated with decreased vocal fremitus? Name some common diseases that can cause these pathological changes.

Answer:

Reduced or absent fremitus; bronchial obstruction, chronic bronchitis, pleural thickening and effusion, pneumothorax, and a large infiltrating lung cancer.

Learning Activity 14

The table below summarizes the major pathological processes. Indicate the physical signs associated with each process based on the guidelines below:

- *Mediastinal shift*: indicate "yes" or "no". If "yes" state whether "towards" or "away" from the lesion.
- *Chest wall movement*: indicate whether "reduced" or "not reduced".
- *Resonance/fremitus*: indicate whether "reduced", "normal", or "increased".
- *Percussion note:* indicate whether "normal", "dull", or "hyperresonant".
- *Breath sounds:* indicate whether "reduced" or "normal" and whether "vesicular" or "bronchial".

Pathological process	Mediastinal shift	Chest wall movement	Resonance/ fremitus	Percussion note	Breath sounds	Added sounds
Consolidation						
Collapse						
Pneumothorax						
Pleural effusion						

Answer:

Pathological process	Mediastinal shift	Chest wall movement	Resonance/ fremitus	Percussion note	Breath sounds	Added sounds
Consolidation	*No*	*Reduced*	*Increased*	*Dull*	*Bronchial*	*Crackles*
Collapse	*Yes, towards*	*Reduced*	*Reduced*	*Dull*	*Reduced or absent/ vesicular*	*No*
Pneumothorax	*Yes, away*	*Reduced*	*Reduced*	*Hyperresonant*	*Reduced or absent/ vesicular*	*No*
Pleural effusion	*No*	*Reduced*	*Reduced*	*Dull*	*Reduced or absent/ vesicular*	*Pleural rubs*

Answers

Case Study 1

A 66-year-old man who has come to hospital with a 2-month history of cough, haemoptysis, malaise, and weight loss. He has smoked 25 cigarettes a day for the past 40 years. There is a history of chronic winter cough productive of some white sputum, but no other history of note. On examination, he is thin; examination of the lungs shows evidence of collapse in the upper zone of the left lung. There are also some generalized expiratory wheezes over both lung fields. The blood tests show that he has a raised serum calcium level.

1. What is the likely diagnosis for the current 2-month symptoms? What is the likely diagnosis for the chronic winter cough and what sign found on examination supports this diagnosis?

The likely diagnosis for the current symptoms is a carcinoma of the bronchus. The diagnosis of the chronic cough is chronic bronchitis which is confirmed by the presence of expiratory wheezes.

2. What are the underlying mechanisms for the cough, and haemoptysis, malaise, and weight loss?

General malaise and weight loss are common features of malignancy. This may be due to anorexia and rapid utilization of nutrients by tumour cells, particularly if there are extensive metastases.
The cough may be due to infection distal to a blocked bronchus. Haemoptysis is due to ulceration of the tumour in the bronchus.

3. State the pathological basis (mechanisms) for the following:
   • The cough and signs of consolidation:
      Cough originally due to COPD but is likely to worsen due to local cancer spread. Consolidation is due to supervening bacterial infection (pneumonia) probably distal to tumour growth
   • The haemoptysis
      Tumour invasion of blood vessels
4. What is the mechanism for the collapse of the left upper zone? What features would you find on examination that would confirm collapse?

Collapse is due to complete blockage of a main bronchus, but tumour or lymph node metastases. Features on examination would include:
   (a) *Shift of the trachea towards the left. There is also likely to be a shift of the apex beat to the left.*
   (b) *Possibly reduced movement of the left side of the chest.*
   (c) *Reduced tactile vocal fremitus over the collapsed area.*
   (d) *Dullness on percussion over the area.*
   (e) *Absent air entry—possibly some bronchial breathing and crackles.*

5. Why is the plasma calcium raised?

The calcium is commonly raised in cancers with bony metastases. Cancer metastases are usually lytic and tend to stimulate osteoclastic activity.
An even more likely reason is that this is a tumour that is making parathyroid hormone—like substance. These are usually squamous carcinomas.

Case Study 2

A previously healthy 56-year-old woman was admitted to hospital with 6-day history of fever and chills, she also complained of a cough productive of yellow-green sputum, tinged with rusty-coloured blood. On examination, the patient had a temperature of 38.9 C, a pulse rate of 110 beats/min, a respiratory rate of 25 breaths/min. Lung signs of consolidation are found localized to the middle lobe of the right lung. She is commenced on antibiotics, but her symptoms worsen, and she begins to produce large amounts of foul-smelling sputum indicating that she had developed a lung abscess. Following culture of the organism, her antibiotic treatment is changed, and she makes a slow recovery. Pneumonia is the likeliest diagnosis.

(a) Outline the clinical features associated with bacterial (pneumococcal) pneumonia.

Acute onset. Patient presents with fever, which may be very high. Can also experience rigors. Also cough productive of rusty coloured sputum (due to presence of altered blood). Chest pain due to pleural involvement is common—this is sharp and aggravated by movement and coughing.

- Discuss the mechanism for the consolidation of the middle lobe of the right lung.

   Consolidation refers to the alveolar airspaces being filled with fluid (exudate/transudate/blood), cells (inflammatory), tissue, or other material.

   The most common cause is pneumonia. The infection spreads through the right middle lobe between alveoli but is limited from spreading between lobes by the visceral pleura.

- What is lung abscess?

   Lung abscess is defined as a circumscribed area of pus or necrotic debris in lung parenchyma secondary to a microbial infection.

   Most frequently, the lung abscess arises as a complication of aspiration pneumonia.

- List the features that you would expect to find on examination of the respiratory system that would confirm consolidation?

   Lung findings: May elicit signs of consolidation—i.e. decreased movement on affected side, increased tactile vocal fremitus and vocal resonance over area of consolidation, dullness to percussion, bronchial breath sounds over affected area with reduced normal vesicular breathing and crackles. May also get signs of pleural effusion (stony dullness to percussion and reduced/absent vesicular breathing) due to pleural involvement.

   Lower lobes are the most frequently involved. Recovery is usually rapid but mortality high in those who are immunocompromised or severely ill or elderly patients.

- Compare and contrast the terms aspiration pneumonia and inhalation pneumonia. State one cause for each

   Aspiration pneumonia is the term used to denote the aspiration of organisms into the lower respiratory tract. Inhalation pneumonia refers to the con-

sequences of inhaling non-infected matter such as particles, fluid, or irritant gases. Cause of aspiration pneumonia is dental sepsis. A cause of inhalation pneumonia is inhalation of gastric contents, e.g. anaesthesia.

Case Study 3

A 65-year-old teacher was admitted to hospital complaining of severe breathlessness of 1 week and his symptom had come on rapidly over a period of 24 h. He had also experienced severe breathlessness at night and had to sleep propped up with pillows. Over the next days following the onset of his severe breathlessness, his legs and ankles had also become very swollen. He smokes 30 cigarettes a day and has got a 15-year history of a chronic cough productive of sputum and for the last past year he has noticed gradual swelling of both ankles, together with increasing shortness of breath on exertion. For the past 3 months prior to admission, he has had experienced haemoptysis, coughing up small amounts of fresh blood and he has also lost about 3 kg in weight.

On examination, he was very short of breath and cyanosed. The pulse was 130 beats per minute, regular with a very small volume, the blood pressure was 70/40 mmHg and the jugular venous pressure was grossly elevated. The heart sounds were faint, and the apex beat was not palpable. He was barrel chested, and the trachea was central. There was swelling of both legs right up to the groin. The lower one-third of the left lung showed the features of a pleural effusion and liver was enlarged, tender with a smooth edge and surface.

- Comment on the 15-year history of chronic productive cough, the 1-year history of progressive ankle swelling and the barrel chest.

The history suggests chronic bronchitis, since the clinical definition is a cough productive of sputum for at least 3 months of the year for a minimum of 2 years. Chronic bronchitis is related to heavy cigarette smoking. The ankle swelling suggests a slow onset of Cor pulmonale (right-sided heart failure due to chronic obstructive airways disease). The barrel chest indicates that there is also a significant amount of emphysema.

- What is the likely significance of the weight loss and 3 months history of haemoptysis? Discuss the causes of haemoptysis that you should consider in this patient.

The weight loss indicates underlying serious pathology, most likely carcinoma of the bronchus. There could be other causes of weight loss in such a patient, e.g. cardiac cachexia (wasting) associated with severe chronic congestive heart failure related to a history of myocardial infarction or long-standing hypertension. However, there is nothing in the history to suggest this. The cause of haemoptysis is a patient such as this include:
Carcinoma of the bronchus. This is the most likely cause, especially as there is a short history of significant weight loss, together with a history of smoking and chronic obstructive airways disease.

Pulmonary embolus/infarction, which must be excluded in a case such as this. Pulmonary infarction is much more likely to occur if there is underlying disease affecting the bronchi, which is the case in this patient. The characteristic features are sudden breathlessness. It is also associated with the coughing up of fresh blood. However, the swelling of the legs is not typical of a deep vein thrombosis since the rapid increase in swelling came on after the onset of the lung features and there is no history of chest pain.

Pulmonary oedema. From the history, this patient obviously has pulmonary oedema, but it is usually associated with the production of copious amounts of frothy, white sputum, which may be tinged with blood. The haemoptysis is thus unlikely to be due to this.

- Discuss the possible causes and mechanisms for the blood pressure, pulse, faint heart sounds, absent apex beat, and rapid deterioration in the shortness of breath. What is the link with the raised JVP, swollen legs, and liver enlargement?

The low blood pressure, rapid weak pulse, and rapid onset of severe dyspnoea point towards significant left-sided heart failure. Left ventricular failure leads to back-pressure of blood to the lungs resulting in pulmonary oedema, which would lead to rapid deterioration of breathing and to orthopnoea (breathing difficulties when lying flat). Possible common causes include myocardial infarction and long-standing hypertension. However, there is nothing in the presentation to suggest either of these (no history of chest pain or hypertension). The likeliest possibility for these acute symptoms must be a pericardial effusion, which is due to infiltration of the pericardium by a bronchial carcinoma. The raised JVP, enlarged liver, and leg swelling are due to back-pressure of venous blood from the right atrium due to significantly worsening right heart failure as a result of the pericardial effusion. Significant pericardial effusion will severely limit the flow of blood from the left and right ventricles.

- Briefly state the findings on examination of the lungs (inspection, palpation, percussion, and auscultation) that led to the diagnosis of pleural effusion. How might the presence of underlying chronic bronchitis and emphysema affect the classical features of a pleural effusion. What is the likely cause for the pleural effusion?

    (a) *Inspection; evidence of reduced movement on the affected side—although this may be difficult to see, since both sides are likely to be reduced in this patient due to the underlying chronic obstructive airways disease. The trachea may be deviated away from the lesion, but, again, the presence of chronic bronchitis and emphysema in this patient could prevent this, as was noted in the history.*

    (b) *Palpation: confirmation of reduced expansion on affected side, reduced tactile vocal fremitus (but see above comment).*

    (c) *Percussion; stony dullness on percussion.*

    (d) *Auscultation: reduced air entry (decreased normal breath sounds but see comment in section on "inspection"). Possibly a pleural rub.*

    The likely cause of the pleural effusion is a carcinoma of the bronchus infiltrating the pleura.

Bibliography

1. Andersson, S. O., Bardel, A., André, M., & Kristiansson, P. (2020). Consultation skills of final year medical students in Sweden: Video-recorded real-patient consultations in primary health care assessed by Calgary-Cambridge Global Consultation Rating Scale, a pilot study. *MedEdPublish, 8*, 88.
2. Garibaldi, B. T., & Elder, A. (2020). Seven reasons why the physical examination remains important. *Journal of the Royal College of Physicians of Edinburgh, 51*(3), 211–214.
3. Kurtz, S., Silverman, J., Benson, J., & Draper, J. (2003). Marrying content and process in clinical method teaching: enhancing the Calgary–Cambridge guides. *Academic Medicine, 78*(8), 802–809.
4. Schirmer, J. M., Mauksch, L., Lang, F., Marvel, M. K., Zoppi, K., Epstein, R. M., Brock, D., & Pryzbylski, M. (2005). Assessing communication competence: A review of current tools. *Family Medicine, 37*(3), 184–192.
5. Walker, H. K. (1990). The origins of the history and physical examination. In *Clinical methods: The history, physical, and laboratory examinations* (3rd ed.). Butterworth.

Assessing and Diagnosing the Digestive System

6

Learning Objectives

In this part of the chapter, we revisit basic anatomy and physiology of the digestive tract and identify the clinical signs and symptoms diagnostic of diseases and disorders of the digestive tract.

Learning Objectives
By the end of this chapter, you will be able to:

Understand the basic pathophysiology of the digestive tract
Explain the physiological changes and anatomical features present in disease of the digestive tract.
Link symptoms and signs of basic pathology to digestive disease.
Identify general and specific signs and symptoms relevant to the diagnosis of digestive disease and their significance in differential diagnosis.
Undertake a step-by-step physical examination on a patient with symptoms of the digestive tract.
Understand key concepts in digestive conditions.

Common Medical Terms

The list of medical terms below is cited for easy reference and the reader is expected to understand these medical terms before they proceed to read this chapter.

Amylase
Ampulla of Vater
Ascites
Barrett's oesophagus

© The Author(s), under exclusive license to Springer Nature
Switzerland AG 2026
C. Leliopoulou, L. Holman, *Physical Examination and Diagnostic Skills for Nurses and Allied Health Professionals*,
https://doi.org/10.1007/978-3-032-26539-5_6

Celiac disease
Crohn's disease
Chyme
Dysphagia
Epigastric
Falciform ligament
Jaundice
Gastroesophageal reflux disease (GERD)
Hepatopancreatic ampulla
Hemochromatosis.
Haematemesis
Hydroxylation
Islets of Langerhans
Ileocaecal valve
Lingual lipase
Lysozyme
Melena
Oedema
Pepsinogen
Peristalsis
Purpura
Plicae circulares
Palmar erythema
Rugae
Spider naevi
Sphincter of Oddi
Ulcerative colitis

6.1   Part 1: Normal Structure and Function of the Digestive Tract

Food processing begins in the oral cavity, where it is mechanically broken down through chewing and moistened by saliva. Saliva plays a crucial role in the initial stages of digestion, containing a mixture of enzymes, such as amylase, which begins the breakdown of carbohydrates, lingual lipase, which initiates fat digestion, and lysozyme, which has antibacterial properties. Additionally, saliva contains bicarbonate, which helps neutralize acids, creating a more favourable environment for enzymatic activity. The secretion of saliva is facilitated by three primary salivary glands: the parotid, submandibular, and sublingual glands, each contributing to the overall composition and volume of saliva produced.

The process of swallowing, which moves food from the mouth into the oesophagus, is governed by a complex neurological mechanism located within the brain stem. This centre coordinates the integration of sensory and motor functions necessary for swallowing, ensuring that the various stages of the act are synchronized.

The transmission of information to and from the pharynx and oesophagus occurs *via **the glossopharyngeal and vagus cranial nerves***. These nerves are essential for relaying signals that dictate the voluntary and involuntary phases of swallowing, facilitating the seamless transition of food from the oral cavity to the oesophagus.

Once the food is transported to the oesophagus, it encounters a uniquely structured muscular tube that extends from the pharynx to the stomach. The oesophagus is lined with smooth muscle, which has its own intrinsic innervation, allowing it to perform peristaltic movements. *Peristalsis* is a coordinated, wave-like contraction of the smooth muscle that propels the food bolus downward towards the stomach. This involuntary process is critical in ensuring the efficient movement of food through the gastrointestinal tract.

As the food moves through the oesophagus, it is guided toward the stomach by the action of rhythmic contractions. The lower oesophageal sphincter (LES) plays a critical role in this transit, serving as a barrier that helps prevent the regurgitation of gastric contents into the oesophagus. The sphincter must relax to allow the food bolus to enter the stomach, effectively timing its opening with the wave of peristalsis that reaches it. This intricate coordination is vital and any malfunctions in this complex system can lead to digestive issues such as *gastroesophageal reflux disease (GERD)*, where acid from the stomach backs up into the oesophagus.

Learning Point
The anatomy of the digestive system involves:

- Mouth: mechanical (chewing) and chemical (enzyme) digestion begins.
- Oesophagus: moves food from the mouth to the stomach using peristalsis (wave-like muscle contractions).
- Stomach: churns food to form semi-liquid *chyme*, begins protein digestion, and produces acid.
- Pancreas: produces pancreatic juice containing enzymes for digestion.
- Liver: involved in nutrient metabolism.
- Gallbladder: stores, concentrates, and releases bile.
- Duodenum: first part of the small intestine; receives chyme from the stomach and digestive juices from the pancreas and gallbladder.
- Small intestine (ileum): completes digestion; most nutrient absorption occurs here.
- Large intestine (colon): absorbs water and minerals; forms and stores faeces.
- Rectum: stores faeces before elimination.
- Anus: allows passage of faeces out of the body.

6.1.1   The Stomach

The stomach stores, mixes, and begins the digestion of food, particularly proteins. Muscle layers and rugae aid in mechanical breakdown, while gastric juices chemically break down food. The stomach has smooth muscle which allows it to churn the food to prepare it for entry into the duodenum. The parietal cells in the body secrete hydrochloric acid and intrinsic factor. The function of hydrochloric acid is to sterilize the meal and absorb vitamin B12. Pepsinogen is the substance secreted by the chief cells of the stomach and acid in the stomach changes pepsinogen to pepsin, which breaks down proteins in food during digestion. The ant-reflux mechanism at the gastro-oesophageal junction involves the intrinsic muscular sphincter (cardiac sphincter) or lower oesophageal sphincter (LES) and the diaphragm that functions as an external sphincter-like mechanism. Sphincters control the entry and exit of material to prevent reflux and ensure proper timing of digestion.

Learning Point
<u>Muscular layers of the stomach wall</u>:
These layers enable the stomach to churn, mix, and propel food:

- *Longitudinal muscle*: The outermost muscle layer; fibres run lengthwise along the stomach.
- *Circular muscle*: Middle muscle layer; fibres encircle the stomach and help mix contents.
- *Oblique muscle*: The innermost and unique muscle layer in the stomach; fibres run diagonally to enhance the churning action. *Rugae* are folds in the inner lining of the stomach that allow expansion after consuming food and help in mechanical digestion.

<u>Anatomical structure of the stomach</u>

- Oesophagus: The muscular tube that delivers food from the mouth to the stomach.
- Cardiac sphincter or lower oesophageal sphincter is a ring-like muscle at the junction of the oesophagus and stomach. Prevents backflow of acidic stomach contents into the oesophagus.
- Fundus: The dome-shaped upper part of the stomach that stores undigested food and gases released during digestion. This is the central, largest region of the stomach where most digestive activity occurs.
- Pyloric antrum: The lower portion of the stomach that helps grind food and mix it with gastric juices.
- Pyloric sphincter: A muscular valve that regulates the passage of partially digested food (chyme) from the stomach into the duodenum (first part of the small intestine).
- Duodenum: The first section of the small intestine, where chyme is mixed with bile and pancreatic enzymes for further digestion.

6.1.2   The Small Intestine

The small intestine is a crucial component of the human digestive system, consisting of three distinct sections: the **duodenum**, **jejunum**, and **ileum**. Each section plays an essential role in the processes of digestion and nutrient absorption. The arterial supply of the small intestine is primarily from the *superior mesenteric artery*, which branches from the abdominal aorta and provides oxygenated blood to this vital organ. Conversely, venous blood from the intestines is collected by the *superior mesenteric vein*, which merges with other veins to form the portal vein. This **portal vein** transports nutrient-rich blood to the liver before it enters the systemic circulation, enabling the liver to metabolize and detoxify the nutrients absorbed from the digestive tract.

The primary functions of the small intestine revolve around the digestion of food and the absorption of nutrients. To maximize these functions, the small intestine has evolved an extensive surface area, which is accomplished through both macroscopic and microscopic modifications. Large visible folds known as **plicae circulares** line the intestinal wall, while thousands of microscopic **villi** and microvilli increase the absorptive surface area exponentially. This structural complexity facilitates optimal contact between the intestinal lumen and the nutrient-filled chyme, enhancing nutrient absorption.

The duodenum, the first segment of the small intestine, is particularly important in the digestive process, as it is where most of the chemical digestion occurs. Several digestive enzymes are delivered to the duodenum, for example, *amylase*, an enzyme secreted by both saliva and the pancreas, initiates the breakdown of carbohydrates into simpler sugars. This process is fundamental to human nutrition, as carbohydrates are a primary energy source for bodily functions. Further breakdown of carbohydrates into monosaccharides is accomplished by specific enzymes, including lactase, maltase, and sucrase, which are located on the brush border membrane of the enterocytes lining the small intestine. These enzymes act to **hydrolyse** disaccharides into their constituent monosaccharides, which can then be efficiently absorbed through the intestinal lining.

In addition to carbohydrates, lipids undergo a critical step in the small intestine. Fats are primarily broken down by *lipase*, an enzyme secreted from the pancreas. The emulsification of these fats is facilitated by bile acids, which are produced by the liver and stored in the gallbladder. Bile acids function to increase the surface area of fats, allowing lipase to effectively hydrolyse triglycerides into fatty acids and monoglycerides, which can then be absorbed in the intestinal mucosa.

Proteins, another essential macronutrient, begin their digestion in the stomach through the action of pepsin. However, most of the protein digestion occurs within the small intestine, facilitated by a group of enzymes collectively referred to as *peptidases*, which are also secreted by the pancreas. These enzymes further hydrolyse protein molecules into smaller peptide fragments and amino acids, which can be readily absorbed into the bloodstream. The duodenum is primarily focused on breaking down food substances; the jejunum and ileum are chiefly involved in the absorption of nutrients.

The jejunum is particularly adept at absorbing sugars, amino acids, fatty acids, and various vitamins and minerals. The extensive folds, combined with the presence of villi and microvilli, ensure that the absorption process is highly effective. The terminal segment of the small intestine, the *ileum*, uniquely specializes in the *absorption of vitamin B12* and bile acids. Vitamin B12 is vital for red blood cell production and neurological function; thus, its absorption is critical for maintaining overall health. Bile acids, once absorbed, are recycled back to the liver through a process known as ***enterohepatic circulation***, illustrating the efficiency of nutrient utilization in the body.

6.1.3 The Large Intestine

The large intestine, or colon, serves as a critical component of the human digestive system, facilitating the absorption of water and electrolytes, as well as the formation and expulsion of faeces. The anatomy of the large intestine includes several distinct parts: the ***caecum*** (which is also connected to the appendix), ***ascending colon***, right (hepatic) flexure, ***transverse colon***, left (splenic) flexure, ***descending colon***, ***sigmoid colon***, rectum, and ***anus***. Each of these segments plays a unique role in the final stages of digestion.

The journey of indigestible food matter into the large intestine commences at the caecum, a pouch-like structure that sits at the junction of the small intestine and the large intestine. It connects to the ileum, the terminal segment of the small intestine, and is equipped with the ***ileocaecal valve***. This valve is essential as it prevents the backflow of colonic contents into the ileum, thus maintaining the one-way direction of digestive material through the gastrointestinal tract. Daily, approximately 1.5 l of fluid enters the large intestine. This significant volume presents a challenging task for the colon, which must absorb the majority of this fluid to prevent dehydration and maintain the body's fluid balance. The large intestine is not only responsible for fluid absorption but also serves as a site for microbial fermentation, where beneficial bacteria break down indigestible carbohydrates and produce gases and short-chain fatty acids, further aiding in gut health.

As the contents move through the colon, they undergo a transformation into faeces. On average, a Western diet results in the production of approximately 200 g of faecal matter each day. Faeces consist of undigested food residuals, bacteria, cells shed from the intestinal lining, water, and waste products. The process of forming and expelling faeces is critical for the maintenance of health, as it eliminates waste materials and prevents the absorption of harmful substances into the bloodstream.

Mucus production is another vital function of the colonic glands. Mucus serves as an essential lubricant that facilitates the smooth passage of faeces through the large intestine. It protects the inner lining of the colon (the mucosa) from abrasive damage caused by the faecal matter and from the action of bacterial enzymes that may lead to irritation or inflammation. The presence of mucus is crucial in preventing conditions such as colitis and ensuring the overall health of the gastrointestinal tract.

Learning Point

A detailed examination of the components of the large intestine reveals the specific functions of each segment.

- Caecum: This initial pouch-like section initiates the fermentation of incoming material, particularly fibre. It acts as a reservoir before the waste enters the colon proper.
- Vermiform appendix: Although often considered a vestigial structure, the appendix is a small, tube-shaped organ that is thought to play a role in immune function, housing beneficial bacteria that can repopulate the gut flora after diarrhoea or other disturbances.
- Ascending colon: Positioned on the right side of the abdomen, this segment of the colon absorbs water and nutrients, continuing the process started in the small intestine.
- Hepatic flexure: This is the bend located near the liver, where the ascending colon transitions to the *transverse colon*. This area is notable for its anatomical relationship with the liver and is a point where obstruction may occur in certain gastrointestinal conditions.
- Transverse colon: Running across the abdomen, the transverse colon continues the absorption of water and electrolytes, while also transporting waste material downward.
- Splenic flexure: This is the bend near the spleen where the transverse colon shifts direction into the *descending colon*. Like the hepatic flexure, it is another critical area for potential obstruction or other pathologies.
- Descending colon: Located on the left side, this section primarily serves to store the indigestible remnants of food until they are ready to be expelled.
- Sigmoid colon: Shaped like an "S," the sigmoid colon is the section that connects the descending colon to the rectum. It is here that the faeces are stored before being moved into the rectum.
- Rectum: This final segment of the large intestine serves as a storage site for faeces. Upon filling, stretch receptors signal the body that it is time to expel waste.
- Anus: The anus represents the external opening of the digestive tract, through which faeces are expelled, marking the final step of the digestive process.

6.1.4   The Liver and Gallbladder

The liver is the largest organ situated within the abdominal cavity and functions as a fundamental component of the human body's metabolic processes. Anatomically, it is divided into two primary lobes: the larger lobe and the smaller left lobe by the ***falciform ligament*** which is *part of peritoneum* that the liver to the anterior abdominal wall and the diaphragm. In terms of weight, the liver typically ranges from 1.2 to 1.5 kg, solidifying its status as *the largest gland* in the human body, underscoring its critical roles in maintaining homeostasis and contributing to digestive processes. The liver occupies a strategic location in the right upper quadrant of the abdomen, primarily filling the **right hypochondriac region**, while also extending into the **epigastric** and **left hypochondriac** regions. This positioning not only highlights its prominence in the abdominal cavity but also signifies its relevance to various organ systems, particularly those related to digestion, metabolism, and detoxification. To provide a comprehensive understanding of the liver's anatomy and function, we must examine its structure from both anterior and posterior perspectives.

Learning Point
Anterior View of the Liver
From the anterior view, several key features of the liver are identifiable:

- **Right Lobe**: This is the larger of the two lobes, situated on the right side of the body. The right lobe accounts for approximately 60% of the liver's mass and contains a greater proportion of functional tissue, which plays a critical role in metabolic activities.
- **Left Lobe**: The left lobe, being smaller, occupies the left side of the liver's anterior surface. Despite its reduced size, it still performs essential functions, contributing to the liver's overall metabolic capabilities.
- **Falciform Ligament**: This ligament acts as a dividing structure between the right and left lobes and attaches the liver to the anterior abdominal wall. As a critical anatomy feature, the falciform ligament provides structural support while facilitating the liver's movement during respiration and other bodily movements.
- **Gallbladder**: Positioned beneath the liver, the gallbladder is a small, greenish sac that specializes in storing bile. Bile, produced by the liver, plays a vital role in the digestion and absorption of fats. During meals, the gallbladder contracts to release bile into the small intestine, aiding in the emulsification of fats and the overall digestive process.

Learning Point
Posterior View of the Liver
From the posterior perspective, additional structures of the liver become apparent, showcasing its complexity and interconnectivity with other crucial organs:

- **Right lobe and left lobe**: Both lobes are visible from this vantage point, illustrating their significance in the overall liver structure.
- **Caudate lobe**: This smaller lobe is found on the posterior aspect of the liver, situated near the inferior vena cava. The caudate lobe's unique position among the liver lobes often makes it an area of interest, particularly during surgical procedures.
- **Quadrate lobe**: Located near the gallbladder, the quadrate lobe complements the anatomy of the liver, serving as another point of reference for surgeons and physicians alike. This lobe's positioning further exemplifies the liver's intricate architecture.
- **Inferior vena cava**: This large blood vessel runs just behind the liver and is instrumental in returning deoxygenated blood from the lower extremities and the abdominal region back to the heart. Its proximity to the liver highlights the organ's role in filtering and processing blood.
- **Hepatic artery**: This artery is responsible for supplying oxygen-rich blood to the liver, thus supporting its numerous metabolic functions. The flow of oxygenated blood is essential for maintaining hepatic cellular integrity and function.
- **Portal vein**: Serving as a vital conduit, the portal vein transports nutrient-rich blood from the intestines to the liver. This specialized blood supply plays a critical role in liver metabolism, allowing the organ to process nutrients, detoxify harmful substances, and regulate various biochemical processes necessary for maintaining homeostasis.
- **Gallbladder**: Once again, the gallbladder is visible, reinforcing its importance in bile storage and fat digestion. Its location under the right lobe of the liver indicates the coordinated relationship between these two structures in the digestive process.

The liver is one of the most vital organs in the human body, performing numerous essential functions related to metabolism, detoxification, and synthesis of important biomolecules. It is characterized by its smooth superior and anterior surfaces, which lie beneath the diaphragm and are well-protected by the rib cage. Under normal circumstances, this anatomical positioning makes the liver difficult to palpate below the costal margin, reinforcing its sheltered location within the abdominal cavity. An abundant supply of blood is crucial for the liver's proper function. The liver receives oxygen-rich blood from the hepatic artery, which branches from the abdominal aorta. Additionally, it collects venous blood from the digestive organs through the hepatic portal vein. This portal vein transports nutrient-rich blood from the gastrointestinal tract, allowing the liver to process nutrients and other substances absorbed after digestion. The liver efficiently filters and metabolizes these components before they enter systemic circulation.

Once the liver has performed its filtering role, venous blood exits through three main hepatic veins, which drain into the inferior vena cava. This well-organized vascular system ensures that the liver can perform its complex functions while maintaining appropriate blood flow. The liver's blood flow is auto-regulated through the action of vascular sphincters, which manage the volume of blood entering the liver via the hepatic artery. This auto-regulation is essential because it allows the liver to adapt to variations in blood flow including fluctuations via the hepatic portal vein while keeping the total hepatic blood flow consistent and stable. This allows for variations in flow via the hepatic portal vein and keeps total hepatic blood flow constant. Patients with history of abdominal injury or trauma to their liver need close monitoring of their vital signs to detect any changes indicative of internal haemorrhage as liver is highly vascular and any injury to the liver can cause profuse internal bleeding.

Among its many functions, the liver is responsible for the production of bile and the synthesis of bile salts, cholesterol, bilirubin, and glucuronic acid. Bile salts play an essential role in the emulsification and digestion of fats in the small intestine, making it possible for the body to absorb dietary lipids effectively. Cholesterol, while often demonized in popular health discussions, is also an essential component of bile and serves as a precursor for steroid hormone synthesis. Bilirubin, a by-product of the breakdown of haemoglobin from red blood cells, is conjugated in the liver to facilitate its excretion from the body. Glucuronic acid, produced in the liver, assists in detoxifying substances, including drugs and toxins, by making them more water-soluble for easier elimination via urine or bile.

In addition to bile production, the liver plays a significant role in vitamin D metabolism. This is accomplished through the hydroxylation of vitamin D to form 25-hydroxyvitamin D (25-(OH)D), an important biological marker that reflects vitamin D status in the body. This **hydroxylation** process occurs in two stages, with the liver carrying out the first critical conversion step, while the kidney performs the final activation of vitamin D, which is necessary for calcium and phosphate regulation in the body. Following digestion, all products of the digestive process enter the liver via the portal venous system. This unique system allows for nutrient-rich blood from the gastrointestinal tract to be channelled directly into the liver, where it can undergo further metabolic transformations before being released into the systemic circulation. This enables the liver to process and regulate the availability of nutrients, ensuring that the body has the required substrates for energy production and cellular function.

The gallbladder, although a small organ, has a significant role in the digestive process by storing and concentrating bile produced by the liver. When digested fats enter the small intestine, the gallbladder contracts in response to hormonal signals from the hormone *cholecystokinin* (CCK). This contraction expels bile into the cystic duct, which subsequently merges with the pancreatic duct before entering the duodenum at a location known as the **hepatopancreatic ampulla**. The flow of bile into the duodenum is tightly regulated by the **sphincter of Oddi**, which opens to allow bile to flow into the intestine when digestion is occurring and closes to prevent backflow during periods of non-digestion.

Furthermore, the liver functions as a vital storage organ for various nutrients, including carbohydrates, vitamins, and minerals such as iron. Carbohydrates are stored in the form of glycogen, which can be readily mobilized to maintain blood glucose levels when needed. The liver also stores vitamins A and D, which are essential for various physiological processes, including immune function and bone health. Iron, crucial for haemoglobin synthesis, is stored as ferritin and hemosiderin within the liver until it is required for the production of new red blood cells.

However, when the liver is unable to effectively regulate iron levels, it can lead to a condition known as **hemochromatosis**. This disorder arises either from an inability to control iron absorption from the intestine or from excessive iron intake; for instance, through repeated blood transfusions. Excess iron deposition can cause significant organ damage and complications, highlighting the liver's important role in iron metabolism. The liver's capacity to store excessive amounts of certain vitamins can also lead to conditions such as hepatomegaly, which refers to an enlargement of the liver. Hypervitaminosis A or D can result from the excessive intake of these fat-soluble vitamins, exacerbating liver size and potentially leading to further health complications.

Microscopically, the liver cells form *lobules* and the lateral borders of the liver cells form bile canaliculi which converge and eventually form the left and right main hepatic bile ducts. The gallbladder lies beneath the lower surface of the liver in the gallbladder fossa. The cystic duct connects the gallbladder to the common bile duct which then enters the duodenum at the **ampulla of Vater**, together with the pancreatic duct.

Learning Point
The primary metabolic functions conducted by hepatocytes are critical for the organism's well-being. These functions include:

- **Conversion of glucose to glycogen**: The liver plays a key role in glucose metabolism by converting excess glucose into glycogen, a process vital for regulating blood glucose levels and providing energy reserves.
- **Synthesis of a range of proteins**: The liver synthesizes essential proteins, such as albumin and clotting factors, which are critical for maintaining osmotic pressure and facilitating blood coagulation, respectively.
- **Degradation of proteins to amino acids**: The liver is involved in amino acid metabolism, where it breaks down proteins and facilitates the reuse of amino acids in various bodily functions.
- **Synthesis of urea from ammonia**: The liver detoxifies ammonia, a by-product of protein metabolism, converting it to urea, which is then excreted by the kidneys, thus helping to maintain nitrogen balance in the body.
- **Synthesis of cholesterol and bile acids**: The liver is responsible for synthesizing cholesterol and bile acids, which are crucial for fat digestion and absorption as well as serving as precursors for steroid hormone synthesis.

The pancreas is a vital organ located in the upper abdomen, nestled between the stomach and the small intestine. It has a unique anatomical structure consisting of three main parts: the head, body, and tail. The head of the pancreas is positioned within the C-shaped loop of the duodenum, which is the first part of the small intestine, while the tail extends towards the spleen. This strategic location allows the pancreas to effectively fulfil its roles in both digestion and metabolic regulation.

One of the distinguishing features of the pancreas is that it functions both as an *exocrine* and an *endocrine* gland. The exocrine component consists primarily of acinar cells that secrete digestive enzymes, which are critical for the breakdown of carbohydrates, proteins, and fats in food. These enzymes, including amylase, lipase, and proteases, are released into the duodenum to aid in digestion. Additionally, bicarbonate is secreted by the pancreas as part of its exocrine function. This bicarbonate plays a crucial role in neutralizing gastric acid, which enters the duodenum along with the chyme (partially digested food). By raising the pH of the chyme, bicarbonate creates an optimal environment for the activity of digestive enzymes, ensuring efficient nutrient breakdown and absorption. In addition to its exocrine functions, the pancreas also serves essential endocrine functions through clusters of cells known as ***the islets of Langerhans***. These clusters comprise various cell types responsible for the secretion of hormones that regulate blood glucose levels and overall metabolism.

The primary hormones produced by the pancreas include insulin, glucagon, somatostatin, and pancreatic polypeptide. Insulin is perhaps the most well-known hormone produced by the pancreas. It is secreted by ***beta cells*** in response to elevated blood glucose levels, such as after a meal. Insulin facilitates the uptake of glucose by cells throughout the body, particularly in muscle and adipose tissues. In addition to promoting glucose uptake, insulin also stimulates the conversion of excess glucose into glycogen (a storage form of glucose) in the liver, thereby lowering blood glucose levels.

Conversely, glucagon is secreted by alpha cells in the pancreas when blood glucose levels are low. Its primary function is to raise blood glucose levels by stimulating the liver to convert stored glycogen back into glucose and release it into the bloodstream. The interplay between insulin and glucagon is critical for maintaining glucose homeostasis, ensuring that the body has a consistent energy supply.

Somatostatin, produced by delta cells of the islets of Langerhans, serves a regulatory function by inhibiting the release of both insulin and glucagon. This hormone acts as a crucial check on the other hormones, helping to maintain overall balance within the endocrine system. Finally, pancreatic polypeptide, secreted by pancreatic polypeptide or PP cells, is believed to play a role in regulating pancreatic secretions and gastrointestinal motility, although its exact functions are still under investigation.

In contrast to the pancreas, the spleen is located in the upper far left quadrant of the abdomen and is notable for its distinct size and shape. Roughly four inches long and often described as fist-shaped and purple in colour, the spleen is primarily protected by the rib cage, making it difficult to palpate during a physical examination unless it is abnormally enlarged, a condition referred to as splenomegaly.

The spleen is an integral part of the lymphoid system and plays several important roles in the body. One of its primary functions is the regulation and destruction of red blood cells. The spleen helps filter and remove aged or damaged red blood cells from circulation, breaking them down and recycling components such as iron for use in new red blood cell production. This function is essential for maintaining the health of the circulatory system and ensuring an adequate supply of functioning red blood cells, which are vital for oxygen transport.

In addition to its role in red blood cell destruction, the spleen also plays a significant part in the immune response. It acts as a reservoir for lymphocytes, particularly B and T cells, which are crucial for the adaptive immune system. When pathogens invade the body, the spleen can mobilize these immune cells to help respond to infections and foreign particles. Moreover, the spleen filters the blood to remove debris and pathogens, further enhancing its role in protecting the body against infection.

6.2   Symptoms of Digestive Disorders

Dysphagia, the medical term for difficulty in swallowing, is a symptom that can indicate a variety of underlying health issues. Patients often express their experiences related to dysphagia in vague and imprecise terms, which can lead to confusion, particularly when distinguishing between similar symptoms related to the digestive tract, such as indigestion and heartburn. This ambiguity highlights the importance of thorough communication and careful history taking by healthcare providers when assessing patients with swallowing difficulties.

Swallowing is a complex physiological process that involves not only the mouth and throat but also the oesophagus. Disruptions in the various phases of swallowing can result from several factors, including neurological deficits, physical obstructions, tumours, structural damage, and congenital or developmental abnormalities. Understanding the aetiology of dysphagia is crucial for developing appropriate treatment plans and interventions.

Learning Point
Types of dysphagia and common causes

Dysphagia can be categorized into four primary types, each associated with different causes and implications:

- Oropharyngeal (oral) dysphagia
  This type of dysphagia occurs at the level of the mouth and throat. It can arise from mechanical issues or disorders affecting the muscles responsible for swallowing. Common causes include:
  - Bad Teeth: Dental problems can impede chewing and make it difficult to form a bolus of food that can be swallowed.

Jaw Problems: Issues such as temporomandibular joint (TMJ) disorders may hinder the ability to manipulate food effectively within the mouth.

- Oesophageal dysphagia
Oesophageal dysphagia refers to difficulties occurring in the oesophagus. It can be caused by structural or functional problems that obstruct the passage of food. Common causes include:
  - Gastroesophageal reflux disease (GERD): Chronic acid reflux can lead to inflammation of the oesophagus (esophagitis) and subsequent difficulty swallowing.
  - Esophagitis: This inflammation can stem from infections (like candidiasis), chemical irritants, or autoimmune conditions.
  - Achalasia: A condition in which the lower oesophageal sphincter fails to relax properly, leading to difficulty in food passage into the stomach. Tumours in the oesophagus: Benign or malignant growths can block the oesophageal lumen and contribute to swallowing difficulties.
- Complex neuromuscular disorders
Disorders affecting the central and peripheral nervous systems can significantly impact swallowing due to muscle control issues. Conditions include:
  - Dementia: Cognitive decline can affect the swallowing reflex and coordination, leading to difficulties.
  - Stroke: A stroke can affect the brain areas responsible for coordinating swallowing movements, resulting in dysphagia.
  - Brain tumour: Tumours can compress or invade structures involved in swallowing, impacting functionality. Myasthenia gravis: This autoimmune condition causes weakness in voluntary muscles, including those involved in swallowing.
- Functional dysphagia
This type of dysphagia does not have a specific structural or neurological cause but is often associated with psychological factors. Common causes include:
  - Anxiety: Psychological distress can manifest physically, leading to muscle tension and difficulty with swallowing. Stress attacks: High levels of stress can exacerbate symptoms of dysphagia, further complicating a patient's ability to eat and drink comfortably.

Learning Point
Important Questions to Ask During History Taking
When taking a medical history from a patient experiencing dysphagia, it is essential to ask targeted questions that can help narrow down potential causes and guide further evaluation and treatment. Here are some key questions to consider:

- **Where does food stick?**
  This question helps to determine the specific location of the difficulty. If a patient mentions feeling food stick in the throat, the problem may be oropharyngeal dysphagia. If the issue occurs lower in the chest, oesophageal dysphagia might be suspected.
- **Is the dysphagia intermittent or progressive?**
  Understanding the pattern of symptoms can provide insights into underlying conditions. Progressive dysphagia may suggest a more serious issue, such as a tumour, while intermittent symptoms might indicate less critical problems.
- **Has the symptom developed over weeks, months, or years?**
  The timeframe of symptom development can help differentiate between acute and chronic conditions, guiding possible diagnostic approaches. A sudden onset may suggest acute inflammation or neurological events, while longstanding issues might relate to chronic diseases.
- **Are both drink and food equally difficult to swallow?**
  Differentiating between the difficulties associated with solids and liquids can help pinpoint the cause. Difficulty swallowing liquids may suggest a more advanced issue, such as neuromuscular dysfunction.
- **Is there a history of reflex symptoms?**
  Inquiring about symptoms such as heartburn, regurgitation, or coughing during meals can provide clues about the involvement of the oesophagus and the possibility of gastroesophageal reflux disease (GERD).

Patients often describe symptoms related to the digestive tract in vague and imprecise terms, which can complicate diagnosis and treatment. For instance, there is a common confusion among patients regarding the meanings of indigestion and heartburn, two terms that are frequently used interchangeably but represent distinct experiences.

Heartburn is characterized by a burning sensation in the chest, resulting from the regurgitation of stomach acid into the oesophagus. This condition occurs when the lower oesophageal sphincter (LES), which normally functions as a barrier to prevent acidic contents from moving back up into the oesophagus, fails to maintain its proper function. A variety of factors can contribute to this loss of tone in the LES, leading to episodes of heartburn.

Common causes of heartburn include:

- Loss of tone in the lower oesophageal sphincter: Conditions such as pregnancy can lead to hormonal changes that relax the LES, making it more susceptible to allowing acid reflux. Similarly, excess weight and obesity can place additional pressure on the abdomen, contributing to a weakened sphincter and increasing the likelihood of acid regurgitation.

- Loss of the external sphincter-like mechanism of the diaphragm: A hiatal hernia occurs when part of the stomach protrudes through the diaphragm into the thoracic cavity, disrupting the normal functioning of the diaphragm's muscular mechanism. This can compromise the effectiveness of the LES, further facilitating the movement of acidic contents into the oesophagus.

As a result of these factors, individuals may experience heartburn in association with particular activities, such as lying down after eating, engaging in physical activity, or even consuming certain types of food and drink. Heartburn is not merely an uncomfortable symptom; frequent episodes can lead to complications such as esophagitis or Barrett's oesophagus, which increase the risk of oesophageal cancer.

Dyspepsia and Indigestion are terms that describe a collection of nonspecific gastrointestinal symptoms, and they encompass a wide range of subjective experiences. Many patients may use these terms to refer to sensations that include heartburn, epigastric pain (pain in the upper abdomen), a feeling of fullness after meals, belching, and nausea. Unlike heartburn, which is more precisely defined, dyspepsia is a broader term that reflects various potential disorders affecting the gastrointestinal tract.

Dyspepsia typically indicates disorders affecting the lower oesophagus, stomach, duodenum, pancreas, and gallbladder all of which may contribute to gastrointestinal discomfort. Common causes of dyspepsia include:

- Gastritis: Inflammation of the stomach lining can lead to abdominal pain, nausea, and changes in appetite.
- Peptic ulcer disease: Ulcers in the stomach or duodenum can result in dyspeptic symptoms, including burning pain and discomfort, especially after eating.
- Gastroesophageal reflux disease (GERD): While heartburn can be a symptom, GERD encompasses a range of symptoms related to acid reflux, including dyspepsia.
- Functional dyspepsia: This is characterized by chronic dyspeptic symptoms without an identifiable organic cause. It may be related to motility disorders or heightened sensitivity to gastric distention.
- Cholecystitis: Inflammation of the gallbladder can also contribute to upper abdominal pain and dyspeptic symptoms, especially after eating fatty foods.

Ultimately, distinguishing between heartburn, dyspepsia, and other gastrointestinal symptoms requires careful assessment and evaluation by healthcare professionals. Questions about the patient's history, symptom patterns, and potential triggers can guide diagnostics and inform management strategies. Proper understanding of these terms and their associated symptoms can aid healthcare providers in developing clearer communication with patients regarding their gastrointestinal concerns.

Weight loss is a significant symptom observed in numerous digestive tract diseases as well as a variety of other health conditions. It serves as an important clinical indicator, signalling potential pathophysiological issues that require further investigation. Common causes of unintended weight loss include malignancies, chronic infections, and organ failures, among others. These conditions can lead to metabolic changes that result in the body utilizing more energy than it consumes, ultimately leading to a reduction in body weight.

Learning Point

Important Questions to Ask During History Taking

When evaluating a patient presenting with weight loss, a comprehensive history taking is vital to understanding the underlying causes. The following questions may be particularly relevant:

- **Is your appetite increased, decreased, or normal?**
  - Changes in appetite can provide essential clues. Increased appetite with weight loss might suggest malabsorption or hypermetabolic states, while decreased appetite often points to psychological issues or organ dysfunction.
- **Do you enjoy your food?**
  - A loss of interest in food can indicate underlying psychological conditions such as depression or anxiety, or it may signal gastrointestinal diseases that make eating uncomfortable.
- **How long has the weight been lost?**
  - The duration of weight loss is critical for assessing the significance of the symptom. A gradual loss over several months may indicate chronic illness, whereas a rapid loss over a few weeks can be alarming and suggests acute pathology.
- **Meal description: usual breakfast, lunch, and dinner.**
  - Understanding the typical dietary intake can help identify deviations from normal eating habits and pinpoint specific dietary issues or preferences.
- **Associated symptoms such as nausea, vomiting, or abdominal pain?**
  - Coexisting symptoms can provide valuable diagnostic clues. For instance, concurrent nausea and abdominal pain may suggest gastrointestinal obstruction, inflammation, or infections.
- **Changes in bowel habits and appearance of stool?**
  - Changes in bowel habits, such as diarrhoea or constipation, as well as stool characteristics, can indicate digestive malabsorption syndromes or infections.
- **Has there been a fever?**
  The presence of fever can indicate underlying infections or inflammatory processes, further informing the diagnostic pathway.
- **Do you pass excessive volumes of urine?**
  Increased urination may point to conditions such as diabetes mellitus or renal dysfunction, which can also contribute to weight loss through fluid loss and metabolic disturbances.

Nausea and **vomiting** are common symptoms that can signal various issues within the digestive system as well as systemic and metabolic disorders. Nausea, in particular, often serves as a precursor to vomiting but can also occur alone, indicating different underlying conditions.

Nausea is typically described as a feeling of unease or discomfort in the stomach that often comes in waves. Interestingly, nausea without vomiting may point to psychological disorders such as anorexia nervosa, bulimia, or even conditions like depression and anxiety. While nausea itself can be distressing, individuals may find some relief through vomiting, which can clear irritants from the stomach or alleviate pressure.

The aetiology of nausea and vomiting is varied, encompassing a range of triggers, including:

- Unpleasant sights, smells, and tastes: Sensory stimuli can trigger the vomiting reflex in susceptible individuals, particularly in cases of early pregnancy or motion sickness.
- Abnormal stimulation of the inner ear labyrinth: Issues stemming from vestibular dysfunction can lead to motion sickness, vertigo, and the associated feelings of nausea.
- Viral hepatitis and biliary diseases: Inflammation of the liver or issues with bile flow can induce nausea due to the digestive system's response to compromised liver function.
- Medications that stimulate the vomiting centre: Drugs like digoxin, morphine, and certain chemotherapeutic agents can provoke nausea and vomiting as side effects.
- Psychological disorders: As mentioned, conditions such as anorexia and bulimia are associated with significant nausea, often related to distorted body image and food intake.
- Gastrointestinal diseases: Conditions such as gastroenteritis, peptic ulcers, and obstruction can lead to both nausea and vomiting due to underlying inflammation or blockage of the digestive tract.

To better understand nausea and vomiting, particularly in the context of digestive disorders, clinicians should consider asking the following questions:

- **When is the vomiting worse, such as in the morning?**
  - Timing can provide insights into the triggers; for example, morning vomiting may suggest pregnancy or metabolic disorders.
- **Is there associated abdominal pain?**
  - Understanding whether vomiting occurs alongside pain can help identify acute or chronic GI conditions that may require urgent attention.
- **Does the vomiting relate to meals?**
  - Timing of vomiting in relation to food intake may indicate whether it is triggered by particular foods or more systemic issues.

- **Appearance of vomit (e.g. blood, bile stained)?**
  - The presence of blood or bile can suggest serious underlying conditions, such as bleeding ulcers or obstructions requiring immediate medical attention.
- **Any recognizable food or coffee grounds in the vomit?**
  - Coffee ground-like material may indicate the presence of old blood, while recognizable food could suggest delayed gastric emptying or obstruction.
- **Do you take any medications?**
  - Knowing the patient's medication history can help identify potential drug side effects or interactions contributing to symptoms.

Gastrointestinal (GI) bleeding is a critical clinical condition that requires immediate assessment and intervention. Blood can be manifested in different ways, primarily through vomiting or rectal passage. When blood is expelled from the mouth, this phenomenon is referred to as **haematemesis**. Conversely, when blood is passed per rectum, it may present in various forms, depending on its origin, including bright red blood or altered stools.

Altered blood that appears black in colour and has a tar-like consistency is termed **melena**. This condition indicates that the blood has undergone digestion and has been in the digestive tract for some time, typically resulting from bleeding in the upper gastrointestinal tract, including the oesophagus, stomach, and duodenum.

The upper GI tract including the oesophagus, stomach, and duodenum, commonly associates with haematemesis. Several conditions can lead to this serious symptom:

- **Oesophageal varices**: These are enlarged veins in the oesophagus that can rupture due to increased pressure, often associated with liver cirrhosis. This condition frequently results in significant bleeding.
- **Gastric cancer**: Tumours in the stomach can invade blood vessels, leading to bleeding, which manifests as vomited blood.
- **Duodenal ulcer**: Ulcers located in the duodenum can erode blood vessels and cause substantial bleeding. Often, patients may notice blood in vomit as a result.
- **Ulcerated oesophagus**: Conditions causing ulceration in the oesophageal lining can lead to bleeding, resulting in haematemesis.

Rectal bleeding can manifest in various forms, depending on the location of the bleed within the gastrointestinal tract.

- **Bright red blood**: The presence of bright red blood when passing stools typically indicates a source in the lower GI tract. Common causes include:
  - **Inflammatory Bowel Disease (IBD)**: Conditions such as ulcerative colitis and Crohn's disease can cause localized inflammation and bleeding in the rectum.
  - **Haemorrhoids**: Swollen blood vessels in the rectal area can rupture, leading to painless bright red blood during bowel movements.

- **Darker red or maroon blood**: Blood that appears darker red or maroon may originate from the ascending colon, transverse colon, or descending colon. Associated conditions include:
  - **Ischaemic colitis**: This condition arises from reduced blood flow to the colon, leading to an insufficient blood supply and resultant bleeding.
  - **Polyps**: Benign growths in the colon can cause intermittent bleeding, which may present as darker red blood.
  - **Diverticular disease**: This describes small mucosal herniations through the bowel wall which can cause localized bleeding without prior symptoms.
- **Melena**: As mentioned, this is indicative of upper GI bleeding but can also be associated with colonic sources like colon cancer and large bowel polyps, leading to intermittent rectal bleeding.

In terms of inflammatory bowel disease, ulcerative colitis leads to distinctive clinical presentations. This condition is characterized by the passage of blood mixed with mucus upon rectal bleeding. In severe cases of ischaemic colitis and diverticular disease, heavy rectal bleeding can occur. Chronic blood loss from the gastrointestinal tract, whether from haematemesis or rectal bleeding can lead to a condition known as **anaemia**. This can often be occult, meaning the blood loss may not be visible to the naked eye, but can still be detected through stool tests. Chronic anaemia may present its own set of symptoms, including fatigue, weakness, and pallor, further complicating the clinical picture.

Diagnosing the source of gastrointestinal bleeding generally involves a careful and thorough history-taking, as well as a physical examination. Healthcare professionals will often inquire about the characteristics of the blood (e.g. colour, consistency), the frequency of the episodes, associated symptoms such as pain, weight loss, or changes in bowel habits, and medical history, including previous gastrointestinal disease or surgeries.

Diagnostic tests may include:

- **Endoscopy**: An upper endoscopy can identify sources of haematemesis, while a colonoscopy can assess lower GI causes of bleeding.
- **Imaging Studies**: CT scans and abdominal X-rays can help visualize structures within the abdomen and locate bleeding.
- **Laboratory Tests**: Complete blood counts (CBC) and stool tests can assess for anaemia and occult blood.

Constipation is a prevalent gastrointestinal issue that affects individuals of all ages. The diagnosis of constipation is largely dependent on the normal bowel habits of the individual, as what constitutes "normal" can vary significantly from person to person. For instance, individuals following high-fibre diets may find that they require three bowel evacuations per day to feel comfortable and symptom-free. In contrast, those adhering to a typical Western diet may experience satisfactory gut health with just one bowel movement per day, or even less frequently.

When evaluating constipation, it is essential to consider its duration and characteristics. Chronic constipation that has persisted for many years is often classified as "functional." This means that it is typically related to lifestyle factors, including diet and physical activity, rather than an underlying structural disease. On the other hand, constipation that has a recent onset, especially if it represents a change from a previously regular pattern may raise concerns about potential underlying medical conditions. This acute form of constipation may be associated with various diseases and requires further inquiry and evaluation.

Particular attention should be paid when constipation is accompanied by additional symptoms such as colicky abdominal pain and rectal bleeding. These symptoms can indicate more serious underlying issues, including colon cancer or diverticular disease; both of these conditions may present with constipation and are associated with rectal bleeding and abdominal discomfort.

Numerous factors can contribute to constipation, ranging from dietary influences to non-gastrointestinal disorders. Some of the common causes include:

- **Dietary factors**: Inadequate fibre intake is one of the leading contributors to constipation. A diet low in fruits, vegetables, and whole grains, which are high in dietary fibre, can lead to infrequent and difficult bowel movements.
- **Insufficient fluid intake**: Dehydration or insufficient fluid consumption can also lead to hardened stools, making them more difficult to pass.
- **Physical inactivity**: Sedentary lifestyles contribute to slower bowel contractions, leading to constipation.
- **Medications**: Certain medications can have side effects that contribute to constipation. Common culprits include antidepressants, opioids, and iron supplements.
- **Metabolic disorders**: Conditions such as hypothyroidism, hypercalcemia (elevated calcium levels), and hypokalaemia (low potassium levels) can also affect bowel function and lead to constipation.

Learning Point
Important Questions to Ask During History Taking

To assess constipation effectively, healthcare providers often ask patients a series of targeted questions that can shed light on their condition:

- **What is the normal stool frequency?**
  Knowing the usual pattern allows the provider to assess deviations from what the patient considers to be normal.
- **How long have you been constipated?**
  Understanding the duration helps differentiate between functional and organic causes, as well as assess the urgency of intervention.

- **Are the stools large or small and pellet-shaped?**
  The size and shape of the stool can indicate the level of dehydration and the effectiveness of bowel function.
- **Do you strain at stool?**
  Straining to pass bowel movements often signifies obstructed or delayed passage of stools, indicating a higher degree of constipation.
- **Is there associated abdominal pain, distention, nausea, or vomiting?**
  These accompanying symptoms can suggest more serious underlying conditions, warranting further investigation.
- **Do you take any drugs?**
  A review of the patient's medication can reveal potential drug-induced causes of constipation.

The management of constipation often begins with dietary and lifestyle modifications. Increasing fibre intake through fruits, vegetables, and whole grains, along with ensuring adequate hydration, can significantly enhance bowel regularity. Encouraging physical activity is also important, as regular exercise stimulates bowel function.

Diarrhoea is defined by an increase in stool volume and a significant change in stool consistency, typically resulting in loose or watery stools. While it is often viewed as a common ailment, diarrhoea can indicate an underlying health issue that may require medical attention. Understanding the various causes and nuances of diarrhoea is crucial for effective diagnosis and treatment. Diarrhoea can stem from a variety of gastrointestinal and non-gastrointestinal sources, and it can manifest in different patterns based on the underlying cause. One of the lesser-known types is functional diarrhoea, which is often associated with psychological factors such as anxiety or stress. Individuals with conditions like irritable bowel syndrome (IBS) may experience alternating episodes of constipation and diarrhoea, often triggered by stress or dietary factors.

Common causes of diarrhoea can be classified into two main categories: gastrointestinal causes and non-gastrointestinal causes.

Learning Point
Gastrointestinal Causes

- **Infections**: Bacterial and viral infections are among the most frequent causes of diarrhoea. Pathogens such as *Salmonella*, *Escherichia coli* (*E. coli*), and viruses like Norovirus can lead to acute diarrhoea and are often associated with foodborne illnesses or contamination.

- **Inflammatory bowel disease**: Conditions such as **ulcerative colitis** and **Crohn's disease** are characterized by chronic inflammation of the gastrointestinal tract. Patients often experience persistent diarrhoea, abdominal pain, and other systemic symptoms.
- **Malabsorption conditions**: Disorders like **Celiac disease** can result in inadequate absorption of nutrients, leading to significant stool volume and changes in consistency. Patients with celiac disease may experience diarrhoea after consuming gluten-containing foods.
- **Antibiotic use**: The use of broad-spectrum antibiotics can disrupt the normal flora of the intestine, leading to antibiotic-associated diarrhoea. The balance of beneficial bacteria is disturbed, which can result in increased stool output and changes in consistency.
- **Laxative abuse**: Overuse of laxatives can lead to dependency and ultimately disrupt normal bowel function, resulting in diarrhoea.

Learning Point

Non-Gastrointestinal Causes

- *Hyperthyroidism*: An overactive thyroid gland can increase metabolism and lead to frequent bowel movements, often presenting as diarrhoea

Learning Point

Important Questions to Ask During History Taking

When evaluating a patient with diarrhoea, careful assessment through a series of targeted questions can help uncover the underlying cause and guide treatment. Some essential questions include:

- **How long have you had diarrhoea?**
  Understanding the duration is crucial. Acute diarrhoea lasts less than 2 weeks, while chronic diarrhoea persists for 4 weeks or longer.
- **What is the stool frequency?**
  Knowing how many times a day the patient has had bowel movements can help assess the severity and indicate specific underlying causes.
- **What is the consistency of stools?**
  If the stools are watery or loose, this information can help differentiate between various types of diarrhoea.

- **What is the colour of the stools?**
  The presence of specific colours can provide valuable diagnostic clues. For example, yellow or green stools might suggest an infection, while blood-stained stools may indicate more severe underlying issues.
- **Is there blood or mucus present?**
  The identification of blood or mucus in the stool can point towards inflammatory bowel diseases or infections and may require immediate medical intervention.
- **Is there associated pain, nausea, vomiting, or weight loss?**
  Coexisting symptoms can help in diagnosis and management. For instance, significant weight loss and abdominal pain may indicate a more severe underlying condition.
- **Do you take any antibiotics?**
  Inquiring about antibiotic use can highlight the potential for antibiotic-associated diarrhoea, which may necessitate a different treatment approach.

Jaundice is a clinical sign indicative of a dysfunction in bile production, transportation, or excretion. It is characterized by a yellowish discoloration of the skin, sclera (the whites of the eyes), and mucous membranes, resulting from elevated levels of bilirubin in the bloodstream. There exist three primary types of jaundice, each of which points to different underlying mechanisms and potential pathologies.

Types of Jaundice

Learning Point

Prehepatic (haemolytic) jaundice also known as haemolytic jaundice, arises primarily from the excessive breakdown of erythrocytes (red blood cells). This excessive haemolysis leads to increased levels of unconjugated bilirubin that the liver becomes overwhelmed in processing.

Common causes of prehepatic jaundice include:

- **Spleen infections**: Infections can lead to splenic enlargement and increased haemolysis.
- **Drugs**: Certain medications can induce haemolysis, leading to a higher turnover of red blood cells.
- **Incompatible blood transfusions**: Transfusion reactions can cause rapid destruction of transfused red blood cells.
- **Genetic conditions**: Conditions such as thalassemia or sickle cell disease result in increased haemolysis due to defects in erythrocyte structure.

Patients with prehepatic jaundice may experience mild symptoms along with some degree of anaemia. Notably, their urine and faeces may appear very dark and urine will be dark due to increased urobilinogen excretion, while faeces may be dark due to elevated stercobilin levels.

Hepatocellular jaundice occurs due to defects in the liver's ability to transport and conjugate bilirubin. This can occur when liver cells are damaged or inflamed. Common causes include:

- **Hepatitis**: Viral infections, such as hepatitis A, B, and C, can cause significant liver inflammation and disrupt normal bilirubin processing.
- **Alcohol consumption**: Chronic exposure to alcohol can lead to alcoholic liver disease, which damages liver cells.
- **Drug-induced liver injury**: Several medications can lead to hepatotoxicity, resulting in hepatocellular damage and jaundice.

In hepatocellular jaundice, bilirubin levels rise due to an inability of liver cells to properly process bilirubin, leading to elevated bilirubin in the blood, resulting in jaundice. The urine may appear dark, and stools can be normal or pale, depending on the extent of liver dysfunction.

Obstructive (Cholestatic) jaundice also referred to as cholestatic jaundice, arises when there is an obstruction to bile flow. This obstruction can be intrahepatic, such as in cirrhosis, hepatitis, or due to the effects of certain medications. Alternatively, it may be extrahepatic, resulting from blockages in the major bile ducts due to conditions such as:

- **Gallstones**: These can lodge in the common bile duct, obstructing bile flow.
- **Carcinoma of the head of the pancreas**: Tumours in this region can compress bile ducts and impede bile drainage.
- **Bile duct strictures and parasitic infections**: Narrowing or obstruction of the bile ducts can also lead to cholestasis.

With obstructive jaundice, bile flow to the duodenum is obstructed, resulting in *dark urine* due to elevated conjugated bilirubin and *pale stools* due to a lack of stercobilin. Patients often present with skin that has a *greenish tinge* and may report a *metallic taste in their mouth* because of the excess bilirubin.

The initial symptoms of jaundice can be vague and non-specific, often causing patients to present with generalized malaise, fatigue, anorexia, and nausea. Given the potential seriousness of jaundice, it is essential to undertake a thorough history to identify potential causes and associated conditions.

Learning Point
Key questions to ask include:

Any history of alcohol abuse or intravenous drug use?
Identifying substance use can help elucidate potential liver damage or hae-molytic concerns.
Any contact with jaundiced patients?
Contact may raise suspicion of contagious hepatitis viruses.
Any travelling history?
Travel history may suggest exposure to infectious agents that can cause hepatitis.
Any blood transfusions?
Recent blood transfusions may contribute to haemolytic jaundice if incom-patible blood types are involved.
Any prescription or non-prescription drugs used?
Medication histories are critical for identifying drug-induced liver reactions.
Any associated pain or weight loss?
Accompanying symptoms can indicate the severity and nature of liver dis-ease, helping guide conditions requiring urgent intervention.
Any family history of liver disease?
Genetic predisposition plays a significant role in conditions that may cause jaundice.

Abdominal pain is a common and complex symptom that can arise from various sources within the abdominal cavity. It can result from visceral organs, such as the intestines, gallbladder, ureters, and uterus, or can be attributed to irritation of the parietal peritoneum, the tissue lining the abdominal wall. Understanding the charac-teristics of abdominal pain, including its location, nature, and associated symptoms, is crucial for reaching an accurate diagnosis and determining appropriate manage-ment strategies.

Learning Point
Types of Abdominal Pain
Visceral pain originates from internal organs and is typically caused by conditions that involve stretching, distension, or inflammation of these organs. This type of pain is often:

- **Aching or cramp-like**: Patients may describe visceral pain as dull or cramp-like, and it can fluctuate in intensity.

- **Poorly localized**: Visceral pain is generally not well localized, making it difficult for patients to pinpoint the exact source. It is often felt in the midline of the abdomen, irrespective of the organ involved.

Parietal Pain affecting the parietal peritoneum, known as parietal pain, is well localized and typically arises from inflammation or irritation of the peritoneum. This type of pain is characterized by:

- **Localized pain**: The pain is usually specific to the area of inflammation, such as the right lower quadrant in cases of appendicitis.
- **Worsening with movement**: Parietal pain often intensifies with movements like coughing, sneezing, or changing positions, leading to a protective response in the patient.
- **Tenderness and rebound tenderness**: Examination may reveal marked tenderness over the affected area and rebound tenderness, indicating irritation of the peritoneum.

A classic example of the transition from visceral to parietal pain is seen in acute appendicitis. Initially, patients experience visceral pain that is referred to the midline of the abdomen, typically around the umbilical region.

As the condition progresses, the inflammatory process involves the parietal peritoneum that overlays the inflamed appendix, resulting in sharper and more localized pain in the right iliac fossa. Understanding this progression is important for timely diagnosis and intervention.

Learning Point
Important questions to ask during History Taking
When evaluating a patient presenting with abdominal pain, a thorough history and physical examination are essential for determining the underlying cause. Key questions to consider in the assessment include:

- **Site—Where is the location of the abdominal pain?**
  Establishing the precise location helps to narrow down potential causes, as different organs are associated with pain in specific areas of the abdomen.
- **Onset—How long has the pain been present?**
  Understanding when the pain began can provide insights into its aetiology; acute pain may indicate acute illness, while chronic pain may suggest more complex underlying conditions.

- **Character—Can you describe the pain?**
  Patients' descriptions of their pain—such as sharp, dull, cramping, or aching—can offer valuable clues about the underlying cause.
- **Relieved by—Have you noticed any relieving factors?**
  Determining whether certain activities, medications, or positions alleviate the pain can help identify specific conditions. For example, pain relieved by food may suggest a peptic ulcer, while pain alleviated by bowel movements may indicate an intestinal obstruction.
- **Associated features/symptoms—Have you experienced weight loss, nausea, or vomiting?**
  The presence of accompanying symptoms provides critical contextual information. For instance, weight loss might raise suspicion for malignancy, while fever may indicate infection.
- **Timing—Is the pain constant or intermittent?**
  Understanding the timing of the pain can assist in diagnosis. Intermittent pain may suggest conditions like colicky pain in intestinal obstruction, while constant pain may be associated with inflammatory processes.
- **Exacerbated by—Have you noticed any specific aggravating factors?**
  Inquiring about activities or foods that trigger or worsen the pain can further narrow the differential diagnosis by linking symptoms to specific conditions.
- **Severity—Is the pain affected by eating or defecation?**
  The relationship between pain and these activities can provide clues to specific gastrointestinal disorders, such as pancreatitis or gallbladder pathology.

6.3   General Signs of Digestive Tract Diseases

Jaundice

Jaundice is one of the most recognizable signs of liver failure and occurs due to an abnormal accumulation of bilirubin in the bloodstream. In cases of hepatocellular failure, the liver's ability to metabolize and conjugate bilirubin is significantly impaired, leading to elevated levels of unconjugated bilirubin. Additionally, intrahepatic obstruction caused by conditions such as cirrhosis or malignancy can impede the normal flow of bile, contributing to increased bilirubin levels. Clinically, jaundice manifests as yellowing of the skin and sclera (the whites of the eyes) and may be accompanied by darker urine and pale stools.

Ascites

Ascites is the pathological accumulation of fluid in the abdominal cavity and is typically a result of portal hypertension. This condition occurs when increased pressure in the portal venous system leads to fluid extravasation into the peritoneal cavity.

Furthermore, liver failure results in inadequate production of albumin, a key protein responsible for maintaining oncotic pressure. The combination of portal hypertension and decreased oncotic pressure due to low albumin levels leads to water and sodium retention, exacerbating the development of ascites. Patients may present with abdominal distension and discomfort duc to the increased pressure in the abdominal cavity.

Oedema and Coagulation Problems

Oedema, or swelling caused by fluid accumulation in tissues, can also occur as a consequence of liver failure. This condition is primarily attributed to ***hypalbuminaemia,*** or low levels of albumin in the blood, which diminishes the oncotic pressure required to retain fluid within the vascular system. Additionally, liver failure affects the synthesis of various clotting factors, including ***prothrombin***, leading to coagulation problems. As a result, patients may experience increased susceptibility to bleeding, hematemesis (vomiting of blood), and easy bruising. The inability to clot properly can lead to serious complications, particularly gastrointestinal bleeding, which necessitates careful medical management.

Purpura and Clotting Problems

Purpura, characterized by the presence of purple or red spots on the skin resulting from bleeding underneath, is another manifestation related to clotting abnormalities in liver failure. The failure of the liver to produce adequate clotting factors leads to increased bleeding tendencies and is a vital consideration in managing patients with liver disease. In patients with liver failure, the accumulation of toxins in the body often results in abnormal drug reactions, heightening the risk of adverse effects. This issue is particularly serious for elderly patients, who may have decreased liver function and altered drug metabolism.

Gynaecomastia

In liver failure, hormonal imbalances can occur due to the liver's dysfunction in metabolizing endogenous hormones. Accumulation of oestrogen and other hormones can lead to gynaecomastia, the development of breast tissue in males. This condition is often accompanied by other symptoms, such as amenorrhea in women, testicular atrophy, and loss of libido.

Hypoglycaemia or low blood sugar levels can also be observed in patients with liver failure. The liver plays a critical role in glucose metabolism and storage. In liver failure, ***glycogen*** storage may be impaired, leading to inadequate glucose release in response to fasting conditions. The result may be hypoglycaemic episodes that manifest with symptoms such as weakness, confusion, and even loss of consciousness.

Hepatic encephalopathy and coma is a severe complication of liver failure characterized by neurological disturbances due to the accumulation of ammonia and other neurotoxins in the bloodstream. The liver's inability to detoxify these substances leads to cognitive dysfunction, ranging from mild confusion to severe alterations in consciousness and coma. This condition underscores the importance of monitoring and managing metabolic derangements in patients with advanced liver disease.

Hematemesis (vomiting blood) can occur as a result of portal hypertension and *variceal bleeding*. Portal hypertension causes increased pressure in the venous system, leading to the development of *varices* (dilated veins) that can rupture, causing significant blood loss. Hypovolaemia, or reduced blood volume, may result from this bleeding, leading to further complications, including shock.

Hepatomegaly, or liver enlargement, is frequently observed in liver failure and can occur due to inflammation, fatty infiltration, or congestion. Patients may report a sensation of fullness or discomfort in the upper abdomen associated with hepatomegaly.

Asterixis, often referred to as "flapping tremor," is a neurological sign that can be observed in hepatic encephalopathy. It typically occurs when the patient's arms are outstretched and wrists are flexed, leading to involuntary jerking movements of the hands. It serves as an indicator of metabolic disturbances associated with liver dysfunction.

Spider naevi and palmar erythema
Skin manifestations such as spider naevi and palmar erythema are also associated with liver failure. Spider naevi present as red, central lesions with radiating blood vessels and are commonly linked to hormonal changes, particularly elevated oestrogen levels due to impaired metabolism. Palmar erythema, characterized by reddening of the palms, is another cutaneous sign observed in liver disease.

Abdominal Pain is a common complaint in patients with liver failure and may arise from various factors such as distension, inflammation, or associated conditions like cholecystitis or pancreatitis. Assessing the character, location, and severity of abdominal pain helps clinicians determine its aetiology and guide further management.

6.3.1   Part 2: Case Study 1

A 50-year-old teacher complained of a 5-month history of left-sided abdominal pain, colicky in nature and relieved by defecation. During this period, she had experienced episodes of constipation and had occasionally noted streaks of blood in her stool when she had been able to defecate. She had recently seen her doctor who had referred her to the local hospital for further investigations. She had now come to you because of sacral pain. On examination, she was thin, ill-looking, and showed clinical evidence of anaemia. Her blood pressure was 130/90 mmHg, the pulse was 109/min, regular, the respiratory rate was 22 per minute and the temperature was 38.2 °C. There was an ill-defined, tender swelling in the left iliac fossa which appeared to be related to the sigmoid colon.

(a) **What other relevant information would you want to obtain from the history and physical examination to help you in the differential diagnosis?**
(b) **Discuss the possible causes and mechanisms for the constipation and colicky pain in this patient.**
(c) **Discuss the likely causes and differential diagnosis of the rectal bleeding in this patient.**
(d) **Briefly comment on the significance of the sacral pain in this patient.**
(e) **Briefly discuss the significance of the vital signs and the mass in the left iliac fossa.**

6.3.2   Case Study 2

A 65-year-old man complains of trouble with his bowels. For the last 6 weeks, he has been suffering from diarrhoea, which sometimes alternates with constipation. He also complains of intermittent lower abdominal pain, but no weight loss and he has also noted some blood in the faeces. Examination reveals clinical evidence of anaemia, tenderness in the lower abdomen and the suggestion of a possible mass in the left iliac fossa. Anorectal examination (using a proctoscope) shows haemorrhoids but nothing else of note.

(a) **Name the most important disorder presenting with altered bowel habit and left iliac fossa mass that must be considered in a patient of this age.**
(b) **What are the possible causes of the anaemia and what would the red cells look like on microscopic examination of the blood?**
(c) **What further relevant information would you want to obtain from the history and physical examination?**
(d) **Discuss the possible causes and mechanisms of alternating constipation and diarrhoea in this patient.**
(e) **Discuss the likely causes and differential diagnosis of the rectal bleeding.**

6.3.3   Case Study 3

A 75-year-old man with a 40-year history of heavy alcohol consumption presents with jaundice, malaise, and fever. Over the past few weeks, his family has noticed progressive confusion, personality changes, and a marked decline in mobility. He also complains of abdominal swelling, recurrent nosebleeds, and black tarry stools. His liver function tests (carried out on serum) and urinalysis confirm chronic hepatitis with intrahepatic obstruction.

(a) **Outline the main signs and symptoms you would expect to be present when clinically examining this patient.**
(b) **Outline the main urine and stool findings that you would expect to be present, giving briefly the mechanism for these abnormalities.**

(c) **Briefly outline the mechanisms for the development of ascites in cirrhosis of the liver.**
(d) **Discuss the likely causes and differential diagnosis of chronic hepatitis.**

6.3.4   Case Study 4

Mr. William, a 77-year-old pensioner, presented with a 5-month history of progressive difficulty in swallowing. This was associated with some discomfort after meals and occasional regurgitation of food. He denied significant unintentional weight loss but reported persistent heartburn, intermittent hoarseness of voice, and a chronic cough. More recently, he had noticed occasional streaks of blood in his vomit. He now presented to you because of a persistent, unresolved "cold" and cough that had not improved since his last visit to the GP.

On examination, he appeared ill-looking, he was off colour and his blood pressure was 130/90 mmHg, pulse rate 90/min regular, respiratory rate 22/min. There was mild tenderness on deep palpation of the epigastrium, but no palpable abdominal mass was detected.

(a) **What other relevant information would you want to obtain from the history and physical examination to help you in the differential diagnosis?**
(b) **Discuss the possible causes and mechanisms for dysphagia and retrosternal discomfort in this patient.**
(c) **Discuss the likely causes and differential diagnosis of the hematemesis (blood in vomitus) in this particular patient.**
(d) **What investigations would you request to confirm the diagnosis and assess disease extent?**
(e) **Discuss the likely causes of his chronic cough and hoarseness of voice in the context of oesophageal pathology.**

6.4   Part 3: Abdominal Examination

Healthcare professionals rely heavily on a combination of palpation and percussion of the abdomen when diagnosing for abdominal disease. These techniques provide critical insights into the condition of the internal organs. It is important to keep in mind that there is significant variability in the shapes and sizes of patients' abdomens, which may impact the examination findings. To facilitate the assessment, the abdomen can be *systematically segmented into specific areas*, enabling the detection of abnormalities associated with major intra-abdominal organs.

Quadrants and Regions
In clinical practice, professionals commonly divide the abdomen into four quadrants for assessment: the right upper quadrant (RUQ), left upper quadrant (LUQ), right lower quadrant (RLQ), and left lower quadrant (LLQ). This quadrant-based

approach allows us to locate and report symptoms and signs, respectively. Additionally, practitioners may refer to specific areas such as the epigastric region, suprapubic region, left iliac fossa, or right iliac fossa when describing pain or mass locations.

The abdomen is divided into four quadrants if we can imagine we draw a vertical line (midline) through the navel (umbilicus) and a horizontal line (transumbilical line) through the same point.
Each quadrant contains specific organs:

- Right Upper Quadrant (RUQ): This quadrant houses key structures, including the liver, gallbladder, right kidney, parts of the stomach, pancreas, and portions of the intestines.
- Left Upper Quadrant (LUQ): The LUQ includes the stomach, spleen, pancreas, left kidney, and parts of the liver and intestines.
- Right Lower Quadrant (RLQ): The RLQ contains the appendix, cecum, right ovary (in females), right ureter, and sections of the intestines.
- Left Lower Quadrant (LLQ): This quadrant comprises the sigmoid colon, left ovary (in females), left ureter, and portions of the intestines.

For a more comprehensive evaluation, the abdomen can also be divided into nine distinct regions using two vertical lines (mid-clavicular lines) and two horizontal lines (subcostal and transtubercular lines). This more granular approach allows clinicians to pinpoint issues with greater precision and detail:

- Right Hypochondriac Region: Contains the liver, gallbladder, and right kidney.
- Epigastric Region: Houses the stomach, part of the liver, pancreas, duodenum, and adrenal glands.
- Left Hypochondriac Region: Comprises the spleen, stomach, and left kidney.
- Right Lumbar Region: Contains the ascending colon and right kidney.
- Umbilical Region: Encompasses the small intestine and transverse colon.
- Left Lumbar Region: Contains the descending colon and left kidney.
- Right Iliac (Inguinal) Region: Houses the appendix and cecum.
- Hypogastric (Pubic) Region: Contains the bladder, reproductive organs, and sigmoid colon.
- Left Iliac (Inguinal) Region: Comprises the sigmoid colon and part of the descending colon.

This regional classification is particularly beneficial in diagnosing specific conditions. For example, pain associated with appendicitis often originates in the right iliac region, while liver and gallbladder disorders are typically located in the RUQ, and issues related to the stomach and spleen may arise from the LUQ. Recognizing the distinct localizations can simplify the diagnostic process and enhance patient care.

The Examination Process

The examination of the abdomen should follow *a systematic approach* that encompasses four key techniques: inspection, auscultation, palpation, and percussion. Each step provides essential information that collectively leads to a thorough understanding of the patient's condition.

Inspection: This initial step involves visually assessing the abdomen for any abnormalities, such as distension, deformities, or visible pulsations. Observing the abdominal contour, colour, and any scars or lesions gives valuable insight into possible underlying conditions.

Auscultation: After inspection, auscultation is performed to listen for bowel sounds using a stethoscope. Normal bowel sounds can indicate proper gastrointestinal function, while absent or hyperactive sounds may suggest various pathologies like ileus or obstruction.

Palpation: This step entails feeling the abdomen to identify tenderness, masses, or organ enlargement. Palpation can help detect areas of discomfort and assess organ size, which is crucial in evaluating liver or splenic enlargement. *It should be the last part of the abdominal assessment.*

Percussion: Percussion is employed to assess the presence of fluid or gas. By tapping on the abdomen, clinicians can differentiate between hollow organs filled with gas and solid structures, as well as identify potentially abnormal fluid accumulation indicative of ascites.

6.4.1   Inspection

Lie the patient flat and inspect across the abdomen from eye level. Look for scars, striate, dilated veins, rashes, and any signs of peristalsis (only seen in very thin patients or those with suspected intestinal obstruction) or pulsations.

Abdominal Contour is a fundamental aspect of physical examination and provides essential clues about underlying health conditions. In a healthy individual lying supine (on their back) on an examination couch, the abdomen should appear *concave*, symmetrical, and exhibit a gentle movement with respiration. This normal contour is indicative of a balanced distribution of abdominal contents and muscle tone.

Abnormalities in abdominal contour can arise from a variety of factors, leading to different presentations of distension or fullness. Clinicians commonly identify two primary forms of abdominal distension: generalized and localized. ***Generalized abdominal distension*** occurs when the entire abdomen expands due to the accumulation of various substances. This can be described using the "Six Fs":

- Fat: Excess adipose tissue can lead to an outward protrusion of the abdomen.
- Fluid: Conditions such as ascites can cause significant fluid accumulation in the peritoneal cavity, resulting in distension.

- Flatus: Gaseous distention from excessive gas in the gastrointestinal tract can lead to an overall increase in abdominal girth.
- Faces: Faecal impaction can result in localized or generalized distension if the colon becomes overly filled.
- Fibroids: Uterine fibroids can contribute to abdominal distension in females, particularly if they become large.
- Foetus: Pregnancy is a well-known cause of abdominal enlargement due to the growing foetus.

Both fluid and gaseous distention are primary mechanisms involved in generalized abdominal distension. Patients may present with a visibly distended abdomen accompanied by a sense of fullness or discomfort. Depending on the location of the fullness, it can be categorized as:

- *Central abdominal distension*: This may present as midline fullness, particularly in the upper abdomen (epigastric) or lower abdomen (suprapubic). Such fullness could be associated with conditions like an enlarged liver, pancreatic masses, or bladder distension.
- *Peripheral abdominal distension*: This type of distension is found specifically in the right or left iliac fossa. Common causes include appendiceal abnormalities in the right iliac region and conditions affecting the sigmoid or descending colon in the left iliac fossa, such as diverticulitis or tumours.

Abdominal distension is a common clinical condition characterized by a noticeable increase in abdominal girth or discomfort due to various underlying factors. This symptom can arise from a diverse range of causes, some of which are benign while others may require medical intervention. Proper assessment of abdominal distension involves a systematic approach that encompasses inspection, palpation, and percussion.

Healthcare professionals evaluate a patient for abdominal distension by generally employing a methodical process that includes the following steps:

- **Inspection**: The first step in the examination involves visually assessing the abdomen for size, shape, symmetry, and any visible abnormalities such as scars, asymmetry, or bulging. Observations made during inspection can offer critical insights into potential causes of distension.
- **Palpation**: This technique allows clinicians to feel the abdomen in order to identify tender areas, palpable masses, or organ enlargement. It can help determine the presence of specific types of fullness, distinguishing between fluid-filled versus solid masses.
- **Percussion**: By tapping on the abdomen, clinicians can evaluate for fluid accumulation, such as ascites, or gas presence, indicated by tympanic sounds. The characteristics of these percussion notes provide guidance for the clinical impression.

Though abdominal distension can indicate significant medical concerns, it is important to recognize that it is not always associated with serious pathology. For instance, individuals living with functional bowel disorders, such as irritable bowel syndrome (IBS), commonly experience feelings of distension without underlying disease.

Localized abdominal distension suggests specific organ involvement or mass presence. Conditions associated with specific areas can include:

- **Upper abdomen (Central)**: Conditions such as stomach carcinoma, pancreatic cysts, or abdominal aortic aneurysms may present with upper midline fullness.
- **Lower abdomen (Suprapubic)**: An enlarged uterus due to pregnancy or fibroids, ovarian cysts or tumours, and a distended bladder are causes of fullness in the lower abdomen.
- **Right Iliac fossa**: Localized fullness or masses may indicate appendiceal abscesses, Crohn's disease, or caecal carcinoma.
- **Examination of the umbilical area** is a meticulous inspection of the umbilical area is crucial, as it can reveal conditions such as ***umbilical hernias*** or para-umbilical hernias, which may require surgical intervention if they become incarcerated or strangulated.

Additionally, changes in ***skin appearance***, such as ***striae*** or bruising, can provide valuable diagnostic clues. For example, patients with conditions like Cushing's syndrome may exhibit specific skin changes purple striae due to hormonal imbalances. Rapid weight gain or loss can also leave distinct marks on the skin, further informing clinical evaluation. The skin may change appearance and stretch marks on the skin are noted in women after giving birth, patients who were successfully treated for ascites, and patients diagnosed with Cushing's syndrome and weight loss. Furthermore, the presence and distribution of dilated abdominal wall veins should be sought, and the direction of their blood flow should be tested. Blood flow can be demonstrated by expelling blood between two fingers and observe the direction of return.

The blockage of the hepatic portal vein or vascular channels in the liver can interfere with the pattern of venous return from abdominal parts of the gastrointestinal system. Vessels that interconnect the portal and cava systems can become greatly distended and tortuous, allowing blood in tributaries of the portal system to bypass the liver, enter the systemic system, and thereby return to the heart. In vena cava obstruction, the thoraco-epigastric veins open up, connecting the great saphenous vein with the axillary vein and veins become very prominent. In a superior vena cava obstruction and in an inferior vena cava obstruction, the blood flows upward and can be tested using the two finger technique in skin (***a palpatory test*** is discussed later on in this chapter).

The pattern of blood flow in distended abdominal wall veins is contingent upon the underlying aetiology of venous dilation and obstruction. This phenomenon can be attributed to various pathological conditions that alter hemodynamic and impede venous return. To elucidate this concept, it is essential to consider the mechanisms of venous anatomy, the common causes of venous distension, and the physiological effects on blood flow dynamics.

Veins in the abdominal cavity are structured to facilitate the return of deoxygenated blood to the heart. They operate under relatively low-pressure conditions, unlike arteries, which are designed to withstand higher pressures. The smooth muscle in venous walls allows for expansion and contraction, accommodating fluctuations in blood volume. However, when there is an obstruction or dilation, the normal antegrade flow of blood can be disrupted, resulting in a range of consequences. The underlying causes of venous dilation and obstruction can be categorized into ***intrinsic factors***, such as thrombosis or pathological changes in the vessel wall, and ***extrinsic factors***, which may include external compression from surrounding tissues or tumours. For instance, venous thrombosis can lead to the formation of a clot that occludes the vein, preventing efficient blood flow. This blockage causes an increase in venous pressure proximal to the site of obstruction, leading to the enlargement of veins in the abdominal wall region due to the pooling of blood.

Additionally, conditions such as hepatic cirrhosis can induce portal hypertension, wherein elevated pressure in the portal venous system causes ***collateral circulation*** to develop. This collateral pathway often manifests as distended abdominal wall veins, commonly observed as *"**caput medusae**"*. Blood flow in these engorged veins can exhibit retrograde patterns due to the increased venous pressure and compensatory development of alternative drainage routes.

Similarly, tumours or masses situated in the abdomen may exert external pressure on the inferior vena cava or other major abdominal veins, resulting in venous obstruction. The resultant increased pressure can engender altered hemodynamic and distension of superficial veins, consequently changing the direction and flow of blood towards the areas of least resistance.

Moreover, the pattern of flow in dilated veins can be characterized by changes in venous return dynamics. In instances of obstruction, there may be a reliance on collateral vessels to maintain blood flow. This compensatory mechanism may allow for continued perfusion; however, it can lead to significant ***venous hypertension*** and further dilation of the venous network over time.

The venous system comprises various superficial and deep veins that play integral roles in facilitating the return of deoxygenated blood to the heart. Notably, these veins are interconnected through extensive networks known as ***cavo-caval anastomoses***, which significantly enhance venous drainage efficiency and hemodynamic stability. **Cavo-caval anastomoses** refer to the <u>connections between the superficial venous system, primarily located in the subcutaneous tissue, and the deep venous system that resides within the musculature and adjacent to major arteries</u>. These anastomoses establish collateral pathways, allowing for alternative routes of venous return in instances when primary conduits are occluded or compromised. As a result, they serve as crucial mechanisms in regulating venous blood flow during physiological stress or pathological conditions.

The interplay between superficial and deep veins is essential for maintaining venous return, particularly in the lower extremities. For instance, during activities such as walking or running, the deep veins are augmented by muscular contractions, while the superficial veins act as reservoirs that can regulate blood volume through distension. Enhanced venous return during movement is facilitated by the valves present within these veins, which prevent retrograde flow and ensure that blood is directed towards the heart.

Cavo-caval anastomoses are particularly significant in clinical scenarios involving increased venous pressure and obstruction. In conditions such as chronic venous insufficiency, deep venous thrombosis, or external compression due to tumours, the body's ability to divert blood through these anastomoses becomes crucial. They mitigate the potential adverse effects of ***venous hypertension***, such as oedema or ***venous ulceration***, by redistributing increased blood volume to alternative pathways.

Earlier on we referred to the collateral pathway "caput medusae" a clinical manifestation characterized by the appearance of engorged, tortuous veins radiating outward from the umbilicus, resembling the serpentine hair of Medusa, a figure from Greek mythology. This phenomenon is primarily associated with portal hypertension, a condition that arises when there is an abnormal increase in blood pressure within the portal venous system. The pathophysiology of caput medusae is deeply rooted in the underlying mechanisms of ***portal hypertension***, which commonly occurs in conditions such as liver cirrhosis.

In a healthy state, blood flows freely through the portal vein, transporting deoxygenated blood from the gastrointestinal tract, spleen, and pancreas to the liver. However, inflammatory or fibrotic changes in the liver parenchyma restrict this blood flow, leading to increased pressure within the portal vein. The resultant portal hypertension creates a pathophysiological environment in which collateral circulation becomes necessary to relieve the backlog of blood in the portal system. As portal hypertension develops, the paraumbilical veins, which are normally obliterated after birth and subsequently transformed into the ligamentum teres hepatis, re-open due to the elevated pressure. This reopening facilitates the diversion of blood from the compromised portal venous system into nearby systemic veins. The paraumbilical veins create anastomoses with the superficial epigastric veins and thoraco-epigastric veins, ultimately leading to the superior vena cava (SVC) and the inferior vena cava (IVC).

As pressure builds in the paraumbilical veins, the diverted blood flows radially outward from the umbilicus toward the systemic veins. The visibility of these engorged veins around the umbilicus is thus indicative of the underlying venous hypertension. These conditions not only illustrate a key physiological adaptation to increased portal pressure but also serve as a clinical indicator of serious underlying liver pathology.

Evaluating caput medusae through clinical examination techniques, such as palpation or auscultation of the abdominal wall will reveal blood flow moving away from the umbilicus. This observation reinforces the notion of venous diversion from the portal system to the systemic circulation, highlighting the compensatory mechanisms that the body employs in response to hepatic dysfunction. Clinicians must remain vigilant for caput medusae, as its presence not only indicates underlying vascular changes but also points to the potential severity of hepatic disease, warranting further investigation and management.

Obstruction of the *inferior vena cava* (IVC) manifests significant physiological changes in venous return from the lower body, generally due to causes such as tumours or thrombosis. When such an obstruction occurs, the normal pathway for deoxygenated blood to return to the heart is hampered, resulting in increased venous pressure and subsequent engorgement of collateral vessels. Collateral pathways emerge predominantly through superficial veins, which become highly visible due to the increased blood volume attempting to circumvent the obstruction.

The pattern of blood flow in the case of IVC obstruction is characterized by a *caudal-to-cranial* direction, wherein blood seeks alternative routes to reach the superior vena cava (SVC). Specifically, blood from the lower extremities and pelvis is directed upward through the *thoraco-epigastric veins*, which connect to the axillary and subclavian veins before draining into the SVC. Clinically, these collateral veins, particularly those found below the umbilicus, become prominent and engorged, creating a distinctive visual sign of IVC obstruction.

Conversely, obstruction of the *superior vena cava* (SVC) produces a different set of circulatory adaptations. This condition may arise from various aetiologies, including mediastinal masses or thrombosis, and it similarly prevents normal venous return from the upper body. As a result, blood flow is diverted through collateral circulation involving the superficial abdominal wall veins. The pattern of flow in the case of SVC obstruction is oriented from cranial to caudal. Blood travels downward toward the inferior vena cava via the thoraco-epigastric veins and into the femoral veins. Unlike IVC obstruction, the veins above the umbilicus become especially prominent in this scenario, creating a distinct distribution of venous engorgement.

To distinguish the specific patterns of collateral circulation and determine the site of obstruction, whether it is in the IVC or SVC, clinical examination is essential. *A palpatory test* can be employed to discern the direction of blood flow in the superficial abdominal veins. During this test, a segment of the vein is manually compressed using two fingers. Once the compression is released from one finger, the clinician observes how the vein refills. If refilling occurs from above the point of compression, this indicates a downward flow associated with SVC obstruction. Conversely, if the refill is observed from below the compression point, this suggests an upward flow consistent with IVC obstruction.

By recognizing these patterns and employing palpation techniques, clinicians can effectively differentiate between obstructions in the IVC and SVC, as well as those due to portal hypertension. This diagnostic approach is critical, as it not only provides insight into the nature of the obstruction but also guides subsequent management strategies. Understanding the underlying physiology and the functional role of collateral veins is paramount in the clinical assessment of patients with suspected venous obstructions.

6.4.2   Auscultation

Auscultation of the abdomen is an essential component of the clinical examination, serving as a preliminary step that should ideally precede palpation. This sequence is crucial to avoid stimulating the resting bowel activity, which may otherwise obscure the assessment of gastrointestinal sounds. Auscultation should be conducted systematically in all four quadrants of the abdomen to provide a comprehensive overview of both *digestive* and *vascular* sounds.

During auscultation, the professional will focus on identifying sounds that are characteristic of digestive tract activity. The most common abdominal sounds heard are *gurgling* or *rumbling noises*, primarily produced by the movement of gas and fluid through the intestines as a result of *peristalsis*. **Peristalsis** refers to the coordinated, wave-like muscle contractions that propel the contents of the gastrointestinal tract forward. These sounds can vary in frequency, typically occurring several times per minute; therefore, it is advisable to allocate a minimum of 1–2 min for auscultation to accurately capture the intestinal activity and its associated sounds.

Normal bowel sounds are indicative of active intestinal motility. The presence of these gurgling noises suggests that the bowel is functioning appropriately, while the absence of bowel sounds can be clinically significant. For instance, absent bowel sounds, or a markedly diminished presence may hint at an *intestinal obstruction*, wherein the normal flow of contents through the gastrointestinal tract is impeded. Moreover, in cases of obstruction, patients may exhibit tinkling or high-pitched bowel sounds, reflecting the increased pressure build-up in the proximal segments of the bowel, indicating heightened peristaltic activity in an attempt to overcome the obstruction.

In addition to evaluating sounds associated with the digestive tract, clinicians must also be attentive to specific vascular sounds during abdominal examination. One such sound, known as a **bruit,** is akin to a heart murmur and is characterized by a whooshing or swishing noise heard over arteries. Bruits arise from turbulent blood flow caused by narrowed or partially obstructed blood vessels, often resulting from conditions such as **atherosclerosis** or the presence of an **aortic aneurysm**. Detecting a bruit over abdominal arteries can have crucial diagnostic implications, as it suggests the need for further investigation.

It is important to note that bruits are generally not heard over the arteries of individuals who are of thin and normal body habitus; such individuals typically exhibit palpable abdominal arterial pulsations without the presence of abnormal sounds. This absence suggests that blood flow through these arteries is normal and that there is no significant vascular pathology present. In contrast, the presence of a bruit in individuals, especially those at risk for vascular disease due to factors such as age, obesity, or a history of cardiovascular conditions, may warrant additional diagnostic procedures, such as imaging studies, to assess the integrity of the affected vessels.

In clinical practice, auscultation remains a vital tool for detecting both gastrointestinal and vascular abnormalities. It offers essential insights into the underlying physiological processes occurring within the abdomen and aids in the identification of potential pathological conditions. A thorough understanding of the sounds produced by the digestive and vascular systems enables healthcare professionals to form a more comprehensive diagnosis and to develop appropriate management strategies for their patients.

6.4.3   Palpation

Before commencing the abdominal examination, it is essential to engage the patient in a dialogue regarding their experience of pain or tenderness. Specifically, the clinician should ask the patient to indicate the precise location of any discomfort. This initial step is crucial, as it informs not only the areas requiring closer examination but also aids in formulating a systematic and empathetic approach to the assessment process. When the actual palpation begins, it should always commence in an area far removed from the site of pain to minimize discomfort and to establish trust. The examination should start with superficial palpation, before transitioning to deep palpation. Throughout this examination, it is advisable for the clinician to maintain *eye contact* with the patient, observing their facial expressions and any involuntary reactions as palpation progresses to different abdominal regions. Such attentiveness can provide valuable cues about the patient's pain threshold and response to the examination.

The process of *superficial palpation* involves utilizing the palmar aspect of the hands to apply gentle, light pressure *across all four quadrants* or the *nine distinct regions of the abdomen*. This initial palpation serves multiple purposes: it allows the examiner to detect areas of *tenderness*, identify any *guarding*, and observe for signs *of peritoneal inflammation*. When performing superficial palpation, the clinician gently presses down and observes the patient's response. It is important to note both the application of pressure and the release of pressure, as *rebound tenderness*, a sudden increase in pain upon release can indicate peritoneal irritation. The term *"guarding"* refers to involuntary tensing of the abdominal muscles that may occur in response to anticipated pain, and it is crucial for the examiner to recognize these signals throughout the examination.

Once superficial palpation has been completed, the clinician can proceed to *deep palpation,* applying firmer pressure to each quadrant or region of interest. This step is vital for assessing deeper structures, such as organs and any potential masses. To perform deep palpation effectively, the clinician may use one hand to apply pressure while the other hand reinforces this pressure. A systematic approach is essential during deep palpation, particularly when evaluating for any masses, *tenderness*, *guarding,* or *rigidity* in the abdomen. As with superficial palpation, the clinician should continuously monitor the patient's facial expressions and reactions. This initial interaction enables the clinician to ascertain whether the pressure applied is tolerable or causes discomfort.

The effectiveness of deep palpation can be enhanced through specific techniques. *The two-handed technique* is particularly useful when examining patients with tense abdominal walls or those who are obese, as this approach can facilitate the assessment of deep abdominal structures more effectively. The steps involved in this technique are as follows:

1. The clinician places their dominant hand flat on the abdomen, ensuring that it remains relaxed.
2. The non-dominant (reinforcing) hand is positioned atop the dominant hand.

3. While the upper hand exerts steady pressure onto the abdomen, the lower hand should remain sensitive, feeling for any resistance, masses, or organ borders.
4. The clinician systematically palpates each quadrant to ensure comprehensive assessment.

One of the advantages of the two-handed technique method is that it allows the palpating hand to remain relaxed, thereby improving sensitivity to underlying structures while the reinforcing hand provides depth of pressure.

The ***bimanual technique*** is a specialized approach used for palpating the spleen, which is located posteriorly along the ribs on the left side. Unless it is enlarged, the spleen typically cannot be palpated. The steps for performing this technique effectively are:

- The patient is positioned supine, with the clinician positioned on the patient's right side to provide optimal access to the spleen.
- The clinician places their left hand behind the patient's lower left rib cage to apply pressure, pushing it forward and upward. This manoeuvre seeks to displace the spleen anteriorly and downward towards the abdomen.
- The right hand is then placed flat on the abdomen, below the left costal margin, with the fingers pointing toward the left costal margin.
- The clinician instructs the patient to take a deep breath, during which the diaphragm descends, pushing the spleen outward.
- The clinician feels for the edge of the spleen as it descends.

The goal of this technique is to facilitate the palpation of the spleen's edge. If the spleen is enlarged due to a medical condition such as splenomegaly, the notched anterior border of the spleen may be detected against the examining hand, confirming its presence.

Abdominal masses can manifest due to a variety of underlying conditions, each with distinct characteristics, locations, and implications for patient management. Recognizing these differences is essential for accurate diagnosis and treatment. The following outlines several key types of abdominal masses, their potential causes, and typical presentations.

1. **Stomach cancer**:

    Large gastric tumours can present as a palpable mass in the epigastric region. When stomach cancer progresses, it can lead to significant enlargement of the affected area, sometimes described as a hard, fixed mass that may be felt upon examination. Early detection is critical as the prognosis can greatly depend on the stage at which the cancer is identified.

2. **Abdominal aortic aneurysm**:

    A prominent pulsating mass may be detected just above and slightly to the left of the umbilicus in cases of abdominal aortic aneurysm (AAA). This condition results from weakening of the arterial wall leading to an abnormal bulge. On palpation, the mass may exhibit a ***distinctive pulsing*** characteristic that correlates with the patient's heartbeat. It is crucial to identify AAA early as it poses significant risks of rupture, which can be life-threatening.

3. **Crohn's disease or bowel obstruction**:

   Patients experiencing Crohn's disease or bowel obstruction may develop numerous tender, sausage-shaped masses intermittently throughout the abdomen. These masses are often a result of inflamed or obstructed bowel loops and can be quite painful. This presentation underscores the inflammatory nature of Crohn's disease, requiring prompt evaluation and management to prevent further complications.

4. **Colon cancer**:

   Like stomach cancer, colon cancer can give rise to palpable masses that may occur in various locations throughout the abdomen. These masses can vary in size and firmness, depending on the tumour's characteristics and whether it has invaded surrounding tissues. Colon cancer screenings are vital for early detection, especially in individuals with a higher risk profile.

5. **Diverticulitis**:

   In cases of diverticulitis, inflammation occurs in the diverticula of the colon, often resulting in a palpable mass located in the left iliac region. This mass may be tender during examination and can suggest localized infection or abscess formation, necessitating careful diagnostic evaluation, often through imaging, to guide management.

6. **Ovarian cysts in female patients**:

   A smooth, rounded, rubbery mass may be palpated above the pelvis in the lower abdomen due to ovarian cysts. These cysts can vary in size and typically present without significant discomfort unless they rupture or become complicated. The transabdominal or transvaginal ultrasound is often used to confirm the diagnosis and assess the need for intervention.

7. **Bladder distention**:

   Urinary bladder distention can be identified as a firm mass located centrally in the lower abdomen, just above the pelvic bones. In extreme cases, this mass can extend as high as the umbilicus. The distended bladder may result from urinary retention, so identifying this condition is crucial to prevent complications associated with prolonged distention.

8. **Liver cancer and hepatomegaly**:

   Liver cancer can create a firm, lumpy mass in the right hypochondrium, often requiring imaging studies like ultrasound or CT scans to confirm the diagnosis. *Hepatomegaly*, or liver enlargement, can produce an irregular mass that may be palpated under the right rib cage or even on the left side of the abdomen in some scenarios. Both conditions warrant further evaluation due to their association with significant morbidity.

9. **Splenic enlargement (Splenomegaly)**:

   Splenomegaly can be felt as a palpable mass in the left hypochondrium. Depending on the degree of enlargement, the splenic mass may extend into the lower quadrants of the abdomen. The causes of splenomegaly can range from haematological disorders to infections, necessitating a thorough workup to determine the underlying aetiology.

10. **Pancreatic abscess**:

   A pancreatic abscess may manifest as a palpable mass in the upper abdominal epigastric region. Patients may experience symptoms such as fever, pain, and abdominal tenderness, making early diagnosis critical for effective management of potential complications.

11. **Gallbladder tumours**:

   Finally, a tender, irregularly shaped mass may indicate a gallbladder tumour, particularly in the right hypochondrium. This condition often accompanies symptoms of cholecystitis or bile duct obstruction, and imaging studies are crucial for diagnosis.

Liver Palpation

The liver is predominantly located beneath the ribs on the right side of the body, although it does extend across the midline. The lower edge of the liver typically lies parallel to the costal margin, which is the lower edge of the rib cage. A critical aspect of the examination is the fact that the liver descends slightly during inspiration due to diaphragmatic movement. This anatomical feature informs the technique used for palpation. To begin the palpation of the liver, follow these steps:

- **Positioning**: The examination hand should be poised so that the lateral margin of the index finger is aligned parallel to the costal margin. The thumb is extended, thus exposing the lateral margin of the index finger for effective palpation.
- **Starting location**: Palpation should commence well away from the costal margin, typically starting in the right iliac region. This positioning acknowledges the potential for enlarged liver to extend inferiorly and helps avoid missing the liver edge when it is enlarged.
- **Patient instructions**: Ask the patient to take a deep breath. This inhalation manoeuvre elevates the diaphragm, thereby pushing the liver downward and closer to the examining hand, enhancing the potential for palpation.
- **Adjusting position**: If the liver edge is not palpated during the initial deep inhalation, the examining hand should be moved approximately 1 cm closer to the costal margin. Repeat the deep breath request, allowing for another opportunity to palpate the liver.
- **Repetition and assessment**: This sequential process continues until either the liver edge is palpated or until the costal margin is reached. A normal liver is often palpable near the costal margin, while an enlarged liver may be felt further distal to the costal margin. In such cases, the distance from the costal margin to the palpable liver edge can be measured in centimetres, providing a quantitative assessment of enlargement.

The ability to palpate the liver is crucial in clinical practice as it can indicate underlying pathologies such as *liver disease*, *cirrhosis*, or *tumours*. An enlarged liver may suggest congestive heart failure or other obstruction-related issues, and precise measurements assist healthcare professionals in monitoring disease progression and treatment efficacy.

In cases of obstructive conditions or significant underlying pathology, the liver's position may shift, making palpation more challenging. Accordingly, clinicians may need to rely on imaging investigations, such as ultrasound or CT scan, for comprehensive evaluation.

Additionally, when assessing the liver, it is beneficial to palpate for any associated findings, such as tenderness, masses, or enlargement of surrounding structures like the spleen and gallbladder. Palpation of the adjacent organs can also reveal reflections of systemic conditions, including splenomegaly or signs of acute cholecystitis.

Kidney Palpation

The kidneys are vital organs responsible for filtering waste products from the blood, regulating electrolyte balance, and contributing to overall homeostasis. Their anatomical location extends from the twelfth thoracic vertebra (T12) to the third lumbar vertebra (L3) in the retroperitoneal space, which is located behind the peritoneum. While normally these structures are not palpable in most individuals, they may become evident during examination, particularly in thin patients or those with specific pathologies. Understanding the proper techniques for kidney palpation and percussion is essential for healthcare providers to assess renal health effectively.

The kidneys have distinct anatomical features. The right kidney is positioned slightly lower than the left, primarily due to the presence of the liver on the right side of the body. Both kidneys have a firm consistency and smooth surface, and they will typically move downwards toward the pelvis during deep inspiration, allowing for expansion of the diaphragm. This movement is crucial during examination, as it enhances the likelihood of palpating the kidney.

Palpation of the kidneys requires deep **bimanual techniques** to effectively assess this retroperitoneal organ. The following steps provide a systematic approach to palpation:

- Patient positioning: Begin by positioning the patient in a comfortable supine position. This allows for relaxation of the abdominal muscles and facilitates examination.
- Hand placement: To initiate palpation, tuck the palmar surfaces of one hand into the patient's flank area. The fingers should be positioned between the posterolateral costal margin and the spine, just beneath the twelfth rib. This creates a supportive base for palpation.
- Anterior lift: Use the tucked hand to lift the surrounding tissues anteriorly. This manoeuvre creates space for palpation and enhances the clinician's ability to feel the kidney.
- Deep palpation: With the opposite hand, palpate the upper quadrant of the abdomen using deep pressure. The goal is to feel the kidney as it passes between both hands. This exercise is often most effective when the patient takes a deep breath.

- Inspiration technique: Instruct the patient to breathe in deeply. As they do, apply firm pressure with the fingers of both hands together. The rounded lower pole of the kidney may be palpable as it shifts downward with respiration, moving between the opposing fingers.
- Assessing kidney size: It is essential to compare findings on both sides. A normal kidney may not be palpable in most individuals, while an enlarged kidney can often be felt beyond its usual dimensions.

When assessing for enlargements, it is critical to distinguish kidney enlargement from splenomegaly on the left and hepatomegaly on the right. Percussion techniques aid in making this distinction.

Spleen Palpation

The spleen is a vital organ located in the upper left quadrant of the abdomen and plays an essential role in filtering blood, recycling iron from haemoglobin, and supporting the immune system. In young individuals, the spleen is typically about the size of a fist. However, it undergoes considerable atrophy as individuals advance in age, making it less prominent in older adults. Understanding how to effectively palpate the spleen is crucial for clinicians, particularly when assessing for *splenomegaly*, or enlargement of the spleen, which can signal various underlying medical conditions.

Under typical circumstances, the spleen is not palpable upon physical examination due to its anatomical location and size. To detect any abnormalities or enlargement of the spleen, palpation must always commence in the *right iliac fossa*. This is because the spleen, when enlarged, tends to expand in the *inferio-medial direction*. During the examination, a notable feature to identify an enlarged spleen is the presence of a distinct notch on the anterior border. This anatomical landmark aids the healthcare professional in differentiating the spleen from other organs, such as the kidney, which lies posterior to the splenic flexure of the colon. The process of palpating the spleen involves several important steps and considerations: As said earlier the spleen moves inferio-medially during inspiration due to the downward movement of the diaphragm. Consequently, if a normal spleen is assessed, it cannot typically be palpated even during deep inspiration. For the spleen to be felt during palpation, it must enlarge to at least twice its normal size.

As the spleen enlarges, it continues to grow inferio-medially. In cases of significant splenomegaly, the spleen may extend into the right lower abdomen, making it potentially palpable at this location. Notably, when the spleen reaches a massive size, the characteristic splenic notch may become palpable, serving as a helpful identification marker. The following steps provide a systematic approach to palpation:

- Initiating palpation: The examination begins in the right iliac fossa, moving diagonally across the abdomen towards the left upper quadrant where the spleen is located.

- Facilitating palpation: To enhance the ability to palpate an enlarged spleen, place the left hand under and behind the lower left rib cage while applying gentle traction. This technique can bring an enlarged spleen forward during inspiration, potentially causing it to extend beyond the costal margin.
- Alternative positioning: Another technique involves positioning the patient into a right lateral decubitus position (rolling onto their right side). This manoeuvre can aid in mobilizing an enlarged spleen towards the abdominal wall, making it easier to palpate.
- Repetition of the process: The healthcare professional continues the palpation procedure until the spleen is either palpated or until the costal margin is reached. In a normal examination, a clinician should not palpate a healthy spleen; however, if the spleen is enlarged, it may be palpable beyond the costal margin. Distances from the costal margin to the palpable spleen edge are recorded in centimetres.

The differentiation of an enlarged spleen from other abdominal organs is crucial during the examination. A dull percussion note over the surface of the spleen, particularly when contrasted with the resonant sound associated with air-filled structures such as the lungs or the tympanic sounds over the bowel, can assist in distinguishing splenomegaly from other conditions like renal enlargement. This percussion technique complements palpation and enhances the diagnostic accuracy of abdominal examinations.

Understanding the assessment and examination of the spleen is vital in clinical practice for several reasons:

- The spleen is involved in numerous pathological processes, and its enlargement can represent underlying conditions such as infections (e.g. mononucleosis), liver diseases (e.g. cirrhosis), haematological disorders (e.g. haemolytic anaemia), or malignancies (e.g. lymphoma). Timely and accurate assessment of splenomegaly allows for appropriate referrals and interventions.
- The healthcare professional should monitor changes in spleen size over time in patients with known conditions. Documenting the size and shape helps to evaluate disease progression and the effectiveness of therapeutic interventions.

An enlarged spleen may complicate surgical procedures, particularly those in the abdominal cavity. Knowledge of its size and position can help guide surgical planning and avoid inadvertent splenic injury.

Bladder Palpation

The urinary bladder, when filled, can be an important structure to assess during an abdominal examination. Under normal circumstances, the bladder lies beneath the *symphysis pubis* and is generally not palpable. However, when the bladder is full, it may become palpable as a tense suprapubic mass. This prominence can serve as an indication of urinary retention or bladder distention, which requires prompt attention.

When palpating the bladder, the clinician should follow these steps:

- Ensure that the patient is comfortably positioned, typically lying supine.
- Using the palms, the clinician gently palpates the suprapubic area, feeling for any tension or fullness. The bladder, when distended, will present as a firm, rounded mass.
- Upon percussion, a distended bladder typically produces a resonant sound due to the presence of urine within the bladder. This resonance contrasts with the dull sounds heard over solid organs or masses, an important clinical distinction.

Recognizing a distended bladder allows the clinician to identify potential causes of urinary retention, such as obstruction, neurological conditions, or post-surgical complications. Prompt evaluation is critical to prevent further complications, such as bladder damage or infection.

Aorta Palpation

The abdominal aorta is a major blood vessel that transports blood from the heart to the lower parts of the body. Deep palpation is the technique used to assess its pulsations during a physical examination. Notably, identifying aortic pulsations can provide insights into vascular health and potential pathology.

To effectively palpate the aorta, the following steps should be considered:

- Hand positioning: The clinician typically uses the finger pads of both hands, positioning them on either side of the midline in the upper abdomen (below the *xiphoid process* and above the umbilicus).
- Apply gentle yet firm pressure with the fingertips, feeling for pulsations that indicate the presence of the aorta. This technique is often most effective in thinner individuals, as aortic pulsations can be more readily palpable. In larger individuals or obese patients, palpation may prove difficult, and reliance on other diagnostic techniques may be necessary.
- Assessing pulsations: Being mindful of the quality, strength, and rhythm of the aortic pulsations can provide valuable information about vascular integrity. An enlarged or palpable abdominal aorta may suggest the presence of an abdominal aortic aneurysm (AAA), which carries significant risks of rupture and requires immediate medical evaluation.

Recognizing abnormalities such as aortic dilation or irregular pulsations can assist in identifying serious conditions that require further investigation, including imaging studies or referrals to specialists.

6.4.4 Percussion

Liver Percussion

Apart from palpation, percussion techniques can confirm the liver's borders and delineate its size. The examiner taps gently on the abdominal wall and listens for variations in sound. A normal liver will typically produce a dull sound, while a tympanic note might indicate the presence of air-filled structures, such as the stomach.

Percussion of the liver is a valuable clinical skill that assists healthcare providers in assessing liver size and detecting potential abnormalities. This technique is grounded in the principle that the liver, when enlarged or healthy, produces a characteristic dull sound upon percussion, distinguishing it from the surrounding structures such as the lungs and intestines, which contribute to different sound characteristics. To perform liver percussion effectively, two key borders must be identified: the upper border and the lower border of the liver. This assessment is typically conducted using systematic percussion techniques, allowing the clinician to delineate the liver's size accurately.

Technique for percussing the liver

- Identifying **the upper liver border**: Begin by palpating the area near the right upper quadrant of the abdomen. With the patient in a sitting or supine position, use your fingers to lightly percuss the thorax, starting above the right clavicle. Move downwards in a systematic manner, assessing for changes in sound quality. Initially, the clinician will encounter resonance over the lungs (tympanic sound), which will transition to a duller sound as the percussion reaches the liver. The upper liver border is indicated where this change from resonance to dullness occurs.
- Identifying **the lower liver border**: Similarly, to locate the lower liver border, begin percussion from the **iliac fossa**, which is located in the lower right abdomen. Start percussing upwards toward the costal margin, ensuring that you listen for changes in sound. This time, the transition will be from a dull sound (reflecting the presence of the liver) to a tympanic sound over the normal bowel. The point at which the sound changes from dull to tympanic signifies the lower border of the liver.

The identification of the liver borders through percussion provides critical diagnostic information. A normal liver will exhibit clear borders between dullness and resonance. However, patterns of liver dullness can suggest conditions such as hepatomegaly, where the liver enlarges and may extend beyond the typical boundaries. In cases of significant enlargement, dullness may be appreciable at lower levels due to the downward displacement of the bowel. Understanding these variations aids in diagnosing potential liver diseases and guiding further evaluation, including imaging studies. Percussion performed over an enlarged liver or spleen will produce dull sounds. Conversely, percussion over the kidney itself should yield a more resonant sound due to the presence of air overlying the bowel. This difference is crucial in clinical evaluations, as it helps direct further investigation or management of the patient's condition.

Kidney Percussion
In addition to palpation, percussion can be performed to evaluate kidney tenderness, a practice that may reveal underlying renal pathologies. Here's how to conduct kidney percussion:

- Positioning: The patient should remain in the same supine position during percussion.
- Costovertebral angle tenderness: To assess the kidneys via percussion, clinician should "thump" the costovertebral angles using the ulnar surface of a fist. This technique involves applying enough force to elicit a response without causing pain or discomfort to the patient.

A positive response may imply kidney tenderness, which could suggest conditions such as pyelonephritis, stone disease, or other renal inflammatory processes. Further diagnostic evaluation, including laboratory tests and imaging, may be warranted based on these findings.

Renal Pathologies resulting in kidney enlargement, or renal swelling, include polycystic kidney disease and hydronephrosis. These conditions can lead to significant alterations in renal size and function, necessitating proper evaluation.

Examination of Other Abdominal Structures

Ascites is the accumulation of fluid in the peritoneal cavity and is a common clinical finding in various conditions, including liver cirrhosis, heart failure, and malignancies. Detecting ascites during a physical examination can be accomplished utilizing two reliable bedside techniques: ***shifting dullness*** and the ***fluid wave (or thrill)***. Both methods are critical for assessing the presence and extent of abdominal fluid, although they serve distinct purposes and have unique indications.

Shifting Dullness test is grounded in the principle that in ascites, free fluid gravitates to the flanks when the patient is in a supine position, while the air-filled intestines located in the central abdomen produce a tympanic sound upon percussion. This characteristic allows for differentiation between areas filled with fluid (dull) and air (tympanic). When the patient is turned onto one side, the fluid shifts due to gravity. Consequently, the area that was previously dull becomes resonant, while the newly dependent side becomes dull. This observable change in percussion notes evidences the presence of free fluid in the peritoneal cavity.

Steps in performing the shifting dullness test:

- ***Supine Position***: The patient lies flat on their back. The examiner begins percussion from the midline of the abdomen out toward the flanks. The examiner notes the differences: the central abdomen is typically tympanic due to air in the intestines, while the flanks are dull because of fluid accumulation.
- ***Lateral Position***: The patient is then asked to roll onto their side. The examiner reapplies percussion on the abdomen. The previously dull flank, positioned uppermost, will likely become tympanic, while the lower flank will now be dull. This change in percussion notes confirms the presence and movement of ascitic fluid.
- ***Positive Shifting Dullness***: Indicates the presence of free peritoneal fluid, typically greater than 500 ml. Accurate detection often necessitates at least 1 litre of fluid for reliable identification.
- ***Negative Shifting Dullness***: Suggests no significant ascites or fluid volume less than 500 ml.

Fluid Wave (Fluid Thrill) test, also known as fluid thrill, evaluates gross ascites by examining the transmission of a wave across the abdomen. In patients with significant ascites, this method allows the examiner to detect the movement of fluid when the abdomen is tapped.

Steps in performing the fluid wave test:

- The patient lies supine, ensuring relaxation of the abdominal muscles. The patient, or an assistant, places their hand firmly along the midline of the abdomen. This position restricts wave transmission through adipose tissue, allowing only the fluid's movement to be felt.
- The examiner taps sharply on one flank of the abdomen with their fingers. With the other hand, the examiner feels for a transmitted wave on the opposite flank. If a wave is felt, this suggests the presence of ascitic fluid. However, it is noteworthy that significant fluid volume is usually required for a positive result. A fluid wave test may yield false positives in obese patients, as fat can also transmit waves.

Both the shifting dullness and fluid wave tests are integral components in the clinical assessment of ascites. Understanding their differences is crucial to optimize clinical evaluation.

Learning Point

Feature	Shifting dullness	Fluid wave/fluid thrill
Detects	Moderate ascites (>500 ml)	Massive ascites (tense abdomen)
Method	Percussion (tympany $\leftrightarrow$ dullness)	Tapping one flank, feeling other flank
Position change?	Yes, supine to lateral	No, performed in supine only
Limitation	Not useful in tense ascites	May yield false positives in obesity

In practice, clinicians typically begin with the shifting dullness test to assess for moderate levels of ascitic fluid. A negative result may indicate the absence of significant fluid, whereas a positive finding would necessitate further evaluation. If the abdomen is notably tense or distended, indicating large volume ascites, the fluid wave test may be performed. This sequential approach facilitates accurate diagnosis and informs further management strategies.

In summary, both shifting dullness and fluid wave tests are valuable bedside techniques for detecting and assessing ascites. Each has its appropriate application depending on the clinical scenario, and together they enhance the clinician's ability to diagnose this common condition effectively.

In slimmer individuals, it may be possible to palpate certain structures such as the liver edge, the lower pole of the right kidney, the aortic pulsation, a descending colon filled with faeces, the sacral promontory, or a tender cecum. The subtlety required in such examinations necessitates both skilful palpation techniques and an understanding of the normal anatomy underlying these organs. Percussion is frequently employed in conjunction with palpation to assess the liver and spleen. This combined approach can enhance diagnostic accuracy and provide insights into organ size and the presence of any abnormalities. Notably, the terms "hepatomegaly" and "splenomegaly" are used to describe enlarged liver and spleen, respectively, and both conditions carry clinical significance requiring careful evaluation.

The liver is a key organ that warrants careful examination during abdominal assessments. Percussion plays a crucial role when the edge of the liver is challenging to detect, potentially due to various factors such as reduced liver size or a change in its position resulting from diaphragmatic or lung disorders. Kidney health can also reflect systemic conditions. Issues such as hypertension and diabetes mellitus can contribute to chronic kidney disease, necessitating regular examination of kidney size and function.

In acute settings, recognizing signs of kidney tenderness or enlargement can prompt rapid assessment and intervention, potentially improving patient outcomes. Frequent examinations of kidney size and tenderness may be essential for patients with known renal diseases, particularly in ensuring that interventions are effective and monitoring progress over time.

The examination of abdominal structures includes not only the assessment of the liver and kidneys but also the evaluation of the bladder and aorta. Recognizing the characteristics of these structures through proper palpation and percussion techniques is essential for comprehensive clinical assessment.

6.5   Part 4: Focused Learning

Learning activity 1

Exercise 1
Answer the questions below related to structure and function

<u>The mouth and oesophagus</u>

(a) Complete the following:

Food is chewed and moistened with saliva which contains enzymes including ___________, __________ and ___________ as well as bicarbonate. Saliva is secreted by the ___________, ____________ and _____________ glands. Swallowing is controlled by a neurological centre in the _______________. Information to and from the pharynx and oesophagus is conducted via the ____________ and ___________ cranial nerves. In addition, the smooth muscle of the oesophagus has its own intrinsic innervation. Once food is ejected into the oesophagus, it is propelled down by ___________action towards the stomach. The ____________ sphincter assists in preventing regurgitation of the gastric contents, but it must relax before the wave of peristalsis reaches it in order to let the food in.

Answer:

Food is chewed and moistened with saliva which contains enzymes including _ amylase_, _lingual lipase_ and _lysozyme_ as well as bicarbonate. Saliva is secreted by the _parotid_, _submandibular_ and _sublingual_ glands. Swallowing is controlled by a neurological centre in the _brain stem_. Information to and from the pharynx and oesophagus is conducted via *the _ glossopharyngeal_ and _vagus_ cranial nerves. In addition, the smooth muscle of the oesophagus has its own intrinsic innervation. Once food is ejected into the oesophagus, it is propelled down by _peristaltic_ action towards the stomach. The _lower oesophageal_ sphincter assists in preventing regurgitation of the gastric contents, but it must relax before the wave of peristalsis reaches it in order to let the food in.*

The stomach

The stomach has smooth muscle which allows it to churn the food to prepare it for entry into the duodenum.

(b) (i) Name the cells in the body that secrete hydrochloric acid and intrinsic factor. What are the functions of hydrochloric acid and intrinsic factor?

Answer:
  Parietal cells
  Functions:
    Hydrochloric acid-sterilizes the meal
    Intrinsic factor-absorption of vitamin B12

(ii) Name the substance secreted by the chief cells of the stomach and state its function:

Answer:
  Pepsinogen
  Acid in the stomach changes pepsinogen to pepsin, which breaks down proteins in food during digestion.

(iii) State the mechanisms preventing reflux of gastric contents into the oesophagus:

Answer:
  The ant reflux mechanism at the gastro-oesophageal junction: The intrinsic muscular sphincter known as the lower oesophageal sphincter (LES) and the diaphragm that functions as an external sphincter-like mechanism.

<u>The small intestine</u>

(c) Complete the following:

The small intestine consists of the ___________, ___________ and ___________. Arterial blood is supplied to the small intestine by the __________________. Blood from the intestine drains via the ____________ first to the ____________ before returning to the systemic circulation. The main functions of the small intestine are ___________ and ___________. Consequently, the small intestine needs a large surface area which is achieved by visible and invisible _________. Most of the enzymes necessary for breaking down foodstuffs are present in the _____________. The breakdown of carbohydrates is commenced by the enzyme ____________ secreted by the ___________ and __________. The completion of carbohydrate breakdown to monosaccharides is accomplished by enzymes such as _________, ___________ and __________ found on the _________________. The enzyme ____________ from the ___________ breaks down fats to ___________ and ____________. These are emulsified by __________ to aid absorption. Protein breakdown is initiated in the stomach but most is carried out in the intestine by the enzyme ____________, secreted by the ____________. The absorption of most nutrients occurs in the ______________ and ___________, but B_{12} and bile acids are absorbed in the ____________.

Answer:

The small intestine consists of the <u>duodenum</u>, <u>jejunum</u> and <u>ileum</u>. Arterial blood is supplied to the small intestine by the <u>superior mesenteric artery</u>. Blood from the intestine drains via the <u>superior mesenteric vein</u> first to the <u>portal vein</u> before returning to the systemic circulation. The main functions of the small intestine are <u>digestion</u> and <u>absorption</u>. Consequently, the small intestine needs a large surface area which is achieved by visible and invisible <u>folds</u>. Most of the enzymes necessary for breaking down foodstuffs are present in the <u>duodenum</u>. The breakdown of carbohydrates is commenced by the enzyme <u>amylase</u> secreted by the <u>saliva</u> and <u>pancreas</u>. The completion of carbohydrate breakdown to monosaccharides is accomplished by enzymes such as <u>lactase</u>, <u>maltase</u> and <u>sucrase</u> found on the <u>brush border membrane</u>. The enzyme <u>lipase</u> from the <u>pancreas</u> breaks down fats to <u>fatty acids</u> and <u>monoglycerides</u>. These are emulsified by <u>bile acids</u> to aid absorption. Protein breakdown is initiated in the stomach but most is carried out in the intestine by the enzyme <u>peptidases</u>, secreted by the <u>pancreas</u>. The absorption of most nutrients occurs in the <u>jejunum</u> and <u>ileum</u>, but B_{12} and bile acids are absorbed in the <u>terminal ileum</u>.

<u>The large intestine</u>

The large intestine consists of the caecum (plus appendix), ascending colon, right (hepatic) flexure, transverse colon, left (splenic) flexure, descending colon, sigmoid colon, and rectum.

(d) (i) How much fluid enters the large bowel every day?

Answer:
   1.5 l

(ii) Name the valve at the junction of the caecum and ileum. What is its function?

Answer:
   Ileocaecal valve
   It prevents reflux of colonic contents into the small intestine.

(iii) What weight of faeces are passed every day in an average western diet?

Answer:
   200 g

(iv) What important substance do the colonic glands produce and what is its functions?

Answer:
   Mucus
   It provides constant lubrication for the passage of faeces and protects the mucosa from bacterial enzymes.

The liver and gallbladder

The liver is the largest organ in the abdomen and is divided into a large right and small left lobe by the falciform ligament. All the products of digestion will enter the liver via the portal system where they can undergo further metabolic change before reaching the systemic circulation. Microscopically, the liver cells form lobules and the lateral borders of the liver cells form bile canaliculi which converge and eventually form the left and right main hepatic bile ducts. The gallbladder lies beneath the lower surface of the liver in the gallbladder fossa. The cystic duct connects the gallbladder to the common bile duct which then enters the duodenum at the ampulla of Vater, together with the pancreatic duct.

(e) (i) List the main metabolic functions performed by the liver cells (hepatocytes)

Answer:
- *Convert glucose to glycogen*
- *Synthesize a range of proteins*
- *Degrade protein to amino acids*
- *Synthesize urea from ammonias*
- *Synthesize cholesterol and bile acids*

(ii) What is bile composed of?

Answer:
  Bile is composed of bile salts, cholesterol, bilirubin and glucuronic acid.

(iii) Which substances are stored in the liver?

Answer:
  Carbohydrate
  Vitamins
  Mineral e.g. *iron*

(iv) What role does the liver play in vitamin D metabolism?

Answer:
  Hydroxylation of vitamin D to 25-(OH)D

(v) What is the function of the gallbladder?

Answer:
  Stores and concentrates bile.

The pancreas

The pancreas consists of a head, body and tail. The head lies in the C-shaped loop of the duodenum and the tail touches the spleen. The pancreas has both endocrine and exocrine functions. The exocrine glands secrete enzymes for digestion (see small intestine) and bicarbonate:

(f) (i) What is the function of the bicarbonate?

Answer:
  Bicarbonate protects the duodenum from gastric acid ensure an optimum pH for digestive enzyme activity.

(ii) Name the hormones secreted by the pancreas.

Answer:
- *Insulin*
- *Glucagon*
- *Somatostatin*
- *Pancreatic polypeptide*

<u>The spleen</u>

The spleen is part of the lymphoid tissues and is also responsible for controlling red cell destruction.

The descriptions by patients of symptoms related to the digestive tract are frequently vague and imprecise. For example, there is often confusion about terms such as indigestion and heartburn.

Exercise 2
Answer the questions related to the following common symptoms:

<u>Dysphagia</u>

(a) (i) What is meant by dysphagia?

Answer:
  Difficulty in swallowing.

(ii) Use the physiological principles regarding the functions of the oesophagus to explain the major mechanisms of dysphagia. List some common causes:

Answer:
  Swallowing is a complex process and many disturbances in oropharyngeal and oesophageal physiology including neurologic deficits, obstruction, fibrosis, structural damage or congenital and developmental conditions can result in dysphagia.

Dysphagia can be classified into the following four types:

1. Oropharyngeal (oral) dysphagia
   - Bad teeth
   - Problems with the jaw
2. Oesophageal dysphagia
   - Gastroesophageal reflux disease
   - Esophagitis-can be caused by different problems, such as infections
   - Achalasia-muscles in the oesophagus lose their ability to relax and open
   - Tumours in the oesophagus

3. Complex neuromuscular disorders
   - Dementia
   - Stroke
   - Brain tumour
   - Myasthenia gravis-that causes the muscles to become weak
4. Functional dysphagia
   - Anxiety
   - Stress attack

(iii) What questions would you ask a patient with dysphagia?

Answer:
   - *Where does food stick?*
   - *Is the dysphagia intermittent or progressive?*
   - *Has the symptom developed over weeks, months or years?*
   - *Are both drink and food equally difficult to swallow?*
   - *Is there history of reflex symptoms?*

Heartburn

This is the sensation of acid secretions regurgitating from the stomach to the oesophagus.

(b) (i) Use the physiological principles regarding the prevention of reflux to explain the mechanisms of heartburn. List some common causes:

Answer:
   - *Loss of tone in lower oesophageal sphincter, e.g. Pregnancy, Overweight*
   - *Loss of external sphincter-like mechanism of diaphragm, e.g. Hiatus hernia*

(ii) The pain of heartburn may sometimes mimic cardiac ischaemic pain. Complete the table below

	Site	Character	Radiation	Aggravating factors	Relieving factors	Associated Features
Cardiac ischaemia						
Heartburn						

Answer:

	Site	Character	Radiation	Aggravating factors	Relieving factors	Associated Features
Cardiac ischaemia	*Lower part of centre chest*	*Crushing*	*Up to chest into the jaw*	*Exertion*	*Nitrates Rest*	*Shortness of breath, nausea*
Heartburn	*Oesophagus*	*Burning*	*Upward behind the sternum*	*Eating, lying down, bending*	*Antacids*	*Water brash*

Dyspepsia and Indigestion

These are rather vague terms covering a range of subjective symptoms. These terms are often applied to sensations of heartburn, epigastric pain and fullness, belching, and nausea. Dyspepsia usually indicates disorders of the lower oesophagus, stomach, duodenum, pancreas, and gallbladder.

Weight Loss

This is an important symptom associated with digestive tract diseases as well as many other illnesses. Cancer, chronic infections, and organ failures result in significant weight loss.

(c) What questions would you ask a patient with weight loss?

Answer:
- *Is your appetite increase, decrease, or normal?*
- *Do you enjoy your food?*
- *How long has the weight been lost?*
- *Meal description—usual breakfast, lunch, and dinner.*
- *Associated symptoms, e.g. nausea, vomiting, abdominal pain?*
- *Bowel habit changes and appearance of stool?*
- *Has there been a fever?*
- *Do you pass excessive volumes of urine?*

Nausea and Vomiting

Nausea without vomiting usually indicates psychological disorders such as anorexia nervosa, bulimia, depression, or anxiety. Nausea usually comes in waves and may be relieved by vomiting. Nausea and vomiting are common in digestive tract disorders and in many metabolic and systemic diseases.

(d) (i) List some common causes of nausea and vomiting.

Answer:
- *Unpleasant sights, smell and tastes*
- *Abnormal stimulation of the inner ear labyrinth*
- *Viral hepatitis, biliary diseases*
- *Stimulating the vomiting centre, e.g. digoxin, morphine, anti-cancer drugs*
- *Psychological disorders, e.g. anorexia*
- *Gastrointestinal diseases*

(ii) What questions would you ask a patient with vomiting?

Answer:
- *When is the vomiting worse, e.g. morning?*
- *Is there associated abdominal pain?*
- *Does the vomiting relation to meals?*
- *Appearance, e.g. blood, bile stained?*
- *Any recognizable food or coffee grounds in the vomit?*
- *Do you take any drugs?*

Gastrointestinal Bleeding

Blood may be vomited, in which case it is called *haematemesis*, or passed per rectum. If the blood passed per rectum is altered, resulting in black stools with a consistency like tar, it is called *melena*.

(e) (i) Name the parts of the GIT that are likely to be associated with haematemesis. List some common diseases of these parts that cause haematemesis:

Answer:
Oesophagus, stomach, and duodenum
- *Oesophageal varices*
- *Gastric cancer, duodenal ulcer*
- *Ulcerated oesophagus*

(ii) Which parts of the GIT are likely to be associated with bright red blood per rectum? List some common disorders in these parts that cause bright red bleeding:

Answer:
Sigmoid colon and rectum
- *Inflammatory bowel disease*
- *Haemorrhoids*

(iii) Which parts of the GIT are associated with darker red or maroon coloured blood per rectum? List some common disorders.

Answer:
   Ascending colon, transverse colon, and descending colon.
   - *Ischaemic colitis*
   - *Polyp*
   - *Diverticular disease (small mucosal herniations through bowel wall muscle.)*

(iv) Which parts of the GIT are likely to be associated with melena

Answer:
   Oesophagus, stomach, and duodenum.

(v) Which large bowel diseases present with intermittent rectal bleeding?

Answer:
   - *Colon cancer*
   - *Polyps*

(vi) Which large bowel disease is associated with the passage per rectum of blood mixed with mucus?

Answer:
   Ulcerative colitis

(vii) Which conditions can be associated with heavy bleeding per rectum?

Answer:
   - *Ischaemic colitis*
   - *Diverticular disease*

(viii) What is the likely outcome if there is chronic blood loss per rectum, which may be occult (microscopic)?

Answer:
   Annemia

<u>Constipation</u>

The diagnosis depends on the normal bowel habit of an individual. People on high fibre diets may need three evacuations daily. Other individuals on typical Western diets may have one bowel movement a day or even less frequently.

Constipation that has been present for many years is unlikely to be related to structural disease and is called 'functional', in that it is related to lifestyle and diet. Constipation of recent onset is more likely to be related to underlying disease. Particular attention should be paid to constipation associated with colicky pain and rectal bleeding. Sometimes constipation can alternate with diarrhoea.

(f) (i) Which disorders causing constipation are associated with rectal bleeding and colicky pain?

Answer:
- *Colon cancer*
- *Diverticular disease*

(ii) List some non-gastrointestinal disorders (e.g. metabolic diseases, drugs, etc.) associated with constipation:

Answer:
- *Drugs, e.g. Antidepressants*
- *Hypothyroidism, Hypercalcaemia, Hypokalaemia*

(iii) What questions would you ask a patient with constipation?

Answer:
- *What is the normal stool frequency?*
- *How long have you been constipated?*
- *Are the stools large or small and pellet-shaped?*
- *Do you strain at stool?*
- *Is there associated abdominal pain, distention, nausea, or vomiting?*
- *Do you take any drugs?*

<u>Diarrhoea</u>

Diarrhoea is associated with a large stool volume and a change in the consistency of the stools. There are many causes of diarrhoea. Functional diarrhoea is associated with anxiety states and irritable bowel syndrome and may alternate with constipation.

(g) (i) List some common gastrointestinal and non-gastrointestinal causes of diarrhoea:

Answer:
- *Infections-bacterial, viral*
- *Inflammatory bowel-ulcerative colitis and Crohn's diseases*
- *Malabsorption-coeliac disease*
- *Following broad-spectrum antibiotics or laxative abuse*
- *Hyperthyroidism*

(ii) What questions would you ask a patient with diarrhoea?

Answer:
- *How long have you had diarrhoea?*
- *What is the stool frequency?*
- *What is the consistency of stools?*
- *What is the colour?*
- *Any blood and mucus present?*
- *Is there associated pain, nausea, vomiting, or weight loss?*
- *Do you take any antibiotics?*

Symptoms of Liver Disease

Early symptoms are vague and non-specific and include malaise, fatigue, anorexia, and nausea.

(h) What questions would you ask a patient with jaundice?

Answer:
- *Any history of alcohol abuse or intravenous drug abuse?*
- *Any contact with jaundiced patients?*
- *Any travelling history?*
- *Any blood transfusion?*
- *Any prescription or non-prescription drugs has been used?*
- *Any associated pain, weight loss?*
- *Any family history of liver disease?*

Abdominal Pain

Pain may arise from the viscera or from the parietal peritoneum, which has pain fibres (unlike the visceral peritoneum). Visceral pain is due to stretching of a hollow organ, such as the gut, gallbladder, ureter, uterus, and may be aching or cramp-like and is often poorly localized, usually being felt in the midline irrespective of the organ of origin. Pain affecting the parietal peritoneum (peritonitis) is well localized to the area of inflammation and is commonly worse on movement. There is severe tenderness including rebound tenderness. In a disease such as acute appendicitis, the pain is initially visceral (in the appendix) and is perceived in the midline (umbilical area). Subsequently, the pain becomes parietal and becomes localized to the right iliac fossa because the parietal peritoneum lying over the appendix becomes inflamed.

(i) What questions would you ask a patient with abdominal pain

Answer:
  SOCRATES
- *Site-Location of the abdominal pain?*
- *Onset-Has the pain been present for how long?*

- *Character-Can you describe the pain?*
- *Relieved by-Have you noticed any relieving factors?*
- *Associated features/symptoms-Has there been associated weight loss, nausea, vomiting?*
- *Timing-Is the pain constant or intermittent?*
- *Exacerbated by-Have you noticed any specific aggravating factors?*
- *Severity-Is the pain affected by eating or defecation?*

Abdominal examination

Most information related to abdominal diseases is obtained from palpation and percussion of the abdomen. Remember that there is a great variation in the shapes and sizes of abdomens. The abdomen may be divided into segments which provide a schematic approach for detecting changes in the main intra-abdominal organs in disease.

Exercise 3
Match the correct abdominal area (listed below) to the numbers in the drawing.

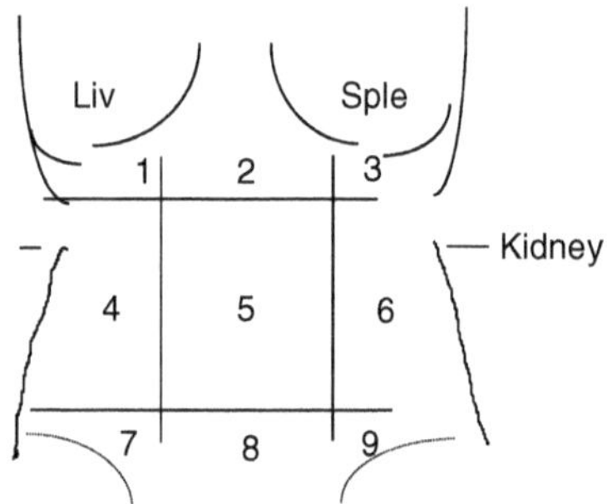

Left Iliac fossa	Hypogastrium	Right lumbar region
Right hypochondrium	Epigastrium	Right iliac fossa
Left lumbar region	Left hypochondrium	Umbilical region

Answer:

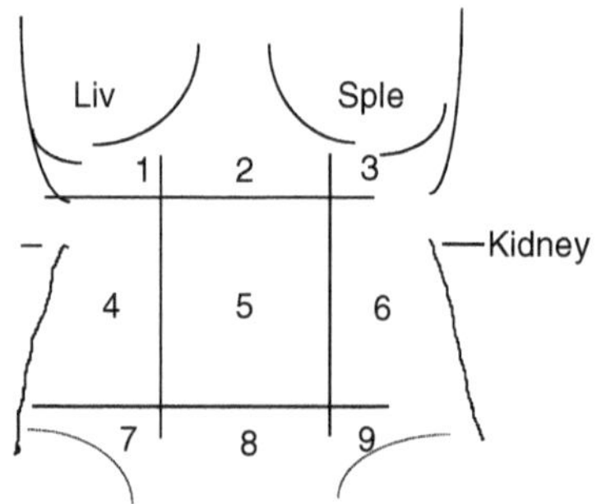

1. *Right hypochondrium*
2. *Epigastrium*
3. *Left hypochondrium*
4. *Right lumbar region*
5. *Umbilical region*
6. *Left lumbar region*
7. *Right iliac fossa*
8. *Hypogastrium (suprapubic region)*
9. *Left iliac fossa*

In practice, however, many physicians divide the abdomen into four quadrants—right upper quadrant, left upper quadrant, right lower quadrant, and left lower quadrant. Sometimes they will describe pain or masses as being in the epigastric, suprapubic, left iliac fossa, or right iliac fossa.

Exercise 4

Answer the questions associated with the major features on inspection listed below:

<u>Contours</u>

The normal abdominal contour alters when there is:

- Generalized abdominal distension
- Localized distension due to fullness or masses. Localized distension may be
  - Central abdominal (midline), either upper abdomen (epigastric) or lower abdomen (suprapubic)
    Peripheral, either right iliac fossa or left iliac fossa

(a) Describe the contour of the normal abdomen in an individual lying on his/her back on the examining couch:

Answer:
   The normal abdomen is concave, symmetrical, and moves gently with respiration.

(b) List the main mechanisms of generalized abdominal distension.

Answer:
   Fluid and gaseous distention

(c) Which organs or structures are associated with central (midline) fullness or masses in the upper abdomen? Can you think of some pathological causes?

Answer:
   - *Stomach-carcinoma*
   - *Pancreas-pancreatic cysts*
   - *Abdominal aorta-abdominal aortic aneurysm*

(d) Which organs or structures are associated with fullness or a mass in the lower abdomen (suprapubic region)?

Answer:
- *Enlarged uterus-pregnancy or fibroids*
- *Enlarged ovaries-cysts or carcinoma*
- *Full bladder*

(e) Which organs or structures are associated with peripheral fullness or masses in the right iliac fossa?

Answer:
- *Appendix mass, Appendix abscess, Crohn's disease*
- *Carcinoma of caecum*
- *Tuberculosis*

What is the importance of inspecting the umbilical area?

Answer:
Umbilical hernia or para-umbilical hernia

List some conditions associated with stretch marks on the skin:

Answer:
- *Women after giving birth*
- *Successfully treated for ascites*
- *Cushing's syndrome*

Distended veins on the abdominal are commonly seen in chronic liver failure and obstruction to the inferior vena cava. What are the mechanisms for both of these?

Answer:
Chronic liver failure: The blockage of the hepatic portal vein or vascular chan-nels in the liver can interfere with the pattern of venous return from abdomi-nal parts of the gastrointestinal system. Vessels that interconnect the portal and cava systems can become greatly distended and tortuous, allowing blood in tributaries of the portal system to bypass the liver, enter the systemic sys-tem, and thereby return to the heart.
The most common cause of abdominal vein distention is obstruction of portal venous drainage (ex. Portal hypertension).
Tortuous veins radiating from or to the umbilicus. This can lead to Caput Medusae.
Obstruction to the inferior vena cava: In vena cava obstruction, the thoracoepi-gastric veins open up, connecting the great saphenous vein with the axillary vein. In a superior vena cava and in an inferior vena cava obstruction, the blood flows upward.

Before palpating the abdomen, it is important to ask the patient to point to the area of pain or tenderness. Palpation should begin in the segment furthest from the site of discomfort. Begin with superficial palpation before proceeding to deep palpation. Always look at the patient's face whenever you move your hand to the next area to note any reactions to palpation.

Exercise 5

In addition to allowing the patient to become used to the examiner's hand, superficial palpation can yield important information if the peritoneum is locally or generally inflamed. Which physical features on superficial palpation would indicate peritoneal inflammation?

Answer:
   Guarding and tenderness and/or rebound tenderness.

Note: the terms for enlarged liver and spleen are *hepatomegaly* and *splenomegaly,*
   respectively.
The liver

Exercise 6

Complete the following table related to alterations in the size of the liver, using the keywords and phrases at the end:

Right heart failure	Metastases	Emphysema/asthma	liver failure (cirrhosis)

Keywords and phrases:

1. Enlarged liver	2. Irregular liver edge and surface	3. Hard edge and surface
4. Lowered right diaphragm on percussion	5. May be normal on palpation	6. Tender
7. Smooth edge and surface	8. Liver edge palpable below abdomen	9. Liver area reduced on percussion
10. Soft liver edge	11. Raised right diaphragm on percussion	12. Enlarged spleen

Answer:			
Right heart failure	**Metastases**	**Emphysema/asthma**	**Liver failure (cirrhosis)**
1. *Enlarged liver* 6. *Tender* 7. *Smooth edge and surface* 8. *Liver edge palpable below abdomen* 12. *Enlarged spleen*	1. *Enlarged liver* 2. *Irregular liver edge and surface* 3. *Hard edge and surface* 6. *Tender* 8. *Liver edge palpable below abdomen* 11. *Raised right diaphragm on percussion* 12. *Enlarged spleen*	4. *Lowered right diaphragm on Percussion* 7. *Smooth edge and surface* 8. *Liver edge palpable below abdomen* 10. *Soft liver edge*	2. *Irregular liver edge and surface* 3. *Hard edge and surface* 5. *May be normal on palpation* 6. *Tender* 9. *Liver area reduced on Percussion*

The Spleen

The spleen is normally the size of a fist in young people, but atrophies considerably by extreme old age. Palpation should always commence in the right iliac fossa since the spleen enlarges in this direction. If the spleen is palpable a notch is felt on the anterior border, which helps to identify it. A dull percussion note over an enlarged spleen distinguishes it from an enlarged kidney, which lies behind the splenic flexure of the colon.

Exercise 7
Look up some causes of splenomegaly under the following headings:

Infective
> *Answer: Infective hepatitis, Subacute bacterial endocarditis, Glandular fever, Malaria*

Congestive
> *Answer: Cirrhosis, Portal and Splenic vein thrombosis*

Related to blood disorders (haematological)
> *Answer: Acute/Chronic Leukaemia, Lymphoma, Thalassaemia*

Infiltrations
> *Answer: Sarcoidosis, Amyloidosis*

Abdominal Distension

Abdominal distension is assessed by inspection, palpation, and percussion. A feeling of abdominal distension is not necessarily related to underlying pathology, since this is commonly experienced by individuals with functional bowel disorders (e.g. irritable bowel syndrome). It is common practice to consider the causes under the "five F's"—fat, faeces, fluid, flatus, and foetus. Some recommend the addition of a sixth F, "fibroids".

Exercise 8

(a) Fat. When obese patients lie flat, the abdomen may show a contour similar to ascites. Briefly describe a procedure that can clinically differentiate obesity from ascites:
Answer: Shifting Dullness

(b) Flatus. Can you think of some physiological and pathological causes of excessive flatus? How can this be clinically detected?
Answer:
   Physiological-Air swallowing, high fibre diets
   Pathological-large bowel obstruction
   Loud rumbling sounds, peristalsis

(c) Faeces. What type of patients are prone to developing accumulations of impacted faeces?
Answer:
   Children-Hirschsprung's disease
   Adults-Demented or psychiatrically disturbed patients

(d) Fluid (ascites). List some common acute and chronic causes of fluid in the abdomen:
Answer:
   Acute-Trauma, Acute pancreatitis, Bacterial peritonitis
   Chronic-Cirrhosis of liver, Heart failure, Abdominal malignancy, Hepatic vein occlusion

<u>Sounds Related to the Digestive Tract</u>

Abdominal sounds heard on auscultation are gurgling noises due to the movement of gas and fluid by peristalsis.

Exercise 9

What is the significance of absent bowel sounds?
   Answer: Up to 2 min no bowel sounds-Bowel complete paralysis
What is the significance of increase in the frequency of bowel sounds?
   Answer: More than 1 bowel sounds/s-Early obstruction and enteritis
What is the significance of bowel sounds with a high-pitched, 'tinkling' quality?
   Answer: Progressive bowel obstruction leading to large amount of gas and fluid accumulate

<u>Sounds Related to the Abdominal Arteries</u>

A bruit is a sound similar to a heart murmur heard over arteries, which is due to turbulent blood flow. It, thus, suggests atherosclerosis or an aortic aneurysm. Bruits are *not* heard over the arteries of thin, normal individuals who have palpable abdominal arterial pulsations.

Case Study 1

A 50-year-old teacher complained of a 5-month history of left-sided abdominal pain, colicky in nature and relieved by defecation. During this period, she had experienced episodes of constipation and had occasionally noted streaks of blood in her stool when he had been able to defecate. She had recently seen her doctor who had referred her to the local hospital for further investigations. She had now come to you because of sacral pain. On examination, she was thin, ill-looking, and showed clinical evidence of anaemia. Her blood pressure was 130/90 mmHg, the pulse was 109/min, regular, the respiratory rate was 22 per minute, and the temperature was 38.2 °C. There was an ill-defined, tender swelling in the left iliac fossa which appeared to be related to the sigmoid colon.

- What other relevant information would you want to obtain from the history and physical examination to help you in the differential diagnosis?

Answer:
   Relevant information from History: Examination
     (i) *Other features of pain—does it radiate? Any aggravating factors.*
    (ii) *Diet—type of food? "Western" style diet (low fibre—high fat). Eating pattern—is there anorexia?*
   (iii) *Change in bowel habit—particularly if recent in origin.*
   (iv) *Lifestyle—any psychogenic factors, emotional and occupational stress factors.*
    (v) *Sacral pain—nature, pattern of radiation, aggravating and relieving factors, time of onset, duration, intermittent, or continuous.*
   (vi) *Physical examination—general, abdominal inspection, palpation, percussion. Auscultation (bowel sounds)—should be referred for sigmoidoscopy.*

- Discuss the possible causes and mechanisms for the constipation and colicky pain in this patient.

Answer:
   Presentation suggests narrowing of colon (left side), i.e. stenosis—possibilities.
     (i) *Carcinoma, especially in a patient who was previously well—also age of patient is relevant.*
    (ii) *Diverticulitis disease—can cause large bowel obstruction with colicky pain—but illness is usually more acute—if no inflammation is present symptoms can mimic irritable bowel syndrome.*
   (iii) *Chronic ischaemia of bowel can lead to stenosis—no evidence in history to support this.*
   (iv) *Crohn's disease—can affect the gut anywhere from mouth to anus, but terminal ilium is commonest site.*

Clinical presentation in this patient shows many of the features of Crohn's disease, i.e. may present if Crohn's is left-sided. Crohn's causes full-thickness lesions which can lead to strictures, presenting with features of obstruction.

 (v) *Ulcerative colitis—risk of cancer association often significant diarrhoea with blood loss—commoner in women and not usually associated with the profound physical changes seen in this patient.*

 (vi) *Haemorrhoids—presents with bright red blood so an unlikely cause of GI haemorrhage. However, haemorrhoids are found in chronic constipation which may be associated with Crohn's disease, colorectal cancer and diverticular disease.*

 (vii) *Strangulated hernia—unlikely—history likely to be much more acute—no evidence on examination. Also, not associated with rectal bleeding.*

- Discuss the likely causes and differential diagnosis of the rectal bleeding in this particular patient.

Answer:
 (i) *Carcinoma colon—colicky pain, recent onset.*
 (ii) *Diverticular disease—left-sided is common—an acute presentation may suggest inflammation.*
 (iii) *Ulcerative colitis—risk of cancer association often significant diarrhoea with blood loss—commoner in women.*
 (iv) *Haemorrhoids—bright red blood.*

- Briefly comment on the significance of the sacral pain in this patient.

Answer:
 Could be due to space-occupying lesion—e.g. tumour of colon, bladder. Could be related to metastases—must exclude history of trauma or degenerative arthritis.

- Briefly discuss the significance of the vital signs and mass in the left iliac fossa

Answer:
 The temperature and pulse rate are high and the blood pressure if slightly elevated, indicating the likelihood of an inflammatory process. While an infective process, such as diverticulitis, must be ruled out, the likeliest cause is inflammatory bowel disease probably Crohn's disease. The mass in the left iliac fossa could be indicative of Crohn's disease but it is essential to exclude colorectal cancer.

Case Study 2

A 65-year-old man complains of trouble with his bowels. For the last 6 weeks, he has been suffering from diarrhoea, which sometimes alternates with constipation. He also complains of intermittent lower abdominal pain but no weight loss and he has also noted some blood in the faeces. Examination reveals clinical evidence of anaemia, tenderness in the lower abdomen, and the suggestion of a possible mass in the left iliac fossa. Anorectal examination (using a proctoscope) shows haemorrhoids but nothing else of note.

- Name the most important disorder presenting with altered bowel habit and left iliac fossa mass that must be considered in a patient of this age.

Answer:
 Carcinoma of the colon
 Another disorder that may present with altered bowel habit and a mass is diverticular disease. Briefly state the major pathological features of diverticular disease and list the common complications that could result:
 Herniations of mucosa and submucosa through the wall of the large bowel. Most commonly at points where blood vessels (arteries) pass through the submucosa. Diverticuli occur due to weakness in bowel wall and increased colonic pressure. Commonest site is sigmoid colon. Rare before the age of 30 years. Complications include:
 Stricture formation
 Perforation of Diverticuli leading to peritonitis.
 Possible fistula formation
 Massive colonic bleeding

- What are the possible causes of the anaemia and what would the red cells look like on microscopic examination of the blood?

Answer:
 Chronic blood loss due to diverticular disease. Possibly haemorrhoids. This is likely to be an iron deficiency anaemia, hence a hypochromic macrocytic anaemia (small, pale red cells, low MCV)

- What further relevant information would you want to obtain from the history and physical examination?

Answer:
 History:
 Detailed description of bleeding (fresh, mixed with stool, or separate).
 Change in stool calibre or frequency.
 Duration and progression of symptoms.
 Family history of colorectal cancer, polyps, or inflammatory bowel disease (IBD).
 Past medical history (diverticulitis, previous bowel disease).
 Systemic symptoms (fatigue, night sweats, fevers).
 Risk factors: diet, smoking, alcohol use.

Examination:
 Full abdominal exam for masses, organomegaly.
 Lymph node exam (inguinal, para-aortic).
 Rectal examination (digital PR) for palpable lesions missed by proctoscope.
 General exam for cachexia, pallor, clubbing.

- **Discuss the possible causes and mechanisms of alternating constipation and diarrhoea in this patient.**

Answer:
 Left-sided colonic cancer:
  Narrowing of the lumen → partial obstruction → alternating bowel habits.
  Tumour ulceration → intermittent diarrhoea.
 Diverticular disease:
  Inflammation and segmental colonic dysfunction.
 Irritable bowel syndrome (IBS):
  Functional disorder with alternating bowel habit (but less likely in elderly with anaemia and blood in stool).
 Stricture formation:
  From prior inflammation or tumour.
  Discuss the likely causes and differential diagnosis of the rectal bleeding.
 Likely cause:
  Carcinoma of the descending or sigmoid colon.
 Differentials:
  Haemorrhoids (not sufficient to explain anaemia and mass).
  Diverticular disease with bleeding.
  Angiodysplasia (usually right colon, but possible).
  Inflammatory bowel disease.
  Anal fissure (unlikely with mass and anaemia).

Case Study 3

A 75-year-old man with a 40-year history of heavy alcohol consumption presents with jaundice, malaise, and fever. Over the past few weeks, his family has noticed progressive confusion, personality changes, and a marked decline in mobility. He also complains of abdominal swelling, recurrent nosebleeds, and black tarry stools. His liver function tests (carried out on serum) and urinalysis confirm chronic hepatitis with intrahepatic obstruction.

- Outline the main signs and symptoms you would expect to be present when clinically examining this patient.

Answer:
 - *On physical examination:*
  General: cachexia, temporal muscle wasting, jaundice, fetor hepaticus (musty odour of breath due to volatile substances).

> *Hands: palmar erythema (vasodilation), asterixis (hepatic encephalopathy), leukonychia (hypoalbuminemia), clubbing.*
> *Skin: spider angiomas ($\uparrow$ oestrogen), bruising and petechiae (coagulopathy, thrombocytopenia), jaundice.*
> *Chest: gynecomastia (altered oestrogen metabolism).*

- *Abdomen:*
  > *Hepatomegaly (initially enlarged, later shrunken and nodular).*
  > *Splenomegaly (portal hypertension).*
  > *Ascites (shifting dullness, fluid thrill).*
  > *Caput medusae (dilated periumbilical veins due to portosystemic collaterals).*
  > *Neurological: drowsiness, confusion, asterixis (flapping tremor) $\rightarrow$ hepatic encephalopathy*

- Outline the main urine and stool findings that you would expect to be present, giving briefly the mechanism for these abnormalities.

Answer:

> *In intrahepatic obstruction there is cirrhosis, which leads to blocking of the bile canaliculi. There is also necrosis of some hepatocytes leading to leakage of cellular enzymes into the blood. Failure to eliminate conjugated bilirubin leads to pale* stools (high fat content) due to lack of urobilinogen.
>
> *Blood findings: In chronic liver disease (e.g. cirrhosis), reduced serum albumin levels and increased prothrombin time (indicating prolonged bleeding). Raised aspartate aminotransferase (AST) and alanine aminotransferase (ALT) levels indicate cellular necrosis. Raises alkaline phosphatase indicting intrahepatic obstruction.*
>
> *Urine findings: Dark brown colour due to increased bilirubin.*
>
> *Stool findings: Steatorrhoea due to inability to excrete conjugated bilirubin. Urobilinogen cannot be formed.*
>
> *Urine Findings*
>> *Dark urine (bilirubinuria): conjugated bilirubin is water-soluble and leaks into urine.*
>> *$\uparrow$ Urobilinogen: reduced hepatic clearance allows more to spill into circulation and urine.*
>
> *Stool Findings*
>> *Pale/clay-coloured stools: less bile pigment reaching the gut due to impaired excretion.*
>> *Occult blood/melena possible: from portal hypertension–related variceal bleeding or coagulopathy.*

- Briefly outline the mechanisms for the development of ascites in cirrhosis of the liver

Answer:

Reduction in plasma protein synthesis by the liver (coupled with malnutrition) leads to a fall in plasma albumin concentration and a fall in colloidal osmotic (oncotic) pressure. This is coupled with a rise in capillary hydrostatic pressure due to increased portal pressure in portal system. This reduces blood volume and renal perfusion leading to secondary hyperaldosteronism with sodium and water retention, which compounds the problem. (Alternative theory, called "overflow theory" developed since most patients have increased cardiac output and peripheral vasodilatation. This suggests that the main problem may be primary hyperaldosteronism keeping water and salt levels high leading to increased cardiac output. Reasons for primary hyperaldosteronism are not clear if this theory is referred to).

- Discuss the likely causes and differential diagnosis of the chronic hepatitis.

Answer:

Alcoholic cirrhosis (primary diagnosis): fits the history of chronic alcohol use, jaundice, ascites, encephalopathy, and GI bleeding.

Hepatocellular carcinoma (HCC): may develop on the background of cirrhosis; sinister features such as weight loss, cachexia, hepatomegaly with irregular nodules suggest possibility.

Chronic viral hepatitis (HBV, HCV): can present similarly with cirrhosis, jaundice, and portal hypertension.

Primary biliary cholangitis/sclerosing cholangitis: cholestatic picture with jaundice, pruritus, and cirrhosis, but less likely in an elderly man with this alcohol history.

Drug-induced liver injury: certain drugs (e.g. isoniazid, methotrexate) may mimic alcoholic hepatitis/cirrhosis.

Decompensated non-alcoholic fatty liver disease (NAFLD/NASH): less likely here, but can mimic advanced cirrhosis.

Extrahepatic obstruction (e.g. pancreatic head carcinoma, cholangiocarcinoma): can cause obstructive jaundice, pale stools, dark urine, but usually without encephalopathy unless secondary liver failure.

Case Study 4

Mr. William, a 77-year-old pensioner, presented with a 5-month history of progressive difficulty in swallowing. This was associated with some discomfort after meals and occasional regurgitation of food. He denied significant unintentional weight loss but reported persistent heartburn, intermittent hoarseness of voice, and a chronic cough. More recently, he had noticed occasional streaks of blood in his vomit. He now presented to you because of a persistent, unresolved "cold" and cough that had not improved since his last visit to the GP.

On examination, he appeared ill-looking, he was off colour and his blood pressure was 130/90 mmHg, pulse rate 90/min regular, respiratory rate 22/min. There was mild tenderness on deep palpation of the epigastrium, but no palpable abdominal mass was detected.

- What other relevant information would you want to obtain from the history and physical examination to help you in the differential diagnosis?

Answer
  History:
    Duration and progression of dysphagia (solids → liquids → saliva).
    History of odynophagia (painful swallowing).
    Details of weight loss and nutritional intake.
    History of reflux disease, chronic smoking, alcohol use, dietary habits (e.g. very hot drinks).
    Family history of gastrointestinal malignancy.
    Presence of persistent cough, hoarseness, aspiration, or haemoptysis.
    Previous history of caustic ingestion or radiation exposure.
  Examination:
    Signs of malnutrition and cachexia.
    Detailed lymph node examination (especially supraclavicular nodes).
    Chest auscultation for aspiration changes or pleural effusion.
    Abdominal examination for organomegaly (liver metastasis).
    Neurological exam if back pain suggests vertebral involvement.

- Discuss the possible causes and mechanisms for dysphagia and retrosternal discomfort in this patient.
  Mechanical obstruction: progressive narrowing of the oesophageal lumen due to tumour growth.
  Infiltration: local invasion of the oesophageal wall causes stiffness and poor peristalsis, worsening dysphagia.
  Inflammation/ulceration: tumour ulceration leads to pain, odynophagia, and sometimes bleeding.
    Reflux/retention: obstruction leads to food stasis, regurgitation, and secondary oesophagitis, contributing to discomfort.
- Discuss the likely causes and differential diagnosis of the hematemesis (blood in vomitus) in this particular patient.

Answer
  Likely causes:
    Tumour ulceration leading to surface bleeding.
    Erosion into submucosal vessels.
  Differential diagnoses:
    Peptic ulcer disease with secondary bleeding.

Severe erosive oesophagitis (e.g. due to reflux or stasis).
Mallory–Weiss tear from repeated vomiting.
Variceal bleed (less likely but important in a patient with underlying liver disease).

- What investigations would you request to confirm the diagnosis and assess disease extent?

Answer
  Diagnostic:
    Upper GI endoscopy with biopsy → histological confirmation.
  Staging:
    Contrast-enhanced CT scan (neck, chest, abdomen) → local spread, lymph nodes, metastases.
    Endoscopic ultrasound (EUS) → depth of tumour invasion and nodal assessment.
    PET-CT (where available) → distant metastasis.
    Bronchoscopy if there is suspicion of tracheobronchial involvement.
  Supportive tests:
    Blood tests (CBC for anaemia, LFTs for liver spread, renal function before contrast).

- Discuss the likely causes of his chronic cough and hoarseness of voice in the context of oesophageal pathology.

Answer
  Cough:
    Aspiration due to oesophageal obstruction and regurgitation.
    Possible tracheo-oesophageal fistula formation.
    Recurrent aspiration pneumonia.
  Hoarseness:
    Invasion or compression of the left recurrent laryngeal nerve by tumour or lymph nodes in the mediastinum.

Bibliography

1. Andersson, S. O., Bardel, A., André, M., & Kristiansson, P. (2020). Consultation skills of final year medical students in Sweden: Video-recorded real-patient consultations in primary health care assessed by Calgary-Cambridge Global Consultation Rating Scale, a pilot study. *MedEdPublish, 8*, 88.
2. Garibaldi, B. T., & Elder, A. (2020). Seven reasons why the physical examination remains important. *Journal of the Royal College of Physicians of Edinburgh, 51*(3), 211–214.
3. Kurtz, S., Silverman, J., Benson, J., & Draper, J. (2003). Marrying content and process in clinical method teaching: Enhancing the Calgary–Cambridge guides. *Academic Medicine, 78*(8), 802–809.

4. Schirmer, J. M., Mauksch, L., Lang, F., Marvel, M. K., Zoppi, K., Epstein, R. M., Brock, D., & Pryzbylski, M. (2005). Assessing communication competence: A review of current tools. *Family Medicine, 37*(3), 184–192.
5. Thomas, J., & Monaghan, T. (2014). *Oxford handbook of clinical examination and practical skills*. Oxford University Press.
6. Walker, H. K. (1990). The origins of the history and physical examination. In *Clinical methods: The history, physical, and laboratory examinations* (3rd ed.). Butterworths.

Assessing and Diagnosing Disorders of the Nervous System

Common Medical Terms
A list of medical terms is cited below for easy reference for the learner to pick up and understand before they proceed to read this chapter.

Articulation of words
Abnormal eye position
Abnormal or asymmetrical pupils
Aphasia
Ataxia
Diplopia
Fasciculation
Facial drop
Gait
Hemianopia

© The Author(s), under exclusive license to Springer Nature Switzerland AG 2026
C. Leliopoulou, L. Holman, *Physical Examination and Diagnostic Skills for Nurses and Allied Health Professionals,*
https://doi.org/10.1007/978-3-032-26539-5_7

Hemiparesis
Hemisensory loss
Meniere's disease
Nystagmus
Plantar reflexes
Ptosis
Sensorineural hearing loss
Strabismus
Tetraparesis
Tinnitus
Vertigo
Vestibular neuronitis

7.1   Part 1: The Brain and the Cortex

The brain has four regions: ***the cerebrum, the diencephalon, the brainstem,*** and ***the cerebellum***.

The cerebral hemispheres constitute the greatest mass of brain tissue. Their outer layers are formed by the cellular grey matter known as ***the cerebral cortex***. There is a common belief that we all have a dominant and a non-dominant cortex. In right-handed people, the left cortex is said to be dominant and most have their language centre in the left cortex. However, this is confusing, since over 70% of left-handed people also have their language function in the left cortex.

Disorders of the dominant cortex cause *aphasia (dysphasia), dysarthria, alexia (dyslexia),* and *agraphia. Aphasia (dysphasia)* is the inability to talk while *dysarthria* is the inability to articulate words. On the other hand, *alexia (dyslexia)* is the inability to read, and *agraphia* is the inability to write. Disorders of the right cortex in right-handed people involve abnormalities of spatial perception (losing one's way in familiar surroundings, or failure to draw simple shapes, etc.).

The brainstem, which continues down to the spinal cord, has three sections: ***the midbrain, the pons,*** and ***the medulla***. The paired cranial nerves (2nd–12th) emerge from the diencephalon and the brainstem (first pair olfactory emerge from the cerebral hemispheres). The *cerebellum* is primarily concerned with ***coordination***. The spinal cord is a cylindrical mass of nervous tissue that is encased within the bony vertebral column. It contains long tracts that connect the brain with the peripheral nervous system.

Learning Point

Spinal Nerves

There are thirty-one (31) pairs of mixed nerves arising from the spinal cord and provide the connections between the CNS and the neck, body, and limbs. They are classified and named by the level at which they leave the spinal cord. Each spinal nerve has two connections with the spinal cord: The motor root with its efferent fibres from the lower motor neurone (LMN) and the sensory root with afferent fibres from the cell bodies in the sensory root ganglion:

- 8 cervical (C1–C8)
- 12 thoracic (T1–T12)
- 5 lumbar (L1–L5)
- 5 sacral (S1–S5)
- 1 coccygeal (C0)

Spinal Root Lesions

Cervical and lumbar disc lesions are common causes of compression of the nerve roots. The pain is referred to the area (*myotome* and *dermatome*) supplied by the nerve and the pain is worsened by stretching the nerve or by pressure in the spinal subarachnoid space (when coughing and/or straining). Pins and needles are also experienced.

The cutaneous branches of a spinal nerve provide sensory innervation to an area of skin known as a dermatome which supplies a horizontal strip of trunk at the approximate level of its exit point. Dermatomes may overlap with each other and therefore that strip of skin may be innervated by two or more spinal nerves so if there is malfunction of a single nerve there may be limited adverse effect on sensation in that strip of skin.

Spinal Cord Compression

This causes spastic weakness with sensory loss below the lesion, together with disturbances of bladder and anal sphincters.

7.2 General Symptoms of Neurological Disease

This chapter explores common symptoms linked to neurological diseases and disorders. Patients with neurological conditions can exhibit a diverse array of symptoms during examination.

Table 7.1 Neurological common symptoms

Headache, facial pain & weakness	*Dizziness & vertigo*	*Walking* & movement *difficulties*
Visual disturbances	Hearing disturbances	Loss of consciousness & *Blackouts*
Limb numbness & paraesthesia	Disturbed higher mental functions	Speech disorders
Swallowing disorders	Gait disorders	Loss of bladder & bowel control

Some common symptoms such as headache, blackouts, dizziness, vertigo, walking difficulties, and visual problems can be ranked by their importance for the physical examination of the neurological system, and they are included in the Table 7.1, highlighted in bold:

(a) Headache
Based on the underlying cause, the patient may experience one of the following types of headaches:

- Tension headache (or psychogenic headache)
- Migraine headache
- Hypertension headache
- Headache caused by extra cranial causes
- Headache due to raised intracranial pressure (ICP)
- Headache due to cranial arteritis

Headaches are common in moderately severe hypertension but are particularly significant in malignant hypertension. Moderately severe hypertension is caused by the constriction of arterioles, while capillary pressure remains normal. In malignant hypertension, blood pressure rises sharply, with systolic pressure reaching 180 mmHg or higher and diastolic pressure reaching 120 mmHg or higher. This increase in capillary pressure can lead to cerebral oedema and elevated intracranial pressure. Headaches, typically classified as tension headaches and migraines (Table 7.2), are common symptoms. Each type of headache has different causes and affects various patient groups, presenting distinct clinical symptoms during examination.

In addition to the classical presentation of migraine, other rarer forms may occur such as:

- Vertebrobasilar migraine—due to ischaemia in the posterior cerebral circulation.
- Hemiplegic migraine—an extremely rare form in which classical migraine is accompanied by hemiparesis (weakness down one side).
- Ophthalmoplegic migraine—in which the third and sixth cranial nerves are affected during a migraine attack.

Table 7.2 Comparison of tension headache and migraine

	Tension headache	Migraine

Epidemiology.
    Who gets it
    Age of onset
	Adults, more often females	Teenagers and adults, more often females

Pathogenesis:	Accompanied by askeletal muscle contraction in neck, face, and jaw Vasodilation of the arterial bed	Aura stage is associated with cerebral vasoconstriction Headache stage is associated with extra cranial and meningeal vasodilation

Clinical pattern (plus associated features)	Unilateral or bilateral
	Ache in temporal, occipital, parietal, frontal regions
	Pain may frequent changes in sites
	Dull, pressure like, a sense of fullness in the head, constricting pain like wearing a tight band.
	Nausea and vomiting, loss of appetite
	Photophobia and phono phobia (rare)
		Aura (15–20 min): variety of visual disturbances, may have numbness or tingling of face and arms, weakness of one side of the body
		Headache(4–72 h):
		    Unilateral or generalized
		    Located in temporal region
		    Throbbing pain in one side of the head
		    Pain worsens with daily activities
		    Feeling sick
		    Sweating, feeling hot or cold
		    Tummy ache and diarrhoea
		    Photophobia and phonophobia

Regarding extra cranial causes, the typical features of a headache following head injury are:

- Unconsciousness
- Persistent headache or worsen headache
- Nausea and vomiting
- Convulsions or seizures
- Clear fluid from ears or nose
- Drowsiness
- Headache made worse by coughing and straining

Some extra cranial disorders that can cause headache can be:

- Nasal and sinus headache
- Dental pain
- Aural pain
- Eye pain

(b) Blackouts

These are recurring episodes of sudden loss of consciousness. In many cases, you will need to obtain essential information from eyewitnesses as well as from the patient. It is important that if we have an eyewitness when someone has a blackout that we ask them the following questions in order to gather information on the nature of the blackout:

- Did they observe colour change?
- What happened when the patient fell?
- How long did the patient lose consciousness?
- Did the patient complain of a headache prior to losing consciousness?

Questions for the patient:

- Did they have any symptoms before losing consciousness?
- Do they remember what happened?
- Are they on any medication?

Blackouts indicate the total dependence of the brain on a continuous supply of oxygen and glucose. It is essential to determine the predisposing factors for attacks of blackouts. The most likely cause responsible for most blackouts is *hypoglycaemia*. And some of the predisposing factors you should consider when taking a history of a blackout are low blood pressure and low blood sugar.

Common causes include:

(a) Epilepsy
(b) Cerebrovascular disease
(c) Syncope
(d) Hypoglycaemia
(e) Severe fluid depletion after severe gastro-enteritis in previously healthy young people
(f) Psychological problems

An epileptic seizure is the result of sudden discharges of impulses from neurones in the brain. About 3% of the population will have two or more epileptic attacks in their lifetime.

Epilepsy is classified as follows:

1. *Generalized seizures*, which implies widespread electrical discharges in the brain:
    (a) *Tonic-clonic seizures*, initially there is rigidity (*tonic phase*) for about 1 min, followed by falling to the ground, which may result in injury and tongue biting. This is followed by convulsions (*clonic phase*), in which there is rhythmic jerking. This usually lasts up to a few minutes, after which the patient lies unconscious for some hours.
    (b) *Absence seizures*, usually seen in children. Normal activity ceases for a few seconds with occasional jerks. Activity is then resumed as if nothing happened.

2. ***Partial seizures***, which are due to activation in a group of neurones in a part of the cerebral cortex. These are also called *focal seizures*. Examples include:
   (a) *Jacksonian seizures*, which affect the motor part of the cerebral cortex, causing jerking movements that originate in the corner of the mouth or the fingers on the opposite side to the focus of the seizure, spreading up the limb.
   (b) *Temporal lobe seizure*, which is associated with odd disturbances of smell, or feelings of unreality or having been in a particular place before. There may also be visual hallucinations.

In contrast to seizures there are the transient ischaemic attacks (TIAs) which can impact the anterior circulation (carotid system) or posterior circulation (vertebrobasilar system) due to emboli lodging in the branches of these circulatory systems. Comparison of the carotid involvement and vertebrobasilar involvement is highlighted in Table 7.3. TIAs can lead to a sudden loss of function in a part of the brain. The associated fainting and symptoms peak within seconds and can last from minutes to hours, typically resolving within 24 h. Cerebrovascular diseases are prevalent, with transient ischaemic attacks (TIAs) being a common manifestation.

Common sources for emboli to the brain which are also common diseases and risk factors that may be associated with TIAs are myocardial infarction, atrial fibrillation, bacterial endocarditis, and atheromatous plaque formation in the internal cerotic artery. Common risk factors on the other hand are diabetes, high cholesterol, high BP, and smoking.

Learning Point
Syncope, or fainting, is due to sudden reductions in cardiac output. It can be due to physiological and pathological factors too. The commonest cause of fainting is emotional shock or pain. Autonomic overactivity in response to emotional shock or pain may cause vasodilation and inappropriate slowing of the pulse and then decrease the blood pressure and cerebral perfusion. Some common heart disorders, such as cardiac arrhythmias can lead to fainting. For example, bradyarrhythmias, tachyarrhythmias, and aortic stenosis are some predisposing factors to syncope.

Table 7.3 Comparison of carotid involvement and vertebrobasilar involvement

Carotid involvement	Vertebrobasilar involvement
Transient loss of vision in one eye due to emboli in the retinal artery	Diplopia, vertigo, nausea
	Choking and dysarthria
Aphasia	Ataxia
Hemiparesis	Hemisensory loss
Hemisensory loss	Hemianopia
Hemianopia	Transient global amnesia
	Tetraparesis

Some patients suffer from a condition called a Stokes-Adams attack. This is a collapse without warning associated with a loss of consciousness. Stokes-Adams attacks are typically associated with complete heart block. Patient's loss of consciousness is abrupt, and the skin colour is pale, they are pulseless, their respiration continues and on recovery the patient becomes flushed. Attack usually lasts for about 30 s.

A typical hypoglycaemic attack also involves dizziness, weakness, hunger, tremor, sweating, palpitations, and a rapid or irregular heart rate. A hypoglycaemic attack is associated with diabetes, gastrointestinal disorders, liver disorders, thyroid disorders, and drug interaction.

(c) Dizziness and Vertigo

The terms *dizziness* and *vertigo* are often used together but have different meanings. *Vertigo* is often accompanied by *deafness, tinnitus* (tinnitus is the perception of abnormal ringing noise within the ear or head) and *nystagmus* (nystagmus is the involuntary oscillation of the eyelids and movement of the eyes. It is accompanied with dizziness and sensitivity to light). *Dizziness*, on the other hand, is an ill-defined sense of disequilibrium, usually without any objective evidence of imbalance. Vertigo can be described as a hallucination of movement and sense of rotation, either of the body or of the environment.

Learning Point
Common causes of vertigo

Meniere's disease
Ethyl alcohol
Migraine
Temporal lobe epilepsy
Vestibular neuronitis (acute labyrinthitis)
Drugs (gentamicin, anticonvulsants)
Multiple sclerosis
Cerebellar and cerebello-pontine angle lesions
Ischaemia of brain stem (see "blackouts")
Benign positional vertigo

Meniere's syndrome is a disorder characterized by recurrent attacks of vertigo, tinnitus, and deafness of unknown cause and is associated with increased pressure in the labyrinths. Attacks recur over months or years resulting in deafness.

(d) Walking Difficulties

Walking difficulties can be caused by various neurological diseases. Common walking difficulties affecting gait and balance include:

Ataxia: This condition involves a loss of muscle control, leading to uncoordinated movements and balance issues.

Parkinson's Disease: Known for causing tremors and slow movements, Parkinson's can also lead to a stiff, shuffling gait.

Multiple Sclerosis (MS): MS can cause muscle weakness and coordination problems, making walking difficult.

Cerebral Palsy: This condition affects muscle tone and movement, often resulting in gait abnormalities.

Disorders of the Cerebellum: Conditions affecting the cerebellum can disrupt balance and coordination, impacting walking ability.

Functional Movement Disorders: These disorders can mimic other neurological conditions but are not caused by a disease of the nervous system.

(e) Visual Problems

Neurological disorders can indeed cause a variety of visual problems. Common conditions and their associated visual issues involved:

Optic Neuritis: This involves inflammation of the optic nerve, often linked to multiple sclerosis. Symptoms include blurry vision, pain when moving the eye, and loss of colour contrast.

Stroke: A stroke can lead to vision problems such as blurred vision, double vision, or loss of visual fields. It can also affect depth perception and visual understanding.

Migraine: Migraines can cause temporary visual disturbances known as aura, which may include flashing lights, spots, or zig-zag patterns.

Parkinson's Disease: This condition can affect the connection between the eyes and the brain, leading to difficulties with visual processing.

Traumatic Brain Injury (TBI): TBI can result in light sensitivity, double vision, blurry vision, or even blindness, depending on the severity and location of the injury.

Diabetic Retinopathy: This is a complication of diabetes that affects the blood vessels in the retina, leading to vision loss.

Below are the short neurological examination lists (Table 7.4).

Learning Point

Table 7.4 The short neurological examination lists

General features and cerebral cortex	Examination of the upper limbs
General demeanour	Posture of outstretched arms
Speech	Wasting, fasciculation
Gait	Power, tone
Arm swinging	Coordination
Examination of the cranial nerves	Reflexes
Fundi	*Examination of lower limbs*
Pupils	Power (especially hip flexion, ankle dorsiflexion) tone
Visual fields	Reflexes
Eye movements	Plantar responses
Facial movements	Co-ordination
Facial sensations	*Sensation*
Tongue movements	Ask the patient to test the area indicated for light touch, pinprick, and position sense

7.2.1 Cranial Nerves

The cranial nerves emerge from the central nervous system within the head rather than from the vertebral column. There are 12 pairs.

The *1st pair of cranial* nerve or the olfactory nerve innervates the tongue. They carry impulses from the epithelium of the nasal cavity to the olfactory cortex in the temporal lobe of the cerebral hemisphere. The 1st cranial nerve pair is sensory, and lesion or damage of this nerve can lead to loss of sense of smell called anosmia.

The *2nd pair of cranial* nerve is the optic nerve which is also sensory and transports visual information to the retina of the eye where the optic nerve is situated and then to the visual cortex in the occipital lobe. They enter the cranial cavity and converge at the optic chiasma, the optic tracts pass through the thalamus to terminate to the visual cortex. Damage to the optic nerves can cause blindness and damage to the optic tracts distal to the chiasma can cause visual field defects. Hemianopia is partial or complete loss of halves of the two visual fields and quadrantanopia is partial or complete loss quarters of the two visual fields. This can be found in physical examination if the patient has a history of optic neuritis which is inflammation of the optic nerve but also in demyelinating-inflammatory diseases such as optic atrophy. In demyelinating-inflammatory diseases there is axon degeneration of the optic nerve and this pathology can be found in multiple sclerosis, ischaemic optic neuropathy, and other conditions.

Papilloedema can also cause problems with visual fields because of optic disc swelling due to raised intracranial pressure. For example, in cerebral tumour and benign intracranial hypertension.

The 3rd cranial nerve (III) or *Oculomotor, 4th* cranial nerve (IV) or trochlear and *6th cranial nerves (VI) or* abducens are motor, somatic, and parasympathetic nerves which originate from the mid-brain. The motor somatic fibres innervate four of the external muscles of the eye and the muscle that raises the upper eyelid. The parasympathetic fibres innervate the muscle that controls the size of the pupil and the shape of the lens. They also control the position of the eyeballs, and the Oculomotor controls the size of the pupils as well as the position of the eyelids. Two conditions that involve the oculomotor or 3rd cranial nerve is *strabismus (squint), diplopia, eyelid drooping (ptosis)*. Strabismus is when the axes of the eyes are no longer parallel and diplopia is when the patient complains of double vision.

The 4th cranial nerve or the Trochlear is motor and innervates <u>superior oblique muscle</u> of the eyeball and the 6th or Abducens (VI) are also motor and arises in the pons varolii and innervates <u>ipsilateral lateral rectus muscle</u>. The 3rd cranial nerve or Oculomotor innervates the rest of the ocular muscles.

The *5th cranial nerve (V)* or *the trigeminal nerve* has both motor and sensory functions. In terms of motor function it innervates the temporalis muscle and the masseter muscles which enable the jaw movement. For example, the jaw opening and clenching. It is the largest cranial nerve and runs from the pons varolii and supplies the head and the face. In terms of sensory function, the trigeminal nerve has three sensory divisions:

(a) The ophthalmic which carries sensory information from the anterior scalp, forehead, lacrimal glands, upper eyelids, nose, cornea, and nasal mucosa.
(b) The maxillary which carries sensory information from lower eyelids, upper gums, teeth, lips and the cheeks.
(c) The mandibular from the lower gums, teeth, chin, and tongue and pinna of the ear.

On physical examination, the main features associated with 5th nerve lesion(s) are selective loss of facial pain, temperature, weak, or absent mastication. For example, trigeminal neuralgia is a condition of unknown cause which can manifest with facial pain, and it may be precipitated by simple stimuli such as brushing teeth, eating, and cold air.

Other types of facial pain are commonly caused by disorders of the teeth, temporomandibular joint, sinuses, and trauma. There are important syndromes that cause facial pain including (Table 7.5):

- Migrainous neuralgia (cluster headaches)—distinct from migraine despite its name
- Trigeminal neuralgia
- Post-herpetic neuralgia
- Temporal arteritis

Temporal arteritis is an important cause of facial pain affecting people over 60 years of age. Temporal arteritis, although it is not due to damage to the trigeminal nerve, is worth considering when assessing a patient with facial pain. Temporal arteritis is due to granulomas (chronic inflammatory lesions) affecting the arteries. This is related to a condition called polymyalgia. Patients may complain of:

Table 7.5 Comparison of migrainous neuralgia, trigeminal neuralgia, and postherpetic neuralgia

Migrainous neuralgia	Trigeminal neuralgia	Postherpetic neuralgia
Severe pain that wakes the patient at night Involves ophthalmic, mandibular, and maxillary areas Occurs in bouts of weeks or months Always unilateral pain Commoner in males in their 30s–40s Freedom of pain between attacks	Shock-like short paroxysms of pain Normally involves mandibular and maxillary area Commoner in middle-aged women Provoked by trivial stimuli (jaw-movements, cold)	Continuous, burning pain Virtually, all patients become depressed

- Headache—over the temporal region
- Pain in the face, jaw, and mouth
- Visual loss due to inflammation of the arteries supplying the retina

Systemic features associated with polymyalgia, including generalized limb pains, proximal limb girdle pain and tenderness, weight loss, sweating, malaise, and joint effusions. It is essential to be aware of this condition, since delay in diagnosis can result in permanent blindness. High-dose steroids appear to be the only treatment that works.

The *7th cranial* nerve or facial nerve (VII) is sensory, motor, and parasympathetic. They also originate from the pons varolii. The sensory fibres carry impulses to the anterior two thirds of the tongue taste and the sensation of the pharynx. The parasympathetic fibres supply the salivary glands, lacrimal glands and the glands of the nasal mucosa. While the motor innervates the facial muscles and controls facial expression except jaw movement.

Bell's palsy is a common lower motor neurone disorder involving the facial nerve on one side of the face. It is believed to be due to a virus and the clinical features include one-sided facial weakness, loss of forehead furrowing, eye closure, mouth elevation, drooping of the face, and drooling.

Upper motor neurone lesion predominantly affects the opposite lower face because there is bilateral innervation of the muscle of the upper part of the face. Lower motor neurone lesion weakness of the upper and lower face on the affected side in the face can help you distinguish between an upper and lower motor neurone lesion of the 7th nerve.

The 8th cranial nerve or vestibulocochlear (acoustic) nerve (VIII) has two main branches, the Vestibular and Cochlear branch. The Vestibular branch carries impulses from the semi-circular canals to the cerebellum and is responsible for balance, posture, and equilibrium. The Cochlear branches carry impulses from the organ of Corti to the auditory cortex in the temporal lobe and it is for hearing.

Common symptoms associated with damage to these branches are also:

- Vertigo
- Nystagmus
- Tinnitus
- Sensorineural hearing loss

The *9th cranial nerve* or the glossopharyngeal (IX) is motor, sensory and parasympathetic and originates in the medulla olongata. The parasympathetic fibres stimulate the secretion of saliva from the parotid glands. The motor fibres innervate the tongue, pharynx and are concerned with swallowing and gag reflex. The sensory fibres transmit taste impulses from the back of the tongue and nasopharynx to the cortex. It is also responsible for the gag reflex and the posterior one third of tongue taste. The 9th supplies the voluntary muscle for swallowing and phonation and the sensation behind ear and part of external ear canal.

The *10th cranial nerves* (X) or vagus nerves are parasympathetic, motor and sensory and they start in the medulla oblongata extend down the neck and innervate muscles and glands to the pharynx, larynx, trachea, lungs, and heart they pass on the abdomen to supply the viscera. The sensory fibres carry impulses to the brain from these structures. Damage to the 9th and 10th nerve is associated with difficulty with swallowing, choking, and phonation.

The 11th cranial nerve (XI) or accessory is motor and originates from medulla oblongata. They innervate the sternomastoid muscle which turns the head and the trapezius muscle which shrugs the shoulders.

The 12th cranial nerve (XII) or the hypoglossal cranial nerves are also motor and controls the tongue appearance and movement.

7.2.2 Part 2: Case Studies

Each individual case study consists of a summary of the patient's clinical presentation starting with a list of diagnostic features and any other clinical details that may be important for a differential diagnosis. Becoming competent at interpreting signs and symptoms depends on seeing as many examples as possible and discussing them with a senior colleague. You may wish to use this chapter as a guide to build a comprehensive collection of your own. We have endeavoured to include commonly encountered case studies as well as less common findings which are of clinical importance. Here we include case studies which feature clinical sign sand symptoms that a competent practitioner should be able to recognize and diagnose.

Case Study 1
Mark is a 68-year-old senior partner in a law firm. While eating dinner Mark experienced sudden onset slurring of speech, had facial droop on his right-hand side with weakness in right side upper and lower limbs. Mark's wife spotted this onset of symptoms and immediately called for an ambulance, which arrived within 10 min.

On presentation in the emergency department, because Mark is still somewhat confused, his wife is asked to provide information on the patient's history. His wife reports that her husband had had an episode of sudden-onset numbness and tingling in the right limb, with slight confusion and slurred speech, 3 days previously. The episode lasted only 5 min. Additional information provided by his wife indicates that Mark has been treated for hypertension for 10 years but notes that he is often not compliant with his antihypertensive medicine, a diuretic. The patient has never smoked, but drinks occasionally, and is of normal weight.

On general examination, he was confused. The pulse was 82 per min regular, the blood pressure was 150/90 mmHg. His speech was slurred.

- Comment on the 10-year history of hypertension and that he is often not compliant with his antihypertensive medicine.

  Answer:

  Patient has two significant risk factors for stroke; one is a long history of hypertension. More than two-thirds of individuals older than 65 years of age are hypertensive, and it is important for individuals with hypertension to have regular blood pressure screening and to maintain a blood pressure of less than 140/90 mmHg. Antihypertension therapy has been found to reduce the incidence of stroke. Patient's noncompliance with his antihypertension medicine indicated that his blood pressure was not controlled.

- Comment on the episode of sudden-onset numbness and tingling in the right limb, with slight confusion and slurred speech, 3 days previously.

  Answer:

  Patient's previous episode of numbness, confusion, and slurred speech appears to be evidence of a TIA, another substantial risk factor for stroke. Research has shown that approximately 5% of patients will have an ischemic stroke within 7 days after a TIA. In addition, the risk of stroke within 7 days is doubled for patients with TIAs who did not seek treatment. As is the case for many individuals who have a TIA, Patient did not seek medical attention because the clinical symptoms resolved quickly. However, research findings indicate that urgent treatment should be provided for TIAs, as early treatment for TIA and minor stroke has been shown to reduce the risk of early recurrent stroke by 80%.

- Based on the results of the history, choose and describe the neurological exams you will perform in order to localize the lesion responsible for the clinical presentation of this patient.

  Answer:

  The patient had the acute onset of right-sided weakness and inability to speak. The temporal profile of his illness is most consistent with a vascular event or a stroke.

  Cranial Nerves: Right CN 7 motor deficit—upper motor neuron.

  Motor System:

  Right pronator drift

  Right side of body weakness and tone change

Right side of body hyperreflexia
Right Babinski
Coordination: Right upper and lower extremity incoordination
Gait: Abnormal spastic gait.

Case Study 2

John, a 32-year-old software engineer, began noticing subtle changes in his motor skills and overall physical condition over the past year. John has no significant past medical history, he is a non-smoker, and occasionally drinks alcohol with his mates at his local pub.

John experienced a slight tremor in his right hand, particularly noticeable when at rest. This tremor often worsened during periods of stress. He also reported a general slowness in movement, making everyday tasks like typing and buttoning his shirt more challenging.

John felt stiffness in his arms and legs, which did not improve with movement. This stiffness was particularly pronounced in the mornings. The past few weeks John had difficulty maintaining his balance, leading to occasional falls and a noticeable stoop in his posture. His colleague noticed that his handwriting had become smaller and more cramped over time.

John also experienced constipation, sleep disturbances, and a reduced sense of smell in the past month or so.

- Comment on the changes in his mobility and speech noted in the past few weeks.
- Comment on the occasional falls and noticeable stoop in his posture, what may be the cause for these?
- Based on the history, choose and describe the neurological exams you will perform in order to localize the lesion responsible for the clinical presentation of this patient.

Case Study 3

Michael, a 48-year-old accountant, experienced sudden onset of neurological symptoms while at work. His colleague, who was with Michael at the office, noticed that Michael had weakness on the right side of his body, affecting his arm and leg and that his right side of the face appeared to droop. Michael had had trouble speaking and his speech was slurred. Michael seemed confused and had difficulty understanding what others were saying.

- Comment on the changes in his face and speech, what do you think the cause may be?
- Michael complained of a sudden, severe headache with no known cause can you think of a possible reason for this?
- Based on the main complaint of this patient, choose and describe the neurological exams you will perform in order to localize the lesion responsible for the clinical presentation of this patient.

Case Study 4

Sarah, a 45-year-old teacher, began noticing progressive weakness and muscle atrophy over the past year. Initially, Sarah experienced weakness in her hands, making it difficult to grip objects and write. She also noticed significant muscle wasting in her arms and legs and reported involuntary muscle twitches, particularly in her arms and legs.

Sarah has also trouble articulating words and often had trouble swallowing, leading to frequent choking and weight loss.

- Comment on the changes Sarah has noticed in her body, what do you think the cause may be?
- Sarah has complained of having trouble articulating herself and trouble swallowing, can you think of a possible reason for this?
- Based on the main complaint of this patient, choose and describe the neurological exams you will perform to localize the lesion responsible for the clinical presentation of this patient.

Case Study 5

Emily, a 52-year-old marketing executive, began experiencing a range of neurological symptoms over the past few months. Emily reported frequent, severe headaches that were different from her usual migraines and a week ago she experienced a sudden seizure while at work, which prompted her colleagues to call emergency services. Emily noticed blurred vision and occasional double vision. She had also found it difficult concentrating and felt increasingly confused. Her speech became slurred, and she had trouble finding words. Emily also experiences weakness on her left side, affecting her arm and leg.

- Comment on the headaches Emily has been suffering in the past few weeks, what do you think is going on?
- Emily has complained of having double vision, is this a significant finding?
- Based on the main complaint of this patient, choose and describe the neurological exams you will perform to localize the lesion responsible for the clinical presentation of this patient.

Case Study 6

James, a 50-year-old construction worker, began experiencing a range of neurological symptoms over the past few months. James noticed progressive weakness in his right arm and leg, making it difficult to perform tasks at work. He experienced increased muscle tone and stiffness, particularly in his right limbs.

- Comment on the changes James has noticed in his body, why do you think he experiences such symptoms?
- James has complained of weakness and stiffness, can you think of a possible reason for this?

- Based on the main complaint of this patient, choose and describe the neurological exams you will perform to localize the lesion responsible for the clinical presentation of this patient.

7.2.3   Part 3: Neurological Physical Examination Technique

The nervous system examination is complex and unlike other systems there are a much larger number of physical signs that may need to be picked upon clinical examination. The problem however for many learners may be the lack of opportunity to acquire and practise the necessary skills and to learn to take a careful and accurate history. A detailed neurological examination can be time-consuming and it may not be indicated in many patients, but if abnormalities are detected in patients they should be referred without delay to a medical specialist.

Upper Nervous System Examination
Introduction (WIPE)
Wash hands
Introduce yourself
Position
Explain the procedure

Mental Status: Assess cognition, orientation, memory, and language during history taking.
Cranial Nerves: Test visual fields, pupil reactions, eye movements, facial strength, and lower cranial nerves if necessary. Please see below detailed physical examination of the cranial nerves.
Motor Examination:
- Inspection: Look for involuntary movements, muscle wasting, and asymmetry.
- Tone: Assess muscle tone for spasticity or rigidity.
- Strength: Test muscle strength through functional tasks.
- Reflexes: Check for hyperreflexia or abnormal reflexes like the Babinski sign.
Tremor (observe muscular movement)

Coordination
Coordination: Evaluate coordination through tasks like finger-to-nose and heel-to-shin tests
Romberg test is used to assess a person's balance and proprioception (the body's ability to sense its position and movement). The test helps determine if balance issues are related to problems with the dorsal column pathway of the brain and spinal cord, which controls proprioception.

The patient stands with their feet together and arms at their sides or crossed in front of them.

The test is performed in two parts: first with the eyes open, and then with the eyes closed.

The healthcare provider observes the patient for any signs of imbalance, such as swaying or falling.

Finger-nose
Heel-shin
Rapid alternating movement

Gait (observe walking)

Gait and Station: Observe the patient's walking pattern and ability to maintain balance

Motor System
Upper limb wasting/fasciculation
Upper limb tone
Upper limb power
Lower limb wasting/fasciculation
Lower limb tone
Lower limb power
Tendon jerks (use the patella)
Plantar responses

Sensory System
Sensory Examination: Focus on areas of reported symptoms, testing for touch, pain, temperature, and proprioception

Upper limb vibration/position sense (use tunic fork for vibration and move the joints for position sense)
Upper limb light touch
Upper limb pinprick
Lower limb vibration/position sense (use tunic fork for vibration and move the joints for position sense)
Lower limb light touch
Lower limb pinprick

Lower Nervous System Examination
Introduction (WIPE)
Wash hands
Introduce yourself
Position
Explain the procedure

Mental Status: Assess cognition, orientation, memory, and language during history taking.

Cranial Nerves: Test visual fields, pupil reactions, eye movements, facial strength, and lower cranial nerves if necessary. Please see below detailed physical examination of the cranial nerves.

Motor Examination

- Inspection: Look for muscle wasting, fasciculations, and asymmetry.
- Tone: Assess muscle tone for spasticity, rigidity, or hypotonia.
- Strength: Test muscle strength in the lower limbs.
- Reflexes: Check for hyperreflexia, hyporeflexia, or areflexia, including the plantar reflex (Babinski sign).

Tremor (observe muscular movement)

Coordination

Coordination: Evaluate coordination through tasks like finger-to-nose and heel-to-shin tests

Romberg test
Finger-nose
Heel-shin
Rapid alternating movement

Gait (observe walking)
Gait and Station: Assess walking pattern, balance, and any signs of foot drop.

Motor System

Upper limb wasting/fasciculation
Upper limb tone
Upper limb power
Lower limb wasting/fasciculation
Lower limb tone
Lower limb power
Tendon jerks (use the patella)
Plantar responses

Sensory System

Sensory Examination: Focus on areas of reported symptoms, testing for touch, pain, temperature, and proprioception in the lower limbs

Upper limb vibration/position sense (use tunic fork for vibration and move the joints for position sense)
Upper limb light touch
Upper limb pinprick

Lower limb vibration/position sense (use tunic fork for vibration and move the
   joints for position sense)
Lower limb light touch
Lower limb pinprick

These steps help in identifying and localizing neurological issues, ensuring a
comprehensive assessment of the nervous system.

7.2.4   Physical Examination Technique for Cranial Nerves

Introduction (WIPE)
Wash hands
Introduce yourself
Position patient (make sure the patient is sitting squarely across you)
Observe the face for:
- Ptosis
- Strabismus
- Facial drop
- Articulation of words
- Abnormal eye position
- Abnormal or asymmetrical pupils

Testing the 1st cranial nerve or the olfactory cranial nerve
- Ask the patient to close their eyes and put in front of them a cup of coffee or
  orange juice. Ask them can they smell it?
- Have they noticed any changes in their smell?

Testing the 2nd cranial nerve or optic nerve
- Optic nerve: check for visual acuity so ask them to read your ID badge.
- Assess their visual fields by asking:
  (a) them to close their L eye and lock their eye with yours.
  (b) Then show them the tips of your fingers pretending there is a glass between
      the two of you. Ask them if they can see the tips of your fingers? Give them
      at least five spooks.
  (c) Then swap eyes and check the other side for visual fields.
- Check for colour vision by using either the Ishihara Charts.

**Testing the 3rd cranial nerve or oculomotor, the 4th or Trochlear and 6th or
Abducens**
- Inspect pupils for size and shape and eyelids.
- Assessing pupil reflexes:
  (a) Shield the other eye effectively.
  (b) Shield the non-examined eye.

- (c) Move light beam abruptly in from the side, or switch on from the front.
- (d) Direct reflex—ipsilateral pupil constricts.
- (e) Consensual reflex—contralateral pupil constricts. Direct response—constriction of pupil to light shone into that eye. Consensual response—constriction of pupil to light shone in the opposite eye.
- Assessing for accommodation:
  - (a) Ask the patient to fix on a distant object and then to focus on finger held about 10 cm from face. Keep target high or eyelids will obscure the pupil.
  - (b) The eyes should converge.
  - (c) The pupils should constrict equally.
- Assessing from the visual fields:
  The "bedside" test: face the patient at a distance of about 1 m. Keep the patient's visual background uncluttered, with light behind the patient.
  To test the right eye:
  - (a) Close or cover your right eye. Say "cover your left eye and look at my left eye". This matches the visual fields.
  - (b) Ensure the patient does not look away from your eye.
  - (c) Keeping in a plane midway between you and the patient, bring a red or white pin head from the extreme of vision (arm's length) in towards the pupil.
  - (d) Test each quadrant using diagonal track bisecting the quadrant. Establish rough boundary then define with slower target movements.
  - (e) Ask the patient to indicate when they first appreciate the red or white ball entering their visual field.
  - (f) Compare this to your own detection.
  - (g) Produce a more detailed "map" of a defect by increasing the number of spokes used.
  - (h) The field is limited superiorly by the supra-orbital ridge and medially by the nose.
  - (i) Any defect should be assessed formally.
- Assessing eye movement
  - (a) Hold a pen or similar object 50 cm from the patient in the midline and on a level with the patient's eyes.
  - (b) Lateral gaze—vertical target. Up/down gaze—horizontal target.
  - (c) Ask the patient to follow object ("with your eyes"), keeping head still, and to report any double vision.
  - (d) Move the object slowly.
  - (e) Side to side.
  - (f) Up and down centrally, then at extremes of lateral gaze.
  - (g) Stay in binocular range.
  - (h) Observe for nystagmus.

Testing for 5th cranial nerve or the trigeminal
- (a) Ask the patient to close their eyes and then take a wisp of cotton and touch their forehead on both sides
- (b) Then on their cheeks and chin on both sides

(c) Ask the patient if they feel the same on both sides?

(d) We may want to check corneal reflex too but this not a routine test nurses do.

Testing for 7th cranial nerve or facial nerve

(a) Ask the patient to scrunch up their eye and gently pull their eyelid to assess strength of muscle tone.

(b) Ask them to say "Aaaa" to see the uvula and determine if there is no pulling on one side, insect the fauna and the dentation of the patient.

(c) Use the orange stick at the back of the throat for gag reflex.

(d) Ask them to stick their tongue and move it side to side and note any changes.

(e) Ask them to purse their lips and keep their tongue between their teeth at the bottom jaw.

(f) Finally, put your two fingers on their jaw and gently apply the patella to see a slight jerk.

Testing for 8th cranial nerve or the vestibulocochlear nerve

Rinne's test

- Place base of tuning fork on mastoid process.
- Confirm it can be heard.
- Then immediately place prongs in front of external auditory meatus.
- Ask the patient which is louder—"behind the ear or in front?" (the latter is normal).
- Use a 512 Hz tuning fork, set it vibrating by gently tapping on your knee.
- Place on the mastoid process (bone conduction).
- Ask the person to tell you when they can no longer "hear" the sound.
- Then place forks in front of ear directly over the auditory meatus (air conduction).
- Ask the patient again if they can hear the sound (normally louder as air conduction is better than bone conduction).

Weber test

- Hold the base of the 512 Hz tuning fork on the vertex of the patient's head.
- Ask which ear seems to hear it louder.

Testing for 9th cranial nerve or glossopharyngeal and 10th cranial nerve or vagus

- Look at the uvula (use tongue depressor if necessary)
- Ask patient to say "Ahh"
- Deviation to one side indicates weakness on the other side (muscle normally "pulls")
- Upper or lower motor neurone lesion
- Does not move on saying "Ahh" or gag
- Bilateral palatal muscle paresis

Testing the 11th nerve or accessory sternomastoid

- Ask patient to turn their head to one side.
- Stabilize patient with shoulder counterpressure.
- Then put your hand against the patient's chin and cheek and ask the patient to resist rotating their head back to midline.

- Watch the opposite sternomastoid contract, and test its power.
- Check the Trapezius so ask the patient to shrug shoulders, push down against movement. Do one side at a time.

Testing the 12th cranial nerve or the hypoglossal
- Put out tongue:

Deviation to one side indicates weakness on that side (tongue muscle "pushes").

Conclusion
- Wash hands
- Review observation chart
- Record examination findings and refer on

7.3   Part 4: The Motor and Sensory Systems

In this part of the chapter, we revisit basic anatomy and physiology of the nervous system and identify the clinical signs and symptoms diagnostic of neurological diseases and disorders. The learning objectives for this part of the chapter are as follows:

Learning Objectives
By the end of the lesson, you will be able to:

Identify the essential structures and functions of the brain, and the cortex.
Discuss general symptoms and signs of diseases and disorders of cranial nerve and the cortex and identify the common symptoms of neurological disorders and diseases associated with cranial nerve and cortical lesions
Compare and discuss common neurological symptoms to help make differential diagnoses.

The Motor System
The motor system includes the following structures:

Motor Cortex: This area of the brain is responsible for generating neural impulses that control the execution of movement. It works closely with the sensory cortex to integrate sensory information and coordinate precise movements.

Basal Ganglia: These structures help regulate voluntary motor movements, procedural learning, and routine behaviours. They influence movement through the extrapyramidal system, which is involved in the modulation and control of motor activity.

Brain Stem Tracts: Some tracts originating in the brain stem are involved in motor control. They play a role in transmitting motor signals from the brain to the spinal cord and muscles and are crucial for maintaining posture and balance.

Cerebellum: The cerebellum is essential for motor control. It does not initiate movement but contributes to coordination, precision, and accurate timing. It receives input from sensory systems and other parts of the brain and spinal cord and integrates this information to fine-tune motor activity.

Learning Point

The motor pathway is a complex network that transmits signals from the brain to the muscles to produce movement.

Motor Cortex: The journey begins in the motor cortex, where motor commands are generated. This area of the brain is responsible for planning, controlling, and executing voluntary movements.

Pyramidal Tracts: These commands travel down through the pyramidal tracts, which include the corticospinal and corticobulbar tracts. The corticospinal tract carries signals to the spinal cord, while the corticobulbar tract transmits signals to the brainstem.

Brainstem and Spinal Cord: In the brainstem, some motor signals are relayed to cranial nerves that control muscles in the face and neck. The corticospinal tract continues down to the spinal cord, where it synapses with motor neurons.

Motor Neurons: These neurons in the spinal cord then transmit the signals to the muscles. The motor neurons release neurotransmitters that bind to receptors on muscle fibres, causing them to contract.

Basal Ganglia and Cerebellum: These structures play a crucial role in refining and coordinating movements. The basal ganglia help regulate the initiation and smooth execution of movements, while the cerebellum ensures precision and timing.

Muscle Contraction: Finally, the signals reach the muscles, resulting in movement. The coordinated activity of multiple muscles allows for smooth and purposeful actions. This pathway ensures that voluntary movements are precise, coordinated, and appropriately timed.

The Pyramidal System

The pyramidal system, also known as the corticospinal tract, is a major neural pathway that controls voluntary motor movements. The pyramidal system originates in the motor cortex, which is located in the precentral gyrus of the brain. The neurons in this system, called upper motor neurons (UMN), send long fibres (axons) that travel through the corona radiata and internal capsule. These fibres then pass through the midbrain, pons, and medulla.

In the medulla, most of these fibres cross over (decussate) to the opposite side of the body. This crossing is why each hemisphere of the brain controls the opposite side of the body.

After crossing, the fibres continue down the spinal cord, forming the lateral and ventral corticospinal tracts. The UMN fibres eventually connect to lower motor neurons (LMN) either directly or through interneurons. These LMN are located in the anterior horn of the spinal cord and the motor nuclei of cranial nerves. The primary function of the pyramidal system is to stimulate LMN to produce voluntary muscle contractions, enabling precise and coordinated movements. The pyramidal system is essential for executing voluntary movements, such as writing, walking, and speaking.

The motor cortex is situated in the precentral gyrus and controls movement in the contralateral half of the body. The neurones of the motor cortex are called *upper motor neurones (UMN)*. They originate in the motor area (precentral gyrus), the premotor area (in front of the precentral gyrus), the sensory area, and part of the sensory association area. UMN have long fibres (axons) that pass through the corona radiata and internal capsule and then the midbrain and pons to reach the medulla. More than 90% of these fibres continue into the spinal cord, where they form the lateral and ventral corticospinal tracts. Most of these fibres (again about 75%) will cross over in the spinal cord to the other side. The majority of UMN fibres then terminate on internuncial (connecting) neurones, which in turn connect to the motor nuclei (neurones) of the cranial nerves and the anterior horn cells in the spinal cord. The motor nuclei of the cranial nerves and the anterior horn cells are called *lower motor neurones (LMN)*. Some UMN fibres bypass the internuncial neurones and connect directly to LMN. The upper motor neurones and the corticospinal tracts are referred to as the *pyramidal system*, which is concerned with stimulating the lower motor neurones to produce *voluntary muscle contraction*.

The Extrapyramidal System

The extrapyramidal system is a network of neurons that is part of the motor system, but it operates outside the pyramidal tracts. Below its components and functions are described in some detail:

Basal Ganglia: Includes structures like the caudate nucleus, putamen, and globus pallidus. These are crucial for regulating voluntary motor movements and procedural learning.

Cerebellum: Although primarily involved in coordination and precision of movements, it also interacts with the extrapyramidal system.

Brainstem Nuclei: Includes the red nucleus, substantia nigra, vestibular nuclei, and reticular formation. These nuclei play roles in motor control and modulation.

Tracts: The main tracts include the reticulospinal, vestibulospinal, rubrospinal, and tectospinal tracts, which connect various parts of the brain to the spinal cord.

Learning Point

The extrapyramidal system contributes to:

Posture Maintenance: Helps maintain and adjust posture.
Movement Coordination: Fine-tunes and adjusts voluntary movements to make them more precise and correct.
Reflex Control: Regulates reflex reactions.
Automatic Movements: Controls automatic voluntary movements like walking and riding a bicycle.
Involuntary Movement Inhibition: Inhibits involuntary movements to ensure smooth and coordinated actions.

The extrapyramidal system is essential for the smooth execution of movements and maintaining balance and posture. It works alongside the pyramidal system to ensure that movements are both voluntary and well-coordinated. In summary, the extrapyramidal system is a term that covers the basal ganglia and consists of:

- The corpus striatum—caudate nucleus and lentiform nucleus (globus pallidus, putamen)
- The substantia nigra
- The thalami
- The subthalamic nuclei

All these structures have interconnections to the cerebral cortex and cerebellum. Consequently, the functions of the extrapyramidal system include the initiation and fine control of movement. Disorders of the extrapyramidal system appear to involve alterations in neurotransmitter levels. For example, Parkinson's disease, the commonest disorder of the basal ganglia, is related to a reduction in dopamine in the substantia nigra and putamen.

The basal ganglia are in the basal forebrain and the midbrain. All of these structures receive connections from the cerebral cortex, the thalamus, and the reticular formation and there are also connections to the cerebellum. Outputs from the basal ganglia pass to the thalamus, pons, superior colliculus, and reticular formation. The major neurotransmitter in the basal ganglia is dopamine.

Consequently, the functions of the extrapyramidal system include the initiation and modification of muscular movement, integrating the components of skilled muscle movement. Disorders of the extrapyramidal system appear to involve alterations in neurotransmitter levels. For example, Parkinson's disease, the commonest disorder of the basal ganglia, is related to a reduction in dopamine in the substantia nigra and putamen.

The Tracts Descending from the Brainstem
These include the vestibulospinal and reticulospinal tracts. The vestibulospinal tracts end on LMN in the cervical spine. The reticulospinal tracts go to lower levels in the spinal cord. Both sets of tracts are responsible for sending signals for initiating movement. The reticulospinal tracts play a major role in the activation of coordinated walking. The vestibulospinal tracts are concerned with balance and their nuclei receive fibres from the cerebellum.

The Cerebellum
The cerebellum is a vital part of the brain located at the back, beneath the occipital lobes and behind the brainstem. The cerebellum structure and functions are:

The cerebellum is situated in the posterior cranial fossa, beneath the occipital lobes and behind the brainstem. It consists of two hemispheres connected by a central region called the vermis. The cerebellum has a highly folded surface, which increases its surface area.

Composed of three layers: the outer molecular layer, the middle Purkinje cell layer, and the inner granular layer. The cerebellum is connected to the brainstem via three pairs of cerebellar peduncles (superior, middle, and inferior), which facilitate communication with other parts of the brain.

Functions of the cerebellum include:

Coordination: The cerebellum is crucial for coordinating voluntary movements, ensuring they are smooth and precise.

Balance: It helps maintain balance and posture by processing sensory information from the inner ear and muscles.

Motor Learning: Involved in motor learning, allowing the body to adapt and refine movements through practice.

Timing and Rhythm: Plays a role in the timing and rhythm of movements, ensuring actions are appropriately timed.

Cognitive Functions: Recent research suggests the cerebellum may also contribute to certain cognitive functions, such as attention and language.

Damage to either hemisphere can result in similar types of motor and coordination problems but affecting different sides of the body.

Disorders affecting the right and left cerebellar hemispheres can lead to distinct symptom:

- Gait and posture disorders such as problems with coordination and balance either on the right or left side of the body and ataxia which is unsteady movements and difficulty with tasks requiring fine motor skills.
- Tremor or shaking during voluntary movements.
- Nystagmus is the involuntary eye movements, which can affect vision.

- Dysarthria—a halting and jerking speech.
- Hypotonia and slow reflexes (not helpful signs for diagnosis of cerebellar disease).

Damage to the vermis can result from various causes, including neurodegenerative diseases, alcohol use, and certain genetic conditions. Disorders of the vermis of the cerebellum will cause:

Loss of equilibrium, with difficulty in standing and sitting unsupported.

Ataxic gait is a type of abnormal walking pattern characterized by unsteady, irregular steps and a lack of coordination. People with ataxic gait often have difficulty walking in a straight line and may appear to stagger or sway. This condition is typically caused by damage to the cerebellum or its connections, which are responsible for coordinating muscle movements.

Vertigo is a sensation of spinning or feeling off balance, often making you feel like you or your surroundings are moving when they are not. It is typically a symptom of an underlying issue with the inner ear or brain.

Learning Point

Causes of Vertigo

***Inner Ear Problems*:**

- *Benign Paroxysmal Positional Vertigo* (BPPV): Caused by tiny calcium particles (canaliths) dislodging and collecting in the inner ear.
- *Meniere's Disease*: Associated with fluid buildup and changing pressure in the ear, leading to vertigo, tinnitus, and hearing loss.
- *Vestibular Neuritis or Labyrinthitis*: Inflammation of the inner ear or vestibular nerve, often due to viral infections.

Brain Issues:

- *Migraine*: Can cause episodes of vertigo.
- *Stroke*: Disruption of blood flow to the brain can lead to vertigo.
- *Tumours*: Growths in the brain can affect balance and cause vertigo.

Other Causes:

- *Head or Neck Injuries*: Trauma can disrupt the vestibular system.
- *Medications*: Certain drugs can have side effects that include vertigo.
- *Stress and Anxiety*: Can trigger vertigo or exacerbate existing symptoms.

Symptoms of Vertigo

- Spinning sensation
- Dizziness
- Nausea and vomiting

- Balance issues
- Abnormal eye movements (nystagmus)
- Ringing in the ears (tinnitus)

The following should be assessed:

Pyramidal system:
- Muscle appearance
- Gait (spastic, foot drop)
- Tone
- Muscle power
- Reflexes

Extrapyramidal system:
- Bradykinesia (reduced movement)
- Involuntary movements
- Gait (Parkinsonian)

Cerebellum:
- Speech (dysarthria)
- Balance and coordination
- Gait (ataxic)
- Eye movements (nystagmus)
- Tone
- Tremor (intention)

Muscle Appearance

An important feature you should look for during the assessment of the motor system is the appearance of muscles. Muscle wasting, fasciculation, and pseudohypertrophy are significant findings. Muscle wasting involves loss of muscle bulk. Fasciculation, on the other hand, is the spontaneous fine flicker or coarse twitch of the muscle fibres belonging to a single motor unit. Fasciculation and muscle wasting can be found in lower motor neurone disease. Pseudohypertrophy is caused by fat and connective tissue which infiltrates the muscle, so on inspection the muscle looks hypertrophic (larger).

Involuntary Movements

During inspection of the nervous system, we also look for tremor. *Physiological tremor* is found in all individuals when the hands are outstretched. In patients suffering from thyrotoxicosis, anxiety and fatigue, emotion, drug side effects, and drug or alcohol withdraw, it is noted that physiological tremor is increased.

Intention tremor is found in certain conditions such as cerebellar dysfunction. Intention tremor appears only when the limb is activated and often gets worse as the target is neared such as multiple sclerosis.

Rest tremors are most prominent at rest and may decrease or disappear with voluntary movement. They are associated with basal ganglia dysfunction such as Parkinson's disease.

Other involuntary movements include *Myoclonus* which is rapid, recurring muscle jerks, sudden, brief, unpredictable shock-like contractions.

Chorea is a brief, random movement that does not have the shock-like quality of myoclonus.

Athetosis is a slower still than chorea and becomes prominent during the performance of voluntary activity, twisting and writhing.

Hemibalismus is violent swing movements involving one side of the body.

Tics are frequent, compulsive, involuntary, stereotyped, and predictable repetition of the same movement.

Muscle Tone

Assessment of muscle tone is one of the most difficult parts of the neurological examination. You can assess the muscle tone by passively moving the patient's limbs and assessing the resistance of the muscle. Pathologically, muscle tone can increase (resistance increase) or decrease (resistance decrease). There are two types of muscle tone increases: spasticity and rigidity. Spasticity is tone increase where the resistance to passive movement initially increased then resistance decreased. This is also called the "clasp-knife phenomenon" and you can see this in upper motor neurone lesions such as stroke. Rigidity is a resistance increase which is uniform throughout the range of movement, and it may be slightly jerky or like "cogwheel" can be found in Parkinson's disease.

Muscle Power

Muscle power is the maximum strength a muscle can exert in a specific movement. When assessing muscle power, we evaluate the strength and/or the weakness of that muscle. With regard to muscle weakness, we should consider the following:

(a) Is the weakness confined to one limb or to one side of the body?
(b) Is the weakness static, progressive, or fluctuant?
(c) Is the weakness accompanied by a feeling of stiffness or is the affected limb floppy?

Some common causes of muscle weakness include:

Central nervous system disorders such as:

- Cerebral cortex stroke
- Brainstem stroke
- Spinal cord trauma
- Basal ganglia Parkinsonism (Parkinson's disease)
- Cerebellar stroke

Peripheral nervous system disorders such as:

- Lower motor neuron disease such as poliomyelitis
- Spinal nerves and Roots-Lumbar disc diseases
- Mononeuropathy trauma
- Polyneuropathy such as diabetes
- Neuromuscular junction such as myasthenia gravis, muscular dystrophy

Reflexes

Tendon reflexes are rapid involuntary motor responses to sensory input and they are controlled by the autonomic nervous system by acting on involuntary muscles. Tendon reflexes operate through spinal cord known as spinal reflexes but there is also some brain involvement through medulla oblongata. Some of the sites on the body where you would test for deep tendon reflexes are:

- Biceps reflex—Biceps tendon (C5, 6)
- Triceps reflex—Triceps tendon (C7, 8)
- Supinator reflex—Styloid process of radius (C5, 6)
- Knee jerk reflex—Patellar tendon (L3, 4)
- Ankle jerk reflex—Achilles tendon (S1,2)

In brackets the spinal cord segments mediating each of these reflexes are indicated.

Other reflexes include:

- Abdominal reflexes, which are cutaneous reflexes and extremely variable on the abdominal wall.
- Cremasteric reflex—elicited by stroking the upper inner aspect of the thigh resulting in upward movement of the testicle on the same side.
- Plantar response—elicited by using an instrument to stimulate the sole of the foot.

Gait (Spastic, Foot Drop)

Here are the five common pathological gaits observed in a physical assessment of the nervous system.

Spastic is the slow walking accompanied with stiff legs, the patient may be dragging his foot and experience weakness and stiffness of one leg if unilateral. This gait may be due to a cerebrovascular disorder (stroke).

The *foot-drop gait* is noted when the patient's leg flexes at hip more than usual while he is walking in order to prevent his toes from catching the floor. When his foot hits the ground, it looks like he is stamping. This gait may be due to peripheral neuropathy (this includes weakness and sensory loss).

Ataxic gait is observed when a patient is unsteady on standing and he adopts a broad base on walking. He also appears to be lurching from side-to-side. The cause of ataxic gait is usually cerebellar disease (tumour).

Waddling on the other hand is the gait that is observed when the patient is unable to tilt the pelvis and he is forced to swing each leg through to take the next step, this patient shows exaggerated lateral trunk movements. Waddling is caused by proximal muscle disorder (thyrotoxicosis).

Parkinsonian gait is associated with a stooped posture, difficulty in initiating movement, and small shuffling steps. Usually, this is caused by Parkinson's disease.

7.3.1   Sensory Pathway

The peripheral nerves carry sensation from nerve endings to the dorsal root ganglion and then to the spinal cord. Sensation is conveyed by two major sets of nerve fibres to the cortex:

- *Posterior columns*—which carry vibration, position, light touch, and two-point discrimination. The fibres travel to the medulla where they cross (decussate) and pass to the thalami and reticular formation. Fibres from these structures then relay the information to the cortex.

The *posterior columns*, also known as the *dorsal columns*, are part of the dorsal column-medial lemniscus pathway (DCML), a major sensory pathway in the central nervous system. Here is a detailed description:

> **Learning Point**
> The posterior columns are located in the dorsal (back) part of the spinal cord. They consist of two main bundles of nerve fibres:
>
> - *Fasciculus Gracilis*: Carries sensory information from the lower half of the body.
> - *Fasciculus Cuneatus*: Carries sensory information from the upper half of the body.

The posterior columns are responsible for transmitting specific types of sensory information:

- *Fine Touch*: Detailed touch sensations, such as texture and shape.
- *Vibration*: Sensations of vibration from the skin and joints.

- ***Proprioception***: Awareness of body position and movement.
- ***Two-Point Discrimination***: Ability to distinguish two closely spaced points on the skin.

Damage to the posterior columns can result in loss of fine touch, vibration, and proprioception, leading to sensory deficits and coordination problems.

- ***Spinothalamic tracts***—which carry pain and temperature. Fibres synapse in the posterior horn of the spinal cord, then cross to the other side of the cord and pass upwards as the spinothalamic tracts to the thalami and reticular formation. The ***spinothalamic tracts*** are part of the anterolateral system, which is crucial for transmitting sensory information related to pain, temperature, and crude touch from the body to the brain. The spinothalamic tracts are located in the anterolateral portion of the spinal cord.

There are two main tracts:

- ***Anterior Spinothalamic Tract***: Conveys crude touch and pressure.
- ***Lateral Spinothalamic Tract***: Conveys pain and temperature.

They are responsible for:

- ***Pain Sensation***: Detects and transmits pain signals.
- ***Temperature Sensation***: Conveys information about heat and cold.
- ***Crude Touch***: Transmits less detailed touch information, such as pressure and general tactile sensations. Damage to the spinothalamic tracts can result in loss of pain and temperature sensation on the opposite side of the body below the level of the lesion.

Interpretation of Symptoms and Signs of Sensory Lesions

The main symptoms of sensory lesions are *pins and needles (parasthaesia), numbness,* and *pain.*

Sensory symptoms include:

- Pain—peripheral nerve injuries cause a burning pain. Pain related to a peripheral nerve usually localizes to the distribution of the affected nerve on the skin (dermatome). In nerve root lesions, the pain follows the distribution corresponding to the muscles (myotome) or other deep structure (sclerotome) supplied by that nerve root.
- Parasthaesia (pins and needles).
- Numbness.

Patients commonly have difficulties in describing sensations such as paraesthesia and numbness and it is often difficult for the examiner to precisely localize the areas of sensory change. This indicates the general difficulty associated with sensory system examinations. Peripheral neuropathies and nerve injuries are the most common causes of pins and needles.

Peripheral Nerve Lesions (Peripheral Neuropathies)

Peripheral nerves contain motor, sensory and autonomic fibres and all of these can be affected in a peripheral neuropathy. The symptoms are felt in the distribution of the affected nerve. The **IMDISTAL** mnemonic is used to remember some common causes of peripheral neuropathies:

- Idiopathic, Inherited neurological disease
- Metabolic, Mechanical such as diabetes
- **Drugs**
- Infections
- Sarcoidosis
- Tumours
- Autoimmune disease
- Lack of vitamins such as Vitamin B_{12}

The Nervous System Examination

There is no doubt that the nervous system is complex and, unlike the other systems, there are a much larger number of physical signs that may need to be picked up on clinical examination. The problem, however, for many students has been the failure to acquire and practise the necessary skills and to learn to take a careful and accurate history—since the diagnosis can usually be made on the basis of the history alone. A detailed neurological examination is time-consuming and is not indicated in many patients. In fact, a short screening examination is all nurses and student nurses will generally need to do if abnormalities are detected, patients should be referred without delay to a medical specialist.

Clinical Applications

We are concerned here with differentiating between upper motor neurone (UMN), lower motor neurone (LMN) disorders, extrapyramidal and cerebellar disorders, and myopathy. In general, the following are assessed with regard to motor disorders:

- Muscle bulk—normal, reduced or evidence of wasting.
- Muscle tone—such as the amount of tension in the muscle at rest (normal muscles always have some tone). In disease the muscle tone is either increased or decreased.

- Tremor—present (intention or rest tremor) or absent.
- Fasciculation—fine "ripples" that can be seen under the skin overlying muscles. May be present or absent in disease.
- Muscle power—either normal or decreased in disease.
- Muscle coordination—may be normal or impaired in disease.
- Limb Reflexes—normal, reduced or absent or increased in disease.
- Plantar reflexes—these are elicited by scratching the underside of the foot with a pointed object. In normal people the plantar is flexor (the toes curl). Extensor plantar (toes go upward) are abnormal.
- Gait—normal or pathological gait.

7.3.2   Part 5: Focused Learning

Learning Activity 1

Can you answer the questions related to the following symptoms?
  Headaches are conveniently classified as follows:

- Psychogenic
- Migraine
- Hypertension
- Raised intracranial pressure (ICP)
- Cranial arteritis
- Extracranial causes

(a) Which of the above groups contain most patients?
  Answer:
  Migraine
(b) Complete Tension headache with Migraine:

  Answer:

	Tension headache	Migraine
Epidemiology; *Who gets it* *Age of onset*	*Adults, more often females*	*Teenagers and adults, more often females*
Pathogenesis:	*Accompanied by askeletal muscle contraction in neck, face and jaw.* *Vasodilation of the arterial bed.*	*Aura stage is associated with cerebral vasoconstriction.* *Headache stage is associated with extra cranial and meningeal vasodilation.*

	Tension headache	*Migraine*
Clinical pattern (plus associated features)	*Unilateral or bilateral* *Ache in temporal, occipital, parietal, frontal regions* *Pain may frequent changes in sites* *Dull, pressure like, a sense of fullness in the head, constricting pain like wearing a tight band* *Nausea and vomiting, loss of appetite* *Photophobia and phono phobia (rare)*	*Aura (15–20 min): variety of visual disturbances, may have numbness or tingling of face and arms, weakness of one side of the body* *Headache (4–72 h):* *Unilateral or generalized* *Located in temporal region* *Throbbing pain in one side of the head* *Pain worsens with daily activities* *Feeling sick* *Sweating, feeling hot or cold* *Tummy ache and diarrhoea* *Photophobia and phono phobia*

(c) Headache is quite commonly found in moderately severe hypertension but is of great significance in malignant hypertension. State the causes and mechanisms of headaches in these two situations:

Answer:

Moderately severe hypertension: arterioles constriction but normal pressure in capillaries.

Malignant hypertension: Blood pressure increases significantly within short time and systolic is 180 mmHg or above and diastolic is 120 mmHg or above, the pressure in capillaries will increase leading to cerebral oedema and increased intracranial pressure.

(d) Regarding extra cranial causes:

(i) Describe briefly the typical features of a headache following head injury.

Answer:

Unconsciousness

Persistent headache or worsen headache

Nausea and vomiting

Convulsions or seizures

Clear fluid from ears or nose

Drowsiness

Headache made worse by coughing and straining

(ii) Look up some extra cranial disorders that can causes headache.

Answer:

Nasal and sinus headache

Dental Pain

Aural Pain

Eye Pain

Learning Activity 2

(a) What questions would you ask an eyewitness if someone has a blackout? What questions would you ask the patient?
Answer:
Did they observe colour change?
What happened when the patient fell?
Did the patient complaint of a headache prior to losing consciousness?

Questions for patient:
Do they remember what happened?
Are they on any medication?

(b) Blackouts indicate the total dependence of the brain on a continuous supply of oxygen and glucose. It is essential to determine the predisposing factors for attacks of fainting. Common causes include:
Epilepsy
Cerebrovascular disease
Syncope
Hypoglycaemia
Severe fluid depletion after severe gastro-enteritis in previously healthy young people
Psychological problems
Which of the above categories is likely to be responsible for most causes of blackouts?
Answer:
Hypoglycaemia

(c) What predisposing factors should you consider when taking a history of a blackout?
Answer:
Low blood pressure
Low blood sugar

(d) Describe the typical symptoms and signs of a tonic-clonic epileptic seizure. List some other types of presentations of epilepsy.
Answer:
Tonic-clonic (grand mal) epileptic seizure:
Patients may have strange feeling or sensation, which is called an aura.
First phase is tonic: consciousness is lost, and the patient falls to the ground. The phase lasts 10–30 s during which the legs become extended, and the arms abducted, flexed at the elbows and wrists.
Second phase is a clonic jerking of the muscles. Incontinence of urine, dribbling from the mouth and tongue-biting. This usually lasts 1–5 min. The movements are initially rapid and then become slower.
Third phase is a coma phase: the patient is deeply unconscious, with complete muscular flaccidity. This state may last up to several hours.
Absence Seizures:
The absences usually last only a few seconds but may occur many times a day.

During the absence the child stops activity and eyes roll upward, eyelids flutter (3 per s), not responding to questions.
The child usually has no recall of the attack.

Learning Activity 3

(a) List some common sources for emboli to the brain and some common diseases and risk factors that may be associated with TIAs.

Answer:

Common sources:

- *Heart: myocardial infraction, atrial fibrillation, bacterial endocarditis*
- *Internal cerotic artery: atheromatous plaque formation*

Risk factors:

- *Diabetes*
- *High cholesterol*
- *High BP*
- *Smoking*

(b) Syncope, or fainting, is due to sudden reductions in cardiac output. It can be due to physiological and pathological factors.

    (i) The commonest cause of fainting is emotional shock or pain. What is the underlying mechanism?

Answer:

Autonomic overactivity in response to emotional shook or pain causes vasodilation and inappropriate slowing of the pulse and then decreases the blood pressure and cerebral perfusion.

    (ii) List some common heart disorders that can lead to fainting

Answer:

Cardiac arrhythmias: Bradyarrhythmias, Tachyarrhythmias

Aortic stenosis

    (iii) Some patients suffer from a condition called a Stokes-Adams attack. Define this and state the cause and typical clinical features.

Answer:

A Stokes-Adams attack is a collapse without warning associated with a loss of consciousness lasting a second not minutes.

Stokes Adams attacks are typically associated with complete heart block.

Patient loss of consciousness is abrupt, and the skin colour is pale and pulseless, respiration continues, on recovery the patient becomes flushed. Attack usually lasts for about 30 s.

(c) Give some reasons why hypoglycaemia may occur. Describe the typical features of a hypoglycaemic attack.

Answer:
Diabetes
Gastrointestinal disorders
Liver disorder
Thyroid disorders
Drug interaction
Typical features: dizziness, weakness, hunger, tremor, sweating, palpitations,
   and a rapid or irregular heart rate.

Learning Activity 4

The terms dizziness and vertigo are often used together, but actually have different
meanings. Vertigo is often accompanied by deafness, tinnitus, and nystagmus

(a) Define the terms, dizziness, vertigo, tinnitus, and nystagmus.
   Answer:
   Dizziness is an ill-defined sense of disequilibrium, usually without any objective
      evidence of imbalance.
   Vertigo is a hallucination of movement sense of rotation, either of the body or of
      the environment.
   Tinnitus is the perception of abnormal ringing noise wither in the ear or head.
   Nystagmus is the involuntary oscillation of the eye lids and movement of the
      eyes. It is accompanied with dizziness and sensitivity to light.
(b) The common causes of vertigo are listed in below:
   - Meniere's disease
   - Ethyl alcohol
   - Migraine
   - Temporal lobe epilepsy
   - Vestibular neuronitis (acute labyrinthitis)
   - Drugs (gentamicin, anticonvulsants)
   - Multiple sclerosis
   - Cerebellar lesions
   - Ischaemia of brain stem
   - Benign positional vertigo
(c) Look up the following causes of vertigo and give brief clinical descriptions:
   (i) Meniere's syndrome
   Answer:
   A disorder characterized by recurrent attacks of vertigo, tinnitus, and deafness
      of unknown cause and is associated with increased pressure in the laby-
      rinths. Attacks recur over months or years resulting in deafness. Orthodox
      treatment is unsatisfactory.
   (ii) Vestibular neuronitis (acute labyrinthitis)
   Answer:
   A common condition associated with vertigo, nystagmus, and vomiting, believed
      to occur following a viral infection of the labyrinth. The disturbance lasts for
      days or weeks and usually resolves completely.

(iii) Benign positional vertigo
Answer:
A disorder in which vertigo is precipitated by head movements. The attacks are transient and last for seconds or minutes. It may follow vestibular neuronitis.

Learning Activity 5

Answer the questions related to the following sections:

The cerebral cortex

(a) Disorders of the left cortex cause *aphasia (dysphasia), dysarthria, alexia (dyslexia)*, and *agraphia*. What do these terms mean?
Answer:
- *Aphasia (dysphasia) is inability to talk*
- *Dysarthria is inability to articulate words*
- *Alexia (dyslexia) is inability to read*
- *Agraphia is inability to write*

Disorders of the right cortex in right-handed people involve abnormalities of spatial perception (losing one's way in familiar surroundings, failure to draw simple shapes, etc.)

Learning Activity 6

Answer the following questions

(a) What is the name of the *1st cranial* nerve. What is meant by the term anosmia?
Answer:
- *Olfactory nerve*
- *Loss of sense of smell*

(b) The *2nd cranial* nerve is called the optic nerve.

(i) What are its major functions?
Answer:
Transports visual information to the retina of the eye where the optic nerve is situated.

(ii) Define the terms hemianopia and quadrantanopia:
Answer:
- *Hemianopia: Partial or complete loss halves of the two visual fields.*
- *Quadrantanopia: Partial or complete loss quarters of the two visual fields.*

(iii) Define the following optic nerve lesions and some common causes:
Answer:
- *Optic neuritis: Inflammation of the optic nerve.*
- *Demyelinating-inflammatory diseases.*
  Optic atrophy:

Answer:
- *Due to any process which axon degeneration of the optic nerve.*
- *Multiple sclerosis, ischaemic optic neuropathy.*

Papilledema:

Answer:
- *There is optic disc swelling due to raised intracranial pressure.*
- *Cerebral tumour, benign intracranial hypertension.*

(c) Give the names of the *3rd, 4th*, and *6th cranial nerves*. What do they supply?

Answer:
- *Oculomotor, Trochlear, and abducens.*
- *They control the position of the eyeballs and Oculomotor controls the size of the pupils as well as the position of the eyelids.*

(i) Define the terms *strabismus (squint)* and *diplopia*

<u>*Answer:*</u>
- <u>*Strabismus: The axes of the eyes are no longer parallel.*</u>
- <u>*Diplopia: Patient complains of double vision.*</u>

(d) The 5th cranial nerve is called the *trigeminal* nerve.

(i)   What are its functions?

Answer:

It has a sensory and motor function.
- *Sensory: Sensation of the face.*
- *Motor: Temporalis and masseter muscles function, e.g. Jaw opening and clenching.*

(ii) List the main features of a 5th nerve lesion

Answer:
- *Selective loss of facial pain and temperature.*
- *Weak or absent of masseter and temporalis muscle function.*
- *Absence of blinking.*

Learning Activity 7

Facial pain is commonly caused by disorders of the teeth, temporomandibular joint, sinuses, and trauma. There are important syndromes that cause facial pain including:

- Migrainous neuralgia (cluster headaches)—distinct from migraine despite its name
- Trigeminal neuralgia (affects Vth cranial nerve)
- Post herpetic neuralgia (affects Vth cranial nerve)
- Temporal arteritis

(i) Complete the table using the keywords provided on page 10:

Migrainous neuralgia	Trigeminal neuralgia	Postherpetic neuralgia

Keywords/phrases

1. Shock-like short paroxysms of pain	2. Severe pain that wakes the patient at night
3. Continuous, burning pain	4. Involves mandibular and maxillary area
5. Involves eye, mandibular and maxillary areas	6. Occurs in bouts of weeks or months
7. Always unilateral pain	8. Virtually all patients become depressed
9. Commoner in males in 3rd and 4th decade	10. Commoner in middle-aged women
11. Provoked by trivial stimuli (jaw-movements, cold)	12. Freedom of pain between attacks

Answer

Migrainous neuralgia	Trigeminal neuralgia	Postherpetic neuralgia
2. Severe pain that wakes the patient at night 5. Involves eye, mandibular and maxillary areas 6. Occurs in bouts of weeks or months 7. Always unilateral pain 9. Commoner in males in 3rd and 4th decade 12. Freedom of pain between attacks	1. Shock-like short paroxysms of pain 4. Normally involves mandibular and maxillary area 10. Commoner in middle-aged women 11. Provoked by trivial stimuli (jaw-movements, cold)	3. Continuous, burning pain 8. Virtually all patients become depressed

Learning Activity 8

Give the name of the 7th cranial nerve.

(i) What does it supply?

Answer:
- *Motor: Movement of facial expression muscles except jaw movement.*
- *Sensory: Anterior* two thirds *of the tongue taste, sensation of pharynx.*

(ii) *Bell's palsy* is a common disorder involving the facial nerve on one side. Briefly describe the clinical features:

Answer:

One side of facial weakness: loss of forehead furrowing, eye closure, mouth elevation, drooping of the face, and drooling.

(iii) What features would you look for in the face to help you distinguish between an upper and lower motor neurone lesion of the 7th nerve?

Answer:

Upper motor neurone lesion predominantly affected opposite lower face because there is bilateral innervation of the muscle of the upper part of the face.

Lower motor neurone lesion weakness of the upper and lower face on the affected side.

The 8th cranial nerve has two main branches:

(i) Name the 8th nerve and the two main branches and state their functions.

Answer:
- *Vestibulocochlear (Acoustic)*
- *Vestibular and Cochlear branches*
- *Vestibular branches: Balance, posture, and equilibrium*
- *Cochlear branches: Hearing*

(ii) List the common symptoms associated with damage to these branches.

Answer:
- *Vertigo*
- *Nystagmus*
- *Tinnitus*
- *Sensorineural hearing loss*

What are the names of the 9th and 10th cranial nerves? What do they supply? What symptoms is someone with 9th and 10th nerve damage likely to complain of?

Answer:
- *Glossopharyngeal:*
  Motor—voluntary muscle for swallowing and phonation.
  Sensory—sensory of nasopharynx, gag reflex, posterior one third *of tongue taste*
- *Vague:*
  Motor—voluntary muscles of phonation and swallowing.
  Sensory—sensation behind ear and part of external ear canal.
- *Difficulty with swallowing, choking, and phonation*

What are the names of the 11th and 12th cranial nerves and what do they supply?
Answer:

- *Accessory:*
  Motor-sternomastoid muscle turn the head trapezius muscle shrug the shoulders
- *Hypoglossal:*
  Motor-tongue appearance and movement

Learning Activity 9

(a) What important features should you look for with regard to the appearance of muscles?
Answer:
Muscle wasting
Fasciculation—Spontaneous contraction of the fibres belonging to a single motor unit, fine flicker or coarse twitch.
Hypertrophy (Pseudohypertrophic muscles)—infiltrated by fat and connective tissue.

(b) Assessment of tone is one of the most difficult parts of the neurological examination. With regard to tone, contrast the terms *spasticity* and *rigidity*?
Answer:
Spasticity—The resistance to passive movement increased initially then resistance decreased, also call it "clasp-knife phenomenon".
Rigidity—A resistance uniform throughout the range of movement, it may be slightly jerky or like "cogwheel".

(c) With regard to muscle weakness:

(i) What would you consider when assessing muscle weakness?
Answer:
Is the weakness confined to one limb or to one side of the body?
Is the weakness static, progressive, or fluctuant?
Is the weakness accompanied by a feeling of stiffness or is the affected limb floppy?

(ii) Look up some common causes of muscle weakness.
Answer:
Central Nervous System Disorders:
Cerebral Cortex, Brainstem—Stroke
Spinal Cord—Trauma
Basal Ganglia—Parkinsonism
Cerebellar—Stroke

Peripheral Nervous System Disorders:
Lower Motor Neuron—Poliomyelitis
Spinal Nerves and Roots—Lumbar disc diseases
Mononeuropathy—Trauma
Polyneuropathy—Diabetes
Neuromuscular Junction—Myasthenia gravis
Muscle—Muscular dystrophy

(d) Name the sites on the body where you would test for deep tendon reflexes. Indicate the spinal cord segments mediating each of these reflexes.
Answer:
Biceps reflex—Biceps tendon (c5,6)
Triceps reflex—Triceps tendon (c7,8)
Supinator reflex—Styloid process of radius (C5,6)
Knee jerk reflex—Patellar tendon (L3,4)
Ankle jerk reflex—Achilles tendon (S1,2)

(e) Tremor is an important involuntary movement.

  (i) *Physiological tremor* is found in all individuals when the hands are outstretched. Which disorders can make this worse?
  Answer:
  Thyrotoxicosis, fatigue, anxiety, emotion, drug side effects, drug or alcohol withdraw, cerebellar or basal ganglia dysfunction.

  (ii) What is an *intention tremor* and which part of the brain is affected?
  Answer:
  Intention tremor appear only when the limb is activated and often get worse as the target is neared.
  Cerebellar disease, e.g. Multiple Sclerosis.

  (iii) What is a *rest tremor* and which neurological disorder is associated with it?
  Answer:
  These tremors are most prominent at rest and may decrease or disappear with voluntary movement.
  Parkinson's disease.

(f) With regard to other involuntary movements, what is meant by the following?

  (i) Myoclonus
  Answer:
  Rapid, recurring muscle jerks, sudden, brief, unpredictable shock-like contractions.

  (ii) Chorea
  Answer:
  Brief, random movements that do not have the shock-like quality of myoclonus.

  (iii) Athetosis
  Answer:
  Slower still than chorea and become prominent during the performance of voluntary activity, twisting and writhing.

  (iv) Hemibalismus
  Answer:
  Violent swing movements involving one side of the body.

  (v) Tics
  Answer:
  Frequent, compulsive, involuntary, stereotyped and predictable repetition of the same movement.

In the table below, match the definition and cause(s) to the appropriate gait.

Gait	Definition	Causes
1. Spastic	(a) Stooped posture, difficulty in initiating movement, small shuffling steps	(i) Proximal muscle disorder (thyrotoxicosis)
2. Foot-drop	(b) Slow walking, stiff legs, may be dragging, weakness and stiffness of one leg if unilateral	(ii) Cerebellar disease (tumour)
3. Ataxic	(c) Flexes leg at hip more than usual to prevent toes catching, stamping as foot hits ground	(iii) Cerebrovascular disorder (stroke)
4. Waddling	(d) Inability to tilt pelvis when swinging each leg through to take the next step, exaggerated lateral trunk movements	(iv) Peripheral neuropathy (weakness, sensory loss)
5. Hypokinetic	(e) Unsteady when standing and adopts a broad base, unsteady when walking, lurches from side-to-side	(v) Parkinson's disease

Answer:

1. Spastic
    (b) Slow walking, stiff legs, may be dragging, weakness and stiffness of one leg if unilateral
    (iii) Cerebrovascular disorder (stroke)
2. Foot-drop
    (c) Flexes leg at hip more than usual to prevent toes catching, stamping as foot hits ground
    (iv) Peripheral neuropathy (weakness, sensory loss)
3. Ataxic
    (e) Unsteady when standing and adopts a broad base, unsteady when walking, lurches from side-to-side
    (ii) Cerebellar disease (tumour)
4. Waddling
    (d) Inability to tilt pelvis when swinging each leg through to take the next step, exaggerated lateral trunk movements
    (i) Proximal muscle disorder (thyrotoxicosis)
5. Parkinsonian
    (a) Stooped posture, difficulty in initiating movement, small shuffling steps
    (v) Parkinson's disease

Learning Activity 10

(i) Look up some common causes of pins and needles.

Answer:

Peripheral neuropathies and nerve injuries.

(ii) Look up some common causes of peripheral neuropathies.

Answer:
Idiopathic, inherited
Metabolic, Mechanical
Drugs
Infections
Sarcoidosis
Tumours
Autoimmune
Lock of vitamins

(iii) Clinical applications

We are concerned here with differentiating between UMN, LMN, extrapyramidal and cerebellar disorders and myopathy. In general, the following are assessed with regard to motor disorders:

Muscle bulk—normal, reduced, or evidence of wasting

Tone—i.e. the amount of tension in the muscle at rest (normal muscles always have some tone). Either increased or decreased in disease

Tremor—present or absent

Fasciculation—fine "ripples" that can be seen under the skin overlying muscles. May be present or absent in disease.

Power—either normal, increased or decreased in disease

Coordination—may be normal or impaired in disease

Limb reflexes—normal, reduced/absent, or increased in disease

Plantar reflexes—these are elicited by scratching the underside of the foot with a pointed object. In normal people the plantar is flexor (the toes curl). Extensor plantars (toes go upward) are abnormal.

Gait—see Exercise 1

Use the above to complete the following table:

	LMN	UMN	Extrapyramidal	Cerebellar	Myopathy
Muscle bulk					
Tone					
Tremor					
Fasciculation					
Power					
Co-ordination					
Limb reflexes					
Plantars					
Gait					

Answer:

	LMN	*UMN*	*Extrapyramidal*	*Cerebellar*	*Myopathy*
Muscle bulk	*Wasting*	*Little or no wasting*	*Normal*	*Normal*	*Wasting*
Tone	*Decreased*	*Spasticity increased*	*Rigidity increased*	*Decreased*	*Decreased*
Tremor	*Absent*	*Absent*	*Present resting*	*Present intention*	*Absent*
Fasciculation	*Present*	*Absent*	*Absent*	*Absent*	*Absent*
Power	*Decreased*	*Decreased*	*Normal*	*Normal*	*Decreased*
Co-ordination	*Normal*	*Normal*	*Normal*	*Impaired*	*Normal*
Limb reflexes	*Reduced/ absent*	*Increased*	*Normal*	*Normal*	*Normal*
Plantars	*Flexor*	*Extensor*	*Flexor*	*Flexor*	*Flexor*
Gait	*Foot-drop*	*Spastic*	*Hypokinetic*	*Ataxic*	*Waddling*

Bibliography

1. Bickley, L., & Szilagyi, P. G. (2012). *Bates' guide to physical examination and history-taking.* Lippincott Williams & Wilkins.
2. Dover, A. R., & Innes, J. A. (Eds.). (2023). *Macleod's clinical examination.* Elsevier.

Assessing and Diagnosing Disorders of the Musculoskeletal System (MS)

8

Learning Objectives
By the end of this chapter, you will be able to:

Outline the relevant structure and functions of selected musculoskeletal regions
Identify appropriate questions to ask regarding bone, joint, and muscle symptoms
List and discuss the major symptoms of bone, joint, and muscle disorders
Interpret relevant signs found on examination of bones, joints, and muscles
Describe the major features of common joint and bone disorders

Common Medical Terms

In this part of the chapter, we revisit basic anatomy and physiology of the musculoskeletal system.

The list of medical terms below is cited for easy reference, and the reader is expected to understand these medical terms before they proceed to read this chapter.

Synovial joints
Hinge joint
Ball-and-socket joint
Cartilage
Bursae
Ligaments
Tendon

Crepitus
Fasciculation
Muscle wasting
Osteoarthritis
Rheumatoid arthritis
Gout
Ankylosing spondylitis
Reiter's syndrome
Systemic lupus erythematosus

8.1   Part 1: Structure and Functions of Skeletal System

The skeletal system includes the bones of skeleton and the cartilages, ligaments, and other connective tissues that connect or stabilize them. The skeletal system provides structural support for the weight of the body, provides attachments for muscles, and protects organs against injury. The bones also house blood-producing cells and store inorganic salts. Bone tissue is a type of connective tissue that is also wrapped by connective tissues, for example, blood vessels and nervous tissue.

Bones are classified by shape as long, short, flat, and irregular. Long bones are long and narrow which are found in the arm, fore-arm, thigh, leg, palms, soles, fingers, and toes. Short bones are boxlike such as wrist bones. Flat bones have thin, broad surfaces and a plate-like shape. Flat bones form the roof of the skull, the sternum, the ribs, and the scapula. Irregular bones have various shapes such as vertebrae. Sesamoid bones are short and rounded, such as the kneecap. Sutural bones are small, flat, irregularly shaped bones between the flat bones of the skull.

Learning Point
The anatomy of the skeletal system involves:
Skeletal System: 206 bones, mainly connective tissue

- **Bone**: Strong, rigid, mineralized (calcium phosphate) connective tissue.
- **Cartilage**: Strong, flexible, protein (elastic/collagen fibres) connective tissue.
- **Fibrous**: Strong, flexible, protein (collagen fibres) connective tissue. Forms tendons and ligaments.

Classification of Bones
According to their shapes:

- Long bones
- Short bones
- Flat bones
- Irregular bones
- Sesamoid bones
- Sutural bones

8.2   Functions of Bones

Learning Point
- **Support:** Provides structural framework and points of attachment for tissues/organs
- **Protection:** Eyes, ears, brain, heart, and lungs
- **Movement:** Some bones act as levers. Movement together with skeletal muscles and joints
- **Mineral storage:** Storage of calcium and phosphorus
- **Blood cell production:** Blood cell production in the red bone marrow
- **Storage of energy:** Yellow bone marrow stores fat

The skeleton is divided into two major portions—an axial skeleton and an appendicular skeleton.

8.2.1   Skeletal Organization

Learning Point
Axial skeleton: Bones of the head, neck, trunk

- Skull (cranium and face)
- Hyoid bone
- Vertebral column consists of 33 vertebrae
- Rib cage (sternum and 12 pairs of ribs)

Appendicular skeleton: Bones of limbs, hip/shoulder blades

- Pectoral girdle (scapula and clavicle)
- Upper limbs (humerus, radius, ulna, carpals, phalanges)
- Pelvic girdle
- Lower limbs (femur, tibia, fibula, tarsals, phalanges)

Types of Joints

The functional junctions between bones are called joints. Joints enable the body to move in response to skeletal muscle contractions. Joints can be structurally grouped by tissue type. Fibrous joints consist of dense connective tissue, which usually do not allow movement. Cartilaginous joints connect the bones with hyaline cartilage or fibrocartilage and they allow a small amount of movement. Synovial joints have a complex structure and they allow free movement. They are presented as a joint capsule, composed of ligaments on the out surface and a synovial membrane on the inside. The synovial membrane secretes a lubricating synovial fluid into the joint cavity. In a hinge joint, the convex surface of one bone fits into the concave surface of another. Ball and socket joint consists of a bone with a ball-shaped head that articulates with the cup-shaped cavity of another bone. They allow the widest range of motion in all planes, including rotation.

Learning Point

- **Fibrous joints:** No movement, e.g. skull.
  Bone ends held together by collagenous tissue.
- **Cartilaginous joints:** Limited movement, e.g. vertebral column, sternum, and ribs.
  Bone ends are bound together by hyaline cartilage or fibrocartilage.
- **Synovial joints:** Freely movable, presence of a joint capsule (spine, knee, shoulder, elbow, and hip).
- **Hinge joint** (knee, elbow).
- **Ball-and-socket joint** (hip, shoulder).

Synovial Joints

Synovial joints are the most common type of joint in the body. They have a fluid-filled joint cavity where the articulating surfaces of the bones contact and move smoothly against each other.

Articular (hyaline) cartilage consists of chondrocytes, matrix, and collagen fibres binding cartilage to the ends of bones where they allow the bones to glide over each other with very little friction. Articular cartilage can be damaged by normal wear and tear or injury.

Synovial membrane is a thin lining of the inner surface of the articular capsule, bursae, and tendon sheaths. Synovial fluid provides lubrication to further reduce friction between the bones of the joint.

Some synovial joints have a fibrocartilage structure located between the articulating bones called an **articular disc** (small and oval-shaped) or **meniscus** (larger and c-shaped).

Bursa is a connective tissue sac filled with lubricating liquid which can reduce friction by separating the adjacent structures. They are usually located near a joint where skin, ligaments, muscles, or muscle tendons can rub against each other.

Tendon is a dense connective tissue structure that anchors a muscle to bone.

Ligaments strengthen the synovial joints by holding the bones together and resist excessive or abnormal movements of the joint.

Fat Pad are large clusters of fat cells that form a protective cushion in areas needing additional help to absorb impact or protect soft tissue from the movement of harder tissues, the knee has several fat pads; the one below the kneecap and behind the patella tendon is called the **Hoffa fat pad**.

Learning Point
- Synovial joints have a capsule
- Joint capsule composed of irregularly arranged collagen bundles
- Joints are covered by "soft tissues"—tendons, bursae, ligaments
- Synovial membrane: specialized connective tissues lining joint capsule, bursae and tendon sheaths
- Synovial fluid is a viscous ultra-filtrate of plasma, functions include lubrication and nutrition of cartilage cells
- Articular (hyaline) cartilage consists of chondrocytes, matrix, and collagen fibres binding cartilage to bone

8.2.2 Function of Skeletal Muscle

There are three types of muscle tissue: skeletal muscle, cardiac muscle, and smooth muscle.

Skeletal muscle produces voluntary movement, maintains posture, protects internal organs, and generates body heat. Skeletal muscle depends on nervous system signals to work properly.

Learning Point
- **Location:** Skeletal muscle attached to skeleton through tendons
- **Functions:** Voluntary movement and posture
  Stabilize body position and posture
  Heat production and thermoregulation

8.2.3 Applied Structure and Functions of Selected Regions

Types of Synovial Joints
Synovial joints are the most common type of joints in the human body. These joints are characterized by a synovial cavity filled with synovial fluid, which lubricates the

joint and reduces friction between the articulating bones. Examples of synovial joints include the spine, knee, shoulder, elbow, and hip joints. Some of the synovial joints are relatively immobile but stable. Other joints have more freedom of movement but are at greater risk of injury. For example, the hinge joint of the knee allows flexion and extension, whereas the ball and socket joint of the hip and shoulder allows flexion, extension, abduction, adduction, and rotation. The knee, hip, and shoulder joints are commonly injured.

The Spine
The spin is a joint complex; each vertebra is joined to the next one by an intervertebral disc and by two posterior facet joints. The differences in the heights of the anterior and posterior aspects of the vertebrae determine the main curvatures of the spine in the thoracic and sacral regions. The differences in the relative heights of the anterior and posterior aspects of the intervertebral discs determine the curvatures in the cervical and lumbar regions.

Shoulder Joint
The shoulder joint is a synovial ball-and-socket joint formed by the articulation between the upper limb and the axial skeleton. This joint has the largest range of motion of any joint in the body. Injuries to the shoulder joint are common, especially during repetitive abductive use of the upper limb such as swimming.

Elbow Joint
The elbow joint connects the upper arm to forearm, where the humerus meets the radius and ulna.

Injuries to the elbow are normally caused by repetitive strain, either from athletic injuries or other forms of overuse.

Hand Joint
There are 27 bones in each human hand. Based on their location and function, there are three types of bones.

Carpal Bones: Comprises eight irregular bones arranged in two rows.
Metacarpal Bones: In the middle part of the hand, there are five metacarpal bones.
Phalanges Bones: There are seven bones forming the fingers in each hand. Based on their location, they are referred to as: *Proximal phalanx, Middle phalanx*, and *Distal phalanx*.

Hand joint injuries are relatively common and can result from a wide variety of causes including infection, overuse, and arthritis.

Hip Joint
The hip joint is a ball-and-socket joint allowing movement in all directions. The hip carries the weight of the body and thus requires strength and stability during

standing and walking. A common hip injury in older adults is a fracture of the head of the femur. Hip fractures are commonly caused by falls.

Knee Joint

The knee functions as a hinge joint that allows flexion and extension of the leg. In addition, some rotation of the leg is available when the knee is flexed, but not when extended.

The knee joint has multiple ligaments that provide support. The lateral collateral ligament is on the lateral side of the knee. The medial collateral ligament runs from the medial side of the femur to the medial tibia. The tibial collateral ligament crosses the knee and is attached to the articular capsule and to the medial meniscus. Inside the knee joint are the anterior cruciate ligament and posterior cruciate ligament.

The patella is a bone incorporated into the tendon of the quadriceps muscle, the large muscle of the anterior thigh.

Located between the articulating surfaces of the femur and tibia are two articular discs, the medial meniscus and lateral meniscus.

The knee is vulnerable to injuries associated with hyperextension, twisting, or blows to the medial or lateral side of the joint, particularly while weight bearing.

Ankle Joint

The ankle joint is formed by tibia, fibula, and talus bone. It joins foot to lower leg. It is a synovial hinge joint that allows for plantar flexion, dorsa flexion, inversion, and eversion. Most ankle injuries occur either during sports activities or while walking on an uneven surface that forces the foot and ankle into an unnatural position.

8.2.4 Types of Joint Movements

Anatomical position is defined as if the body is standing erect, head facing forward, the arms by the sides, the palms facing forward, and the feet parallel and together.

Flexion is the movement of the body or limbs that the angle between them decreases and the parts come closer together.

Extension is the movement of the body or limbs that the angle between them increases and the parts move further apart.

For the vertebral column, flexion (anterior flexion) is an anterior (forward) bending of the neck or body, while extension involves a posterior-directed motion, such as straightening from a flexed position or bending backward.

Lateral flexion is the bending of the neck or body towards the right or left side.

Dorsiflexion is the movement at the ankle joint that brings the foot towards the shin.

Plantarflexion is the movement at the ankle that lifts the heel of the foot from the ground or points the toes downward.

Abduction is moving a part laterally away from the midline of the body.

Adduction is moving a part toward the body or across the midline.

For example, abduction is raising the arm at the shoulder joint, moving it laterally away from the body, while adduction brings the arm down to the side of the body. Similarly, abduction and adduction at the wrist move the hand away from or towards the midline of the body. Spreading the fingers or toes apart is also abduction, while bringing the fingers or toes together is adduction. For the thumb, abduction is the anterior movement that brings the thumb to a 90° perpendicular position, pointing straight out from the palm. Adduction moves the thumb back to the anatomical position, next to the index finger.

Rotation is the movement of a body part around an axis. Internal rotation is the turning of the anterior surface of a limb towards the midline. External rotation is the turning of a limb in the opposite direction. Rotation of the neck or body is the twisting movement.

Circumduction is the movement of a body part in a circular manner, in which one end of the body part being moved stays relatively stationary while the other end describes a circle. For example, moving the finger in a circular motion without moving the hand.

Supination is the movement of the forearm so the palm is upward or facing anteriorly.

Pronation is the movement of the forearm so the palm is downward or facing posteriorly.

Inversion is the turning of the bottom of the foot toward the midline.

Eversion is the turning of the bottom of the foot away from the midline.

Protraction is the movement of a body part forward. Protraction of the scapula occurs when the shoulder is moved forward.

Retraction is the opposite motion, with the movements of a body part backward, in this case the scapula being pulled posteriorly and medially, towards the vertebral.

For the mandible, protraction occurs when the lower jaw is pushed forward, to stick out the chin, while retraction pulls the lower jaw backward.

Depression is downward movement of the body part. These movements are used to droop the shoulder.

Elevation is upward movement of the body part. These movements are used to shrug the shoulder.

Elevation of the mandible is the upward movement of the lower jaw used to close the mouth or bite on something, and depression is the downward movement that produces the opening of the mouth.

Opposition is the thumb movement that brings the tip of the thumb in contact with the tip of a finger. Returning the thumb to its anatomical position next to the index finger is called **Reposition**.

Learning Point
- Anatomical position
- Flexion and extension
- Dorsiflexion and plantar flexion
- Abduction and adduction
- Rotation and circumduction
- Supination and pronation
- Inversion and eversion
- Protraction and retraction
- Depression and elevation
- Opposition and reposition

8.2.5 Anatomical Movements at Individual Joints

Learning Point
Anatomical movements at individual joints are listed in Table 8.1.

Table 8.1 Anatomical movements

Joint	Movement
Temporomandibular joint (TMJ)	Elevation
	Depression
	Protraction
	Retraction
Cervical spine	Flexion
	Extension
	Lateral flexion
	Rotation
Thoracic spine	Flexion
	Extension
	Lateral flexion
	Rotation
Lumbar spine	Flexion
	Extension
	Lateral flexion
	Rotation
Acromioclavicular joints	Elevation
	Depression
	Protraction
	Retraction

(continued)

Table 8.1 (continued)

Joint	Movement
Glenohumeral joint	Flexion
	Extension
	Abduction
	Adduction
	Internal rotation
	External rotation
Elbow	Flexion
	Extension
	Pronation
	Supination
Wrist	Palmar flexion
	Dorsi flexion
	Ulna deviation
	Radial deviation
Fingers	Flexion
	Extension
	Abduction
	Adduction
	Opposition
Hip	Flexion
	Extension
	Abduction
	Adduction
	Internal rotation
	External rotation
Knee	Flexion
	Extension
Flexed only	Internal rotation
Flexed only	External rotation
Ankle	Plantar flexion
	Dorsi flexion
	Inversion
	Eversion
Toes	Flexion
	Extension

8.2.6   Part 2: Musculoskeletal Case History Taking

Competent case history taking is the key to make accurate diagnosis. It is important to identify those cases where the problem. For example, pain may appear to arise from the joint, but is in fact referred pain, left shoulder pain which might in fact be referred pain from neck, diaphragm, or heart.

Musculoskeletal symptoms lasting more than 6 weeks are generally described as chronic. The way in which symptoms evolve can be import guide in making a diagnosis. Was the onset sudden or gradual? Chronic disease may start insidiously and may have a variable course with remissions. Was the onset associated with trauma or infection?

The main symptoms of musculoskeletal conditions are pain, stiffness, and joint swelling.

Pain needs to record the location, onset, character, radiation, aggravation, and relieving factors. The pain may feel radiating from the joint or even from an adjacent joint, for example, pain from the knee may be felt in the knee but can sometimes be felt in the hip or ankle. Also, the tennis elbow, pain will usually be felt on the outside of the elbow joint. Pain due to pressure on nerves often has numbness and tingling but the character of musculoskeletal pain can be very variable. Non-inflammatory pain is more directly related to use and pain caused by inflammation is often present at rest as well as on use. Ask whether the pain is constant (probably inflammatory) or intermittent (probably mechanical). The activity or positions make the mechanical joints disorder worse and rest relieves the pain. Bone pain may be localized or diffuse but muscle pains are difficult to localize and are usually continuous and deep. Another major symptom of muscle disorder is weakness which may be generalized or localized and may be associated with wasting. Tendon or bursa pains are usually localized, often accompanied by signs of inflammation.

Stiffness and joint swelling are common to many joint problems; both may have been noticed by the patient and volunteered during history taking. If the patient has noticed, licit for how long they have been present, prolonged morning stiffness or short-lasting (less than 30 min), whether they are associated with pain.

Learning Point
History of presenting complaint:

- Timing of symptoms: Onset, frequency, duration, pattern
- Mode of onset
- Initiating, aggravating, and relieving factors
- Quality, intensity, and severity of symptoms
- Associated manifestations
- Life events preceding and/or at onset
- Previous episodes of similar symptoms
- Diagnosis and/or treatment by other healthcare practitioners

Also consider:

- Occupation
- Hobbies
- Exercise
- Lifestyle
- Ethnicity

8.2.7 Subject Matter for Case History Questioning

Learning Point
Joint

- Pain
- Discomfort
- Swelling
- Stiffness
- Temperature
- Deformities
- Trauma including repetitive strain
- Family history of autoimmune, rheumatic, or connective tissue disorder
- Drug history

Muscle

- Pain
- Stiffness
- Cramps
- Weakness
- Involuntary movements
- Claudication
- Osteoporosis
- Generalized anorexia, malaise, or fatigue
- Skin manifestations

Each individual case study consists of a summary of the patient's clinical presentation starting with a list of diagnostic features and any other clinical details that may be important for a differential diagnosis. Becoming competent at interpreting signs and symptoms depends on seeing as many examples as possible and discussing them with a senior colleague. You may wish to use this chapter as a guide to build a comprehensive collection of your own. We have endeavoured to include commonly encountered case studies as well as less common findings which are of clinical importance. Here we include case studies which feature clinical sign sand symptoms that a competent practitioner should be able to recognize and diagnose.

Using the enhanced Cambridge-Calgary (Kurtz et al. 2003) consultation model, the practitioner should collect data on the patient's presenting complaint and taking the patient-centred approach should assess and diagnose the problem. This consultation model enables health care practitioners to communicate the patient's problem and plan for a safe and effective management plan. The Calgary-Cambridge model also focuses on the patient's perspective on the problem and builds on the rapport with patients.

The dividing line between history taking and clinical examination is an artificial one since the examination begins from the moment the patient walks into the room. The practitioner uses their observational skills to inspect and assess the general appearance of the patient and uses verbal and non-verbal skills to assess the patient's physical health but also engage with the patient and observe their tone of speech, mood, and orientation for time, place, and person. Throughout the physical examination, we need to be aware of the patient's body language and use our senses of hearing, sight, and touch to communicate and listen to the patient.

Make sure that you apply the principles of the Cambridge-Calgary consultation model and note key findings before you proceed with the physical examination of the patient to maximize patient-centred care and utilize quaternary prevention.

Case Study 1
A 55-year-old female visits your clinic. She has recently returned from holiday. Since when she reports suffering from "left hip and thigh pain", the pain during and after prolonged standing and walking.

(a) What question concerning the pain would be particularly useful with this history?
(b) What might you be looking for in the clinical examination?

Case Study 2
A 60-year-old male presents with 8 months of pain and paraesthesia noticed in the right hand (particularly in the thumb, index, and middle fingers). Last month he started to have difficulty using his right hand for gripping and it is starting to affect his work. The pain is now extending up the forearm and it is waking him up during the night sleep.

(a) In addition to a musculoskeletal examination which other examination should be carried out on a patient complaining of paraesthesia?
(b) When observing a patient before performing a musculoskeletal examination, give four factors that you would specifically observe for when looking at his general appearance.
(c) Give four signs that a practitioner aims to identify during palpation.
(d) Give two factors that the practitioner should specifically observe for during active range of movement testing.
(e) What other features would you look for on clinical examination?
(f) List the main symptoms seen in muscle disorders.

Case Study 3
A 42-year-old woman presents with foot and hand pain, neck stiffness, and worsening fatigue over the last 3 months.

(a) What findings on your physical examination of a patient complaining of multiple joint pain would help you differentiate between osteoarthritis and rheumatoid arthritis?
(b) When palpating bones and joints, give two specific things for each that you would palpate for.
   Following for bones:
   Following for joints:

(c) What general signs and symptoms may you expect to elicit in a cartilage pathology?

Case Study 4
A 78-year-old woman presenting to you for evaluation of her "arthritis pain" in both her hands, knees, and hips. She states that she has had arthritis pain for 5 years, but it has progressively gotten worse in the last 6 months. Her right knee is stiff for 10–15 min most mornings and often feels stiff after prolonged sitting. Her pain is typically worse when she is more active and improves somewhat with rest.

(a) What are the risk factors for osteoarthritis?
(b) What non-pharmacologic treatment modalities should be recommended?
(c) List at least four risk factors for hip fractures.

8.2.8   Part 3: Symptoms and Signs of Bone Muscle and Joint Disorders

The main symptom of bone disorders is pain.
   The cardinal symptoms and signs of joint disorders are:

- Pain
- Skin colour change
- Swelling and crepitus
- Stiffness
- Locking
- Clicking noises
- Loss of function

The main symptoms of muscle disorders are:

- Pain and stiffness
- Weakness
- Wasting and fasciculation
- Cramps

Pain

Bone pains are probably the most common presenting symptom. Bone pain is usually described as deep and boring, although the pain of a fracture is usually very sharp and made worse by movement. Bone pain may be localized or diffuse. Pain is the most significant complaint in joint disorders and it is important to determine the site, severity, the effect of movement and rest, and whether the onset was acute or chronic. Acute joint pains are constant and chronic joint pain usually has period of exacerbation.

Muscle pains are difficult to localize and are usually continuous and deep. Another major symptom of muscle disorder is weakness which may be generalized or localized and may be associated with wasting. Tendon or bursa pains are usually localized, often accompanied by signs of inflammation.

Skin Colour

Redness of the overlying skin suggests inflammation and bruising suggests trauma or systemic condition.

Swelling and Crepitus

Swelling is common to many joint problems; the location and texture of swelling is often indicative of cause. Nodal osteoarthritis causes bony, hard, and non-tender swelling in the proximal interphalangeal (PIP) and distal interphalangeal (DIP) joints of the fingers. Joint effusion is a sign of joint inflammation, in which effusion fluid is displaced from one part to another. Swelling of the knee usually occurs with trauma and in OA. Ankle swelling is more commonly due to oedema than to swelling of the joint.

Crepitus is a grinding sensation that may suggest damage to articular surfaces or tenosynovitis.

Stiffness

Stiffness means a restriction in the range of movement of a joint or the inability to move the joint smoothly.

Inflammatory arthritis is associated with prolonged stiffness after a period of immobility (early-morning), which is generalized and may last for several hours, its duration being directly proportional to the severity of the inflammatory process. Non-inflammatory arthritis, such as osteoarthritis, tends to cause localized stiffness which may last only a few moments (less than 30 min) but can recur after sitting for short periods.

Locking

Suggest a loose body in the joint space, which may be a symptom of articular surface degeneration.

Clicking Noises

Noises coming from joints are not always pathological but if the joints accompanied by pain are very significant, they may suggest a loose body in the joint space.

Muscle Wasting and Fasciculation

Muscle wasting suggests that muscle is not being used. Fasciculation is a small number of muscle fibres' spontaneous contraction, often causing a flicker of movement under the skin.

Cramps

Cramp is a sudden tightening of one or more muscles. Common causes include forced muscle contraction and dehydration.

> **Learning Point**
> - **Pain**—bone pains are deep and boring; muscle pains are difficult to localize and are continuous and deep
> - **Skin colour**
>   - Bruising suggests trauma or systemic condition
>   Red skin suggests inflammation
> - **Swelling**—texture of swelling is often indicative of cause
> - **Crepitus**—grinding sensation, may suggest damage to articular surfaces or tenosynovitis
> - **Stiffness**—restriction in the range of movement of a joint or inability to move joint smoothly
> - **Locking**—suggest a loose body in the joint space, may be a symptom of articular surface degeneration
> - **Clicking**—may suggest a loose body in the joint space, clicking without pain usually has no clinical significance
> - **Change in movement**—hyper or hypo mobility, may be due to either joint or muscle dysfunction
> - **Wasting**—suggests that muscle is not being used, and fasciculation is a small number of muscle fibres' spontaneous contraction
> - **Cramp** is a sudden tightening of one or more muscles

8.3   Local Musculoskeletal Conditions

> **Learning Point**
> - **Strain**—damage of muscle fibre
> - **Sprain**—damage of ligament
> - **Tendonitis/tenosynovitis**—inflammation

8.3.1 Joint Pathologies

Learning Point
- Signs and symptoms of acute or chronic inflammation
- Loss of muscle and or joint function
- Swelling and/or nodules
- Deformity
- Palpable/audible crepitus/locking
- Point tenderness

Cartilage Pathologies

Learning Point
- Signs and symptoms of acute or chronic inflammation
- Joint instability
- Loss of muscle and or joint function
- Deformity
- Palpable/audible crepitus/locking
- Point tenderness

8.3.2 Bursae and Fat Pad Pathologies

Learning Point
- Signs and symptoms of acute inflammation
- Loss of or painful joint function
- Point or diffuse tenderness

8.3.3 Muscle Pathologies

Learning Point
- Signs and symptoms of acute or chronic inflammation
- Poorly localized pain
- Loss of muscle/joint function
- May or may not have indentation at lesion site
- Bruising
- Most strains occur at musculotendinous junction

8.3.4   Tendon Pathologies

Learning Point
- Signs and symptoms of acute or chronic inflammation
- Loss of muscle and or joint function
- Deformity
- Palpable has audible crepitus in sheathed tendons

8.4   Ligament Pathologies

Learning Point
- Signs and symptoms of acute or chronic inflammation
- Joint instability
- Joint deformity
- Proprioception issues
- Often a history of trauma

8.5   Part 4: Clinical Problems

Arthritis

Arthritis is a condition which causes joint pain, swelling, and stiffness with inflammation. There are more than 100 different types of arthritis. Some types are long-term conditions, including osteoarthritis and rheumatoid arthritis.

Learning Point
- Joint disease associated with inflammation
- Arthritis produces pain, stiffness, and loss of function in one or more joints
- Classified as either **Seronegative Arthritis** or **Seropositive Arthritis** dependent upon presence of rheumatoid factors in blood

Seronegative Arthritis:
A group of inflammatory conditions affecting spin and peripheral joints

- Ankylosing spondylitis
- Psoriatic arthritis
- Arthritis associated with inflammatory bowel disease

> **Seropositive Arthritis:**
>
> - Vague-associated symptoms: malaise, anorexia
> - Pain or swelling of one or more joints
> - Specific associated symptoms according to underlying cause
>
> May also be described as systemic or non-systemic dependent upon involvement of other organ systems
>   **Systemic**—Seropositive-Rheumatoid Arthritis (RA), Gout
>   **Non-systemic**—Seronegative-Osteoarthritis (OA)

8.5.1   Osteoarthritis and Rheumatoid Arthritis

An estimated 10 million people in the UK are said to be affected by osteoarthritis (OA) and it can be detected in 50% of those over 60 years of age. OA is a degenerative disease and causes erosion of the articular cartilage which becomes progressively thinner as the disease progresses. The hips and knees are most commonly involved, leading to severe disability. OA is thus a *degenerative disease*. OA is found throughout the world and is said to be more common in women. The incidence is low in black populations.

Rheumatoid arthritis (RA) is a chronic inflammatory disease of younger people involving many joints and is known as a multisystem disorder, since it can affect other body systems. There is progressive damage to the joints resulting in severe disability. RA affects about 2% of the population worldwide and is three times commoner in women, usually starting in the fourth decade.

Osteoarthritis
Sometimes the term, *primary OA* is used to distinguish those cases with no apparent cause from *secondary OA*, where an underlying pre-existing disorder is present. Some secondary causes include:

- Past joint infections
- Congenital dislocation of the hip
- Intra-articular (within the joint) fractures
- Disorders of the hip
- Previous inflammatory arthritis
- Acromegaly

Aetiological factors that could operate in primary OA include:

- *Age*—OA affects middle-aged and elderly people predominantly.
- *Genetics*—there is a strong family history and genetic abnormalities of cartilage could be implicated.
- *Obesity, lifestyle, and hormonal factors*. OA of the knees is strongly associated with obesity. Sex steroids and growth hormone may influence the articular cartilage.

OA is a disease of articular cartilage. The two most likely stimuli are:

- Mechanical trauma
- Abnormalities of the cartilage

The pathogenesis is not fully understood but may involve:

1. *General ageing.*
2. *Inflammatory processes in the joint.*
3. *Abnormal weight bearing.*
4. *Enzyme destruction of cartilage*. The chondrocytes (the cells responsible for laying down the collagen and matrix of cartilage) may release enzymes that damage cartilage and matrix. The broken collagen fibres swell and split, releasing crystals into the joint leading to inflammation and cartilage destruction. Attempts at repair lead to bone remodelling resulting in the production of spurs (outgrowths) of bone in the joint called **osteophytes.**
5. *Alterations in the muscle and nerve function around the joint* leading to reduced shock-absorbing capacity.

Pathogenesis of Osteoarthritis

Learning Point
- General ageing
- Inflammatory processes in joints
- Abnormal weight bearing
- Crystal deposits in joints
- Enzyme destruction of cartilage
- Alteration in muscle, nerve function around joint reducing shock-absorbing ability

Pathological Features of Osteoarthritis

Learning Point
- Increase in proteoglycan turnover and change in composition
- Increase in collagen production
- Thinning, erosion, fibrillation, and loss of cartilage
- Sclerosis and increased vascularity of underlying bone; later formation of cysts
- Proliferation of cartilage to form osteophytes

Clinical Features of Osteoarthritis

Learning Point
<u>**Symptoms**</u>

- Joint Pain—Involves the DIP, first carpometacarpal (CMC) and PIP joints, knee joints and spin, hip, and knees. Pain, worse in the evenings, aggravated by use and relieved by rest
- Morning stiffness less than 30 min and stiffness later in the day
- Joint instability
- Loss of function

<u>**Signs**</u>

- Crepitus on movement
- Limitation of movement
- Joint deformities and instability
- Effusion in joint
- Osteophytes (bony swellings)
- Muscle wasting

Diagnostic Criteria for Osteoarthritis

> **Learning Point**
> - **History** of joint pain worsened by movement
> - **Physical exam** findings such as tenderness, swelling, and redness
> - **Osteophyte formation** (small abnormal bony outgrowth or spur)
> - **Blood tests** to rule out other causes for symptoms
> - **Imaging tests** like **x-rays** or **magnetic resonance imaging (MRI), the** presence of joint space narrowing
> - **Increased density** of subchondral bone and pseudocyst in the subchondral bone

Treatment for Osteoarthritis

OA is usually treated by simple analgesia and non-steroidal anti-inflammatory drugs (NSAIDs). Physical therapy is often used, such as heat application, exercises to maintain muscle power, hydrotherapy, etc. Surgery involves joint replacement, with good results regarding the hip and knee, although these have limited life.

8.5.2 Rheumatoid Arthritis

The cause of RA is unknown, although viruses and bacteria have been implicated. The following immunological changes have been described:

1. *Autoantibodies.* IgG and IgM can be detected in the blood. Collectively, these are called *rheumatoid factor.* For this reason, RA is *seropositive arthritis* which distinguishes it from other inflammatory joint disorders (like OA and ankylosing spondylitis) which are termed *seronegative arthritis.*
2. *Immune (antigen-antibody) complexes.* RA is said to be a type III hypersensitivity reaction.
3. *Abnormal cell-mediated immunity.*
4. *Association with other autoimmune disorders*, such as primary hypothyroidism and pernicious anaemia.
5. *Locally synthesized IgG and cytokines* are found in the synovial fluid.

Since the causative agent cannot be removed (persistence of the virus and immune complexes), chronic inflammation ensues, resulting in the formation of fibrous tissue that protrudes from the synovial membrane into the joint space. This tissue is called a *pannus*, which leads to further joint destruction.

Pathological Features of Rheumatoid arthritis

Learning Point
- Chronic inflammation of synovium
- Pannus formation (proliferation of chronic inflammatory tissue into joint space)
- Formation of rheumatoid nodules over bony prominences, tendons, in lungs, pleura, and pericardium
- Articular cartilage and underlying bone destruction with local osteoporosis
- Lymphadenopathy

Clinical Features of Rheumatoid arthritis

Learning Point
<u>**Symptoms**</u>

- Pain, stiffness of MCP, PIP, DIP in hands and MTP joints in feet
- Wrist, elbows, and knees also involved
- Morning stiffness lasting for hours, limitation of movement and function
- Generally unwell
- Peak onset 30–40 years. Commoner in women

<u>**Signs**</u>

- Joint soft swelling
- Joints warm and tender
- Limitation of movement
- Muscle wasting
- Deformities (swan-necked, ulnar deviation, and boutonniere)

Diagnostic Criteria for Rheumatoid Arthritis

Learning Point
- Arthritis of three or more joints (soft tissue swelling or fluid)
- Arthritis of wrist and hand joints (MCP and PIP joints)
- Symmetrical swelling of same joint areas
- Serum rheumatoid factor
- X-ray features of RA
- Signs must have been present for at least 6 weeks

Extra-articular Features for Rheumatoid Arthritis

Learning Point
- Scleritis
- Sjogren's syndrome (dry eyes and mouth)
- Lymphadenopathy and splenomegaly
- Pericarditis
- Pleurisy, effusions, and fibrosing alveolitis
- Anaemia
- Carpal tunnel syndrome
- Tenosynovitis, bursitis, RA nodules, and tendon sheath swelling
- Renal amyloidosis
- Nailfold lesions, leg ulcers, and ankle oedema

Treatment for Rheumatoid Arthritis
- Lifestyle change
- Medication
    - NSAIDs—Nonsteroidal anti-inflammatory drugs: Reduces inflammation
    - DMARDs—Disease-modifying antirheumatic drugs: Relieves pain and slows down the progression
    - Corticosteroids: Reduce pain, swelling, and slow down damage to joints Biologics: Suppress the immune system

8.5.3   Crystal Deposition Arthritis

Three types of crystals can be deposited in joints:

- Uric acid (urate)
- Calcium pyrophosphate
- Hydroxyapatite

Gout is the most important of these and we will not consider the other two here.

Gout

Gout is an abnormality of uric acid metabolism, resulting in the deposition of uric acid crystals in joints, soft tissues, and urinary tract. In the West, about 0.2% of the population are affected, and gout is usually associated with heavy alcohol drinkers, obesity, sedentary lifestyle, red meat eaters, a family history, and being a male.

Pathogenesis
Increased uric acid in the blood (hyperuricaemia) is due to:

Table 8.2 Causes of gout

Increased production	Decreased excretion
1. Increased purine turnover (leukaemia, advanced) Cancer, psoriasis—cancer cells are very active 2. Increased purine production—Rare enzyme disorders	1. Drugs (thiazide diuretics and low-dose aspirin) 2. Hypertension 3. Primary hypothyroidism 4. Primary hypoparathyroidism 5. Alcohol and starvation (increased lactic acid) 6. Chronic renal disease 7. Lead poisoning

- Excessive production
- Decreased excretion

Uric acid is the final product formed in the breakdown of purines and is completely filtered by the glomerulus. Most cases of gout are *primary (idiopathic)* in which no underlying disease can be detected. Primary gout is usually due to increased uric acid production, although impaired renal secretion can also contribute. Table 8.2 lists the causes of gout.

Clinical Features

Gout commences with recurrent acute attacks of arthritis. After some years, the attacks do not resolve completely and deposits of uric acid crystals collect in the joints and in the soft tissues around the joints and on the ear lobes, where they are called *tophi*. The acute attack affects the big toe in 75% of cases, but other joints of the lower limb may be affected in the remaining 25% of cases, e.g. ankles, knees, and other toes. Some patients develop uric acid deposits in the kidneys, which can lead to urinary tract stones and, eventually, renal failure. There is also a strong association with cardiovascular disease and hypertension.

Learning Point
- Clinical condition produced by deposition of uric acid crystals in joints characterized by episodes of acute arthritis usually affecting only one joint
- Sudden onset of shiny, acutely inflamed joint often in early hours, the patient is irritable and anorexic.
- In 10–15% patients with ulcerative colitis and Crohn's disease
- Symmetrical arthritis affecting mainly lower limb joints
- HLA B-27 association

These are a series of disorders characterized by certain common features. They are often termed seronegative, since they show no immunological changes in the blood. They include:

- Ankylosing spondylitis
- Reiter's syndrome
- Enteropathic arthritis (associated with inflammatory bowel diseases)

All have a common genetic marker, the HLA-B27 gene. Some patients may have several different syndromes from this group, and these disorders are also known to occur in families.

8.5.4   Ankylosing Spondylitis

Learning Point
- Usually male
- Spinal pain and stiffness (improving with exercise)
- Loss of spinal mobility-thoracic kyphosis, lumbar lordosis
- Seronegative arthritis
- Affects young adults—almost as common in women but much milder
- Associated with HLA B27 gene
- Sacroiliac joint affected first; back pain, morning stiffness
- Iritis, urethritis
- Asymmetrical peripheral joint involvement
- Inflammation of costochondral junction in chest causes chest pain
- Increasing kyphosis, reduced flexion (bamboo spine)

8.5.5   Reiter's Syndrome

Learning Point
- Arthritis, non-specific urethritis, and conjunctivitis
- Follows a non-specific urethritis or bacterial gastrointestinal infection
- Knee, ankle, and foot most commonly involved
- Acute onset, resolves after some months
- Link with HLA B-27 gene
- Heel pain, MTP joint synovitis, knee effusion, plaques and pustules on skin

8.5.6   Enteropathic Arthritis

Learning Point
- In 10–15% patients with ulcerative colitis and Crohn's disease
- Symmetrical arthritis affecting mainly lower limb joints
- HLA B-27 association

Prolapsed Intervertebral Disc

Learning Point
- Back pain with very limited movement
- Usually in a fit young adult
- Sudden onset while lifting or stooping
- Inability to straighten up
- Worsened by coughing and straining
- May be paraesthesia or numbness in the leg or foot
- Tenderness in the midline of the lower back
- Pain may be worsened by foot dorsiflexion

8.5.7   Connective Tissue Disease

This term is applied to three types of disorders:

- Systemic lupus erythematosus (SLE)
- Systemic sclerosis (scleroderma)
- Polymyositis and dermatomyositis

All three are associated with arthritis, vasculitis, immunological abnormalities, and multisystem involvement.

Systemic Lupus Erythematosus

SLE is the commonest of the three and is characterized by the presence of antibodies to nuclear components in the serum. It affects about 0.1% of the population and is due to a widespread vasculitis (inflammation of the small blood vessels). It affects the joints (but less severely than RA), skin ("butterfly" rash on the cheeks), lungs (pleurisy, pleural effusions), heart (pericarditis with effusions), kidneys, nervous system (psychiatric disturbances, epilepsy, ataxia, peripheral neuropathy, meningitis, etc.), eyes, and GIT. The course of the disease involves attacks and remissions in most cases.

8.6   Differential Diagnosis

Learning Point
Rheumatoid Arthritis

- Symmetric involvement of small hand joints (PIP, MCP), wrists, and foot joints
- Joint pain
- Morning stiffness lasting for hours, limitation of movement and function
- Soft swelling, wasting
- Deformities, ulnar deviation of the fingers

Osteoarthritis

- Involves the DIP, first carpometacarpal (CMC) and PIP joints, knee joints and spin, hip, knees
- Symmetry of involvement
- Bony swelling
- Pain, worse in the evenings, aggravated by use and relieved by rest
- Morning stiffness less than 30 min
- Joints deformities

Tendonitis-Bicipital

- Complaints of pain in the anterior aspect of the shoulder and arm
- Pain by palpating the tendon or contracting the muscle

Cervical Radiculopathy

- Affects the fifth nerve root
- Muscle weakness
- The biceps and supinator reflexes are depressed

Carpal Tunnel Syndrome

- Seen in hypothyroidism, diabetes mellitus, pregnancy, RA
- Nocturnal tingling and pain in the hand followed by weakness of muscles
- Sensory loss of the palm and radial three and one half fingers
- Tapping pain on the carpal tunnel

Back Pain

- Causes: Infection-TB, discitis
- Malignancy-spinal tumour, metastases
- Referred pain
- Inflammatory-Ankylosing spondylitis
- Disc disease-disc prolapse
- Osteoarthritis
- Bone disease-Paget's disease
- Mechanical problem-posture, pregnancy, obesity
- Soft tissue problem-strains
- Psychogenic

8.6.1   Part 5: Musculoskeletal Examination

The orthopaedic surgeon, Apley, recommended the following procedure for examining the musculoskeletal system:

- Look (inspect)
- Feel (palpate)
- Move
- Assess function

First introduce yourself, explain to the patient what you are going to do, gain verbal consent to examine. It is important to make the patient feel comfortable about being examined.

Inspection
Always observe before touching a patient. Talk to your patient, explain in appropriate language what you are doing.

Ask the patient to walk a few steps, turn, and walk back. Observe the patient's gait for symmetry, smoothness, and the ability to turn quickly. With the patient standing in the anatomical position, observe from front and behind and compare one side with the other, checking for symmetry, also look specifically for skin changes, muscle bulk, and swelling in and around the joint. Look also for deformity of the joint, alignment of muscles and joints. Observe coordination and muscle function.

Palpation
Feel for skin temperature by using the back of your hand across the joint line and at relevant sites. Gently palpate bones, joints, muscles, and surrounding tissue for swelling, tenderness, deformities, and crepitation.

Assess tenderness (pain) and swelling always compare one side with the other. With regard to tenderness, palpate the joint margins, bony prominences, and surrounding tendons and ligaments to determine whether tenderness is inside or outside the joint and whether it is localized or generalized. Acute inflammation causes generalized tenderness. Degenerative diseases are associated with tenderness in adjacent structures and knee cartilage damage produces localized tenderness at the margin of the cartilage. Tenderness is an important clinical sign—both in and around the joint. Hard-bony swellings are normally due to osteoarthritis, and soft, rubbery swellings could be due to inflammatory joint disease.

Move

With regard to movement, both active (that done by the patient) and passive movement (that carried out by the examiner) must be assessed. Compare one side with the other. Observe the quality and equality of motion bilaterally. Note any limitation, pain, or crepitus with movement. Reduced active movement compared to passive movement is usually related to muscle disorders, whereas joint disorders usually lead to reductions in both. Always assess the full range of movements and look for abnormal movement positions produced by joint instability. In certain cases, joints may move further than expected—this is called hypermobility. It is also important to assess whether there is any abnormal change in bone angle whether there is shortening. Always compare one side with the other.

Function

It is important to make a functional assessment of the joint.

Hand and wrist: Ask the patient to grip your two fingers to assess power grip. Ask the patient to pinch your finger, this assesses pincer grip, which is very important functionally.

Elbow: Function of the elbow includes moving the hands to reach the mouth and behind head.

Shoulder: Function of the shoulder includes getting the hands behind the head and back. This is important in washing and grooming.

Hip: Observe the patient's gait for a limping or a "waddling" walk.

Knee: Looking for any varus or valgus deformity.

Foot and ankle: Observe the patient's gait and watch for the normal cycle of heel strike, stance, and toe-off.

8.6.2   Necessities for Musculoskeletal Examination

Learning Point
Knowledge base

- Surface anatomy
- Posture and gait observation
- Anatomical movements
- Muscles and innervation
- Bony landmarks
- Myotomes

Equipment

- Couch
- Towels to cover patient
- Pillows
- Tape measure

8.6.3   Physical Examination Structure

Learning Point
- General observation whilst taking history
- Prepare self, patient, and area
- General examination
- Focussed system examination, e.g. musculoskeletal system
- Consider need for additional system examination, e.g. nervous system, cardiovascular system

Remember at all times

- Hygiene and safety
- Patient comfort and dignity

8.7   General Observation

Learning Point

Patient may not be unaware of that they are being looked at:

- Walking
- Standing
- Seated
- Lying
- Mobility aids
- Responses
- Body position

8.7.1   General Examination

Learning Point
- Non-specific observation/palpation/testing
- Identify signs that may be associated with other conditions especially systemic

Pitfalls

- Looking but not seeing
- Palpating but not registering

8.7.2   Musculoskeletal System-Specific Observation

Learning Point
- General appearance
- Posture and anatomical position
- Limb symmetry
- Deformity
- Joint: open and closed
- Muscles: loaded and unloaded resistant
- Fat distribution
- Bony contours
- Nodules
- Skin and scars
- Gait—specifically watch turning
- Specific observation depends upon symptoms

8.7.3   Musculoskeletal System-Specific Palpation

Learning Point
Skin

- Temperature
- Hydration
- Texture

Soft tissue and muscle

- Tone
- Nodules
- Presence of tenderness

Bone

- Shape
- Outline
- Prominences
- Presence of tenderness

Joints

- Capsule
- Ligaments
- Bursae
- Presence of tenderness

Palpation Pitfalls

- Moving too fast
- Non-systematic examination
- Failure to observe the patient's face

8.7.4   Musculoskeletal System Testing

Learning Point
Range of Motion (ROM):
Active range of motion (AROM)

- Patient moves joint through range of motion without assistance from the practitioner
- To observe "what the patient can do unaided"
- To assess quality and range of movement

Passive range of motion (PROM)

- To assess quality of joint function and end feel of movement
- Practitioner moves the joint through full ROM without assistance from the patient whilst simultaneously palpating the target joint
- Contraindicated in acute inflammatory states: palpate joint during active range of motion

Resisted range of motion (RROM)

- To test power of a muscle or group of muscles. Muscle power may be reduced due to abnormalities of nerves, muscles, tendons, ligaments, or joints
- Patient moves joint through full ROM against resistance from the practitioner
- Contraindicated in acute inflammatory states

Pitfalls in Range of Motion Testing
  Active range of motion

- Poor explanation and/or demonstration of range of motion
- Substitution movement
- Failure to complete full range of motion

  Passive range of motion

- Failure to palpate joint
- Failure to move joint through full range of motion
- Joint between hand moving target joint and target joint

  Resisted range of motion

- As active range of motion plus failure to load muscle correctly

8.8   Using Range of Motion as an Aid to Diagnosis

Learning Point
Active range of motion

- Utilizes patients' joints, nerves, and muscles

Passive range of motion

- Utilizes patients' joints—bypasses muscle and nerve activity

Resisted range of motion

- As active range of motion with sequential loading of muscle

Basic pattern—must be considered in combination with case history and results of other techniques

- Joint problems—pain on AROM, PROM, and RROM. AROM tends to equal PROM.
- Muscle and/or tendon problems—pain on AROM and RROM concentric contraction of target muscle plus pain on PROM of opposite anatomical movement when lengthening target muscle. AROM tends to be less than PROM.

8.8.1   Musculoskeletal System Joint Stability Testing

Learning Point
Testing ligament integrity

- Pressure is applied to contralateral side of joint through a fulcrum towards target ligament
- Unstable target ligament demonstrated by excessive movement or abnormal separation of joint

8.8.2   Musculoskeletal System Functional Movement Testing

Learning Point
- It is prudent to observe a patient performing the movement that causes discomfort rather than relying on isolated anatomical movements.
- Ask the patient perform a relevant action, e.g. comb their hair or put their coat on.

8.8.3   Examination Hints

Learning Point
Remember at all times

- Hygiene and safety
- Patient comfort and dignity
- Use your equipment correctly
- Eyes first, hands last
- You will notice that different sources recommend different ways of examining. The key to examining effectively and efficiently is to be able to rationalize the need for the technique itself
- Examine side to side: key to detecting pathological signs is asymmetry
- Consider need for additional system examination
- Recognize the range of normal movement
- Test functionally if isolated movements are negative

8.8.4   Basic Joint Examination Routines

Learning Point
Basic joint examination routines are listed in Table 8.3.

Table 8.3   Joint testing (including cartilage, fat pads, and bursae)

- Observe all aspects: anterior, posterior, lateral, and medial—symmetry, deformity, colour
- Palpation—swelling and characteristics, nodules, temperature, general and point tenderness
- Range of motion (ROM)
  - Active range of motion (AROM)—smoothness, lack of substitution movement, +/− pain
  - Passive range of motion (PROM)—end feel, +/− pain, crepitus/locking
- Examine structures on normal side before abnormal side to establish what is usual for the patient
- Examine structures side to side

Knee	
Observation	Joint in flexion and extension, weight bearing and non-weight bearing, gait
Palpation	Joint (open and closed), muscle and associated structures, move patella
Testing Routine	
AROM, PROM, RROM	Flexion
	Extension
	Internal rotation
	External rotation
Fluid	Patella effusion and patella tap: Slide your hand down the thigh, pushing down any effusion over the suprapatellar pouch behind the patella, keep your hand and maintain pressure on the upper pole of the patella. Use fingers of the other hand to push the patella down gently. If it bounces and "tap", this indicates the presence of an effusion.

(continued)

Table 8.3 (continued)

Spine	
Observation	Postural assessment, gait
Palpation	Patient prone, seated or standing, palpate spinous processes, paraspinal structures and superficial muscles of back and pelvis.
Testing Routine	
AROM: Cervical and lumbar	Flexion
	Extension
	Lateral Flexion
	Rotation
AROM: Thoracic	Rotation—seated
	Expansion
Hip	
Observation	Joint in flexion and extension, weight bearing and non-weight bearing, gait
Palpation	Joint, muscle, and associated structures
Testing Routine	
AROM, PROM, RROM	Flexion
	Extension
	Internal rotation (flexed and extended)
	External rotation (flexed and extended)
Shoulder	
Observation	Joint, muscle and associated structures
Palpation	Shoulder Girdle
Testing Routine	
AROM	Elevation
	Depression
	Protraction
	Retraction
PROM, RROM	Glenohumeral joint Flexion
	Extension
	Abduction
	Adduction
	Internal rotation
	External rotation
Elbow	
Observation	Joint in flexion and extension
Palpation	Joint (open and closed), muscle, and associated structures
Testing Routine	
AROM, PROM, RROM	Flexion
	Extension
	Pronation
	Supination

8.8.5   Muscle Testing (Includes Tendon)

Learning Point
- **Observation**—static and dynamic, muscle relaxed and contracted
- **Palpation**—whole muscle—depth of palpation depends upon location. If tendon is sheathed, palpate tendon in stretched and relaxed position
- **Range of motion (ROM)**
  Active range of motion (AROM)—smoothness, lack of substitution movement, +/− pain
  Passive range of motion (PROM)—end feel, +/− pain and site
  Resisted range of motion (RROM)– loss of power, +/-pain and site

8.8.6   Ligament Testing

Learning Point
- **Observation**—static and dynamic, symmetry, deformity, colour
- **Palpation**—attachments, course of ligament

8.8.7   Considerations

Learning Point
Pain or dysfunction of the following areas warrants nervous system examination

- Cervical spine
- Lumbar spine
- Upper limbs
- Lower limbs
- Cramping of lower limb muscles initiated by exercise and relieved by rest warrants cardiovascular system examination

8.8.8 Caution

Learning Point
- One single technique should not be used to make a diagnosis
- The case history will yield up to 80% of information required to make a working diagnosis
- Musculoskeletal symptoms may be indicative of systemic disease
- Joint pain in children warrants referral
- Consider the possible contraindications of each technique, e.g. acutely inflamed joint

8.8.9 Examination of the Knee

Learning Point
The examination of the knee checklist is showed in Table 8.4.

Table 8.4 Examination of the knee

Technique	
General examination	
Observation	Patient standing and seated; joint in extension and flexion
	Gait
Palpation	Joint open and closed
	Muscle and associated structures
	Move patella
Range of Motion	
Extension	AROM
	PROM
	RROM
Flexion	AROM
	PROM
	RROM
Int. rotation	AROM
	PROM
	RROM
Ext. rotation	AROM
	PROM
	RROM
Fluid	Patella effusion Patella tap

Part 8: Learning Activity 1
Answer the questions related to the following regions of the body:
   The spine

(a) List the movements that can take place at the spine.

   The shoulder

(b) List the movements that can take place at the shoulder
(c) Name the two joints involved in movements at the shoulder. Functionally, what type of joints are they?

   The elbow

(d) The elbow has two joints. Name the bones involved in the main joint and the bones involved in the second joint. Functionally, what type of joint is the main elbow joint
(e) List the movements that can take place at the elbow

   The wrist and hand

(f) Give the overall names of the bones that comprise the wrist and hand.
(g) List or describe the movements that can take place at the
      (i) Wrist
      (ii) Fingers
      (iii) Thumb

   The hip

(h) Functionally, what type of joint is the hip joint? What advantage does the structure of the hip joint have over that of the shoulder?
(i) List the types of movements that can take place at the hip.

   The knee

(j) Functionally, what type of joint is the knee joint?
(k) List the types of movements that can take place at the knee

   The ankle and foot

(l) Functionally, what type of joint is the ankle joint?
(m) List the types of movements that can take place at the ankle and foot.

Learning Activity 2
Define the following terms:

(a) Polyarthritis
(b) Oligoarthritis

(c) Monoarthritis
(d) Migratory (flitting) arthritis
(e) Seropositive and seronegative arthritis

Learning Activity 3
(a) List some causes of localized and generalized bone pain to complete the following table:

Generalised	Localised

(b) What questions would you ask someone with joint pain?
(c) What is meant by the term, crepitus?
(d) Why do you think that a joint might lock?

Learning Activity 4
(a) What questions would you ask someone with back pain?
(b) What important points would you note when assessing weakness of the hands?
(c) What questions would you ask someone presenting with knee pain?

Learning Activity 5
(a) Using your knowledge of the structures of joints, give some reasons why joints might swell.
    (i) A hard swelling
   (ii) A fluctuant swelling (swelling displaced from one part of the joint to another).
  (iii) A spongy swelling
(b) Give two reasons hy joints can become deformed:
(c) What changes are you trying to detect when you inspect and palpate the skin overlying a joint? What is the likely cause of these changes?

Learning Activity 6

(a) Muscle wasting can be a significant finding in joint diseases (e.g. rheumatoid arthritis). Why do you think that this occurs?

(b) What is meant by the term, fasciculation? What might be the reason for it?

Fasciculations are a hallmark symptom of diseases that affect the lower motor neurons, like amyotrophic lateral sclerosis (ALS).

(c) What is the significance of muscle cramps?

Learning Activity 7

(a) Joint disorders are classified into traumatic, infective, inflammatory, and mechanical. Complete the following table using the keywords below:

Inflammatory	Infective	Mechanical

Keywords:

1. Osteoarthritis	2. Tuberculosis	3. Ankylosing spondylitis
4. Gout	5. Pyogenic arthritis	6. Rheumatoid arthritis
7. Systemic lupus erythematosus	8. Reiter's disease	9. Osteochondritis

(b) Compare and contrast the features of the following joint disorders using the keywords provided:

Rheumatoid arthritis	Osteoarthritis

Keywords:

1. Younger people	2. Middle-aged and older	3. Male & female equally affected
4. Mainly women	5. Symmetrical presentation	6. Asymmetrical presentation
7. Metacarpophalangeal joints	8. Distal interphalangeal joints	9. Proximal interphalangeal joints
10. Mainly affects spine, knees, hips	11. Initially affects fingers, wrists	12. Morning stiffness
13. Later affects large joints	14. Stiffness later in day	15. Systemic involvement

(c) Two types of hand deformities are associated with rheumatoid arthritis, swan-necked and ulnar deviation. Describe them:

Learning Activity 8
Look up the definitions of the following:

1. Osteoporosis
2. Osteomalacia/Rickets
3. Paget's disease

Part 8 Answers: Case Study 1
A 55-year-old female visits your clinic. She has recently returned from holiday. Since when she reports suffering from "left hip and thigh pain". The pain during and after prolonged standing and walking.

(a) What question concerning the pain would be particularly useful with this history?

Answer:

- Where is the pain?
- Did the pain come on suddenly or gradually?
- How would you describe the pain?
- Does the pain spread elsewhere?
- Are there any other symptoms that seem associated with the pain?
- Is the pain worse at a particular time of day?
- Does anything make the pain better or worse?
- On a scale of 0–10, how severe is the pain, if 0 is no pain and 10 is the worst pain?

(b) What might you be looking for in the clinical examination?

Answer:

Inspection

- General appearance
- Posture and anatomical position
- Lower limb symmetry
- Deformity
- Muscles
- Fat distribution
- Bony contours
- Nodules
- Skin and Scars
- Gait—specifically watch turning

Palpation

Skin

- Temperature

Soft tissue and muscle

- Presence of tenderness

Bone

- Shape
- Outline
- Prominences
- Presence of tenderness

Joints

- Capsule
- Ligaments
- Bursae
- Presence of tenderness

Move: Range of Motion (ROM):

- Joint problems—pain on AROM, PROM, and RROM. AROM tends to equal PROM.
- Muscle and/or tendon problems—pain on AROM and RROM concentric contraction of target muscle plus pain on PROM of opposite anatomical movement when lengthening target muscle. AROM tends to be less than PROM.

Function

- Hip: Observe the patient's gait for a limping or a "waddling" walk.
- Knee: looking for any varus or valgus deformity.
- Foot and ankle: Observe the patient's gait and watching for the normal cycle of heel strike, stance, and toe-off.

Case Study 2

A 60-year-old male presents with 8 months of pain and paraesthesia noticed in the right hand (particularly in the thumb, index, and middle fingers); last month he started to have difficulty using his right hand for gripping and it is starting to affect his work. The pain is now extending up the forearm and it is waking him up during the night sleep.

(a) In addition to a musculoskeletal examination which other examination should be carried out on a patient complaining of paraesthesia?
Answer:
Nervous system

(b) When observing a patient before performing a musculoskeletal examination, give four factors that you would specifically observe for when looking at his general appearance.
Answer:
- Symmetry.
- Deformity.
- Joint attitude.

(c) Give four signs that a practitioner aims to identify during palpation.
Answer:
- Relative temperature of the structure compared to surrounding tissue.
- Nature of swelling, e.g. oedema.
- Tissue thickening or effusion relative tissue texture, e.g. skin, connective, muscle, and bone.
- Compared to surrounding tissue, abnormal structures, point of maximum tenderness.

(d) Give two factors that the practitioner should specifically observe for during active range of movement testing.
Answer:
Actual range of movement and substitution movements.

(e) What other features would you look for on clinical examination.
Answer:
Grip strength assessment.

(f) List the main symptoms seen in muscle disorders.
Answer:
- Pain.
- **Stiffness.**
- Weakness.

- Wasting.
- Fasciculation.

Case Study 3

A 42-year-old woman presents with foot and hand pain, neck stiffness, and worsening fatigue over the last 3 months.

(a) What findings on your physical examination of a patient complaining of multiple joint pain would help you differentiate between osteoarthritis and rheumatoid arthritis?

Answer:

Osteoarthritis	Rheumatoid arthritis
Joint swelling without redness or warmth	Joint pain, stiffness, and warmth
Capsular fibrosis, bone remodelling, crepitus, muscle	Symmetrical swelling of peripheral
Atrophy	Joints. Joints are hot, effusions more likely, bulge test
Weight-bearing joints affected	Joint instability and subluxation
No systemic symptoms	Deformity. Muscle atrophy
Heberden's nodes more than	Peripheral joints affected
Bouchard's nodes	Systemic symptoms: Pericarditis, anterior eye structure
Square-shaped fingers	inflammation, erythema nodosum
Muscle wasting and weakness	Lymphadenopathy
-ve Rheumatoid factor	Rheumatoid nodules and Bouchard's nodes more than
Joint x-rays	Heberdon's
Bone scan	Spindle-shaped fingers
	Swan neck deformities
	Ulnar deviation
	Pannus over MCP
	Signs of anaemia
	Muscle wasting and weakness
	FBC
	ESR, Hb
	+ye Rh factor 80%.
	HLA B27
	Synovial fluid analysis

(b) When palpating bones and joints, give two specific things for each that you would palpate for.

Answer:

Following for bones:

- Shape
- Outline
- Prominences
- Presence of tenderness

Following for joints:

- Capsule
- Ligaments
- Bursae
- Presence of tenderness

(c) What general signs and symptoms may you expect to elicit in a cartilage pathology

Answer:

- Signs and symptoms of acute or chronic inflammation
- Joint instability
- Loss of muscle and or joint function
- Deformity
- Palpable/audible crepitus/locking
- Point tenderness
- Any other reasonable answer

Case Study 4

A 78-year-old woman presenting to you for evaluation of her "arthritis pain" in both her hands, knees, and hips. She states that she has had arthritis pain for 5 years, but it has progressively gotten worse in the last 6 months. Her right knee is stiff for 10–15 min most mornings and often feels stiff after prolonged sitting. Her pain is typically worse when she is more active and improves somewhat with rest.

(a) What are the risk factors for osteoarthritis?

Answer:

- Female sex is associated with an increased risk of osteoarthritis, especially osteoarthritis of the hand, foot, and knee.
- Advancing age is by far the most well-known risk factor for osteoarthritis.
- Overweight is also a risk factor.
- Certain occupations that involve repetitive motion of a joint, like typing, can worsen osteoarthritis symptoms.

(b) What non-pharmacologic treatment modalities should be recommended?

Answer:

- Weight loss.
- Reduce periods of physical inactivity as sustained periods of rest can worsen osteoarthritis symptoms; therefore, promoting simple activity (e.g., every 20–30 min) may reduce osteoarthritis pain and stiffness.
- Physical activity programs encourage her to discuss specific exercises with physical therapist that will target the osteoarthritis in her both her hands, knees, and hips.

(c) List at least four risk factors for hip fractures.
   Answer:

- Age. The risk for hip fractures increases as aging.
- Sex. About 70% of hip fractures occur in women. Women lose bone density at a faster rate than men do, in part because the drop-in oestrogen levels that occurs with menopause accelerates bone loss. However, men also can develop dangerously low levels of bone density.
- Medications, such as Cortisone, can weaken bone if taken for long term. Rabeprazole (Aciphex) and methotrexate (Amethopterin) could cause dizziness and more prone to falling.
- Physical inactivity. Weight-bearing exercises, such as walking, help strengthen bones and muscles, making falls and fractures less likely. Not participating in regularly weight-bearing exercise, may lead to lower bone density and weaker bones.
- Smoking can interfere with the normal processes of bone building and maintenance, resulting in bone loss.

Learning Activity 1
Answer the questions related to the following regions of the body:
The spine
   (n) List the movements that can take place at the spine.
Answer:
Cervical spine: Flexion, Extension, Lateral flexion, and Rotation
Thoracic spine: Flexion, Extension, Lateral flexion, and Rotation
Lumbar spine: Flexion, Extension, Lateral flexion, and Rotation
The shoulder
   (o) List the movements that can take place at the shoulder.
Answer:
Flexion, Extension, Abduction, Adduction, Circumduction (It consists of a combination of adduction, abduction, flexion, and extension), Horizontal abduction, Horizontal adduction, Internal rotation, and External rotation.
   (p) Name the two joints involved in movements at the shoulder. Functionally, what type of joints are they?
Answer: The glenohumeral and acromioclavicular joints. They are a synovial ball-and-socket joint.
The elbow
   (q) The elbow has two joints. Name the bones involved in the main joint and the bones involved in the second joint. Functionally, what type of joint is the main elbow joint
Answer:
Humerus involved in the main joint and radius and ulna involved in the second joint. The elbow is a synovial joint.
   (r) List the movements that can take place at the elbow.

Answer:

Flexion, Extension, Pronation, and Supination.

The wrist and hand

   (s) Give the overall names of the bones that comprise the wrist and hand.

Answer:

Carpal bones (proximal): A set of eight irregularly shaped bones located in the area of the wrist.

Metacarpals: A set of five bones, each one related to a digit, located in the area of the palm.

Phalanges (distal): The bones of the digits. Based on their location, they are referred to as:

Proximal phalanx, Middle phalanx, and Distal phalanx. The index to little finger has three phalanges each, while only two are in each thumb.

   (t) List or describe the movements that can take place at the

      (i) Wrist

Answer:

Palmar *flexion*, Dorsi flexion, Ulna deviation, and Radial deviation.

      (ii) Fingers

Answer:

Flexion, Extension, Abduction, and Adduction

      (iii) Thumb

Answer:

Flexion, Extension, Abduction, Adduction, and Opposition.

The hip

   (u) Functionally, what type of joint is the hip joint? What advantage does the structure of the hip joint have over that of the shoulder?

Answer:

The *hip* and the shoulder are both ball and socket joints. In the hip the socket is deeper, allowing a smaller range of movement but providing greater stability so the hip is much more constrained or inherently stable than the shoulder.

   (v) List the types of movements that can take place at the hip.

Answer:

Flexion, Extension, Abduction, Adduction, Internal rotation, and External rotation.

The knee

   (w) Functionally, what type of joint is the knee joint?

Answer:

The knee *functionally* is a hinge joint.

   (x) List the types of movements that can take place at the knee

Answer:

Flexion and extension of the leg. In addition, some rotation of the leg is available when the knee is flexed, but not when it extended.

The ankle and foot

   (y) Functionally, what type of joint is the ankle joint?

Answer:

It is a *synovial* hinge joint.

(z) List the types of movements that can take place at the ankle and foot.
Answer:
Plantar flexion, Dorsa flexion, Inversion, and Eversion.

Learning Activity 2
Define the following terms:

(f) Polyarthritis
   Answer:
   Polyarthritis means five or more of joints have arthritis at the same time.
(g) Oligoarthritis
   Answer:
   Oligoarthritis is joint stiffness and swelling that diagnosed in children and teens
   who are less than 16 years old. The arthritis is most commonly affecting one or
   both knees. This form of arthritis is often mild and is the most likely to go away
   and leave little or no damage to the joints.
(h) Monoarthritis
   Answer:
   Monoarticular arthritis is an inflammation of one joint that may later involve
   other joints of the body.
(i) Migratory (flitting) arthritis
   Answer:
   Migratory arthritis pain spreads from one joint to another. Conditions like
   osteoarthritis, gout, and rheumatoid arthritis can cause migratory arthritis.
(j) Seropositive and seronegative arthritis
   Answer: Seropositive arthritis means there are certain antibodies present in the
   blood. The presence of anti-CCPs and RF antibodies can help diagnose seropositive RA. The antibodies are not detectable in people with another, less common type of RA, known as seronegative RA.

Learning Activity 3
(e) List some causes of localized and generalized bone pain to complete the following table:

Generalised	Localised

Answer:

Generalized	Localized
Health conditions that weaken bones	Traumas
Metastatic cancer	Sports injuries and other injuries
Anaemia	Falls
Leukaemia	Bone infection
Rickets	Bone fractures
Osteoporosis	Benign bone tumours
Bone cancer	Bone cancer

(f) What questions would you ask someone with joint pain?
   Answer:
   Where is the pain?
   Did the pain come on suddenly or gradually?
   How would you describe the pain?
   Does the pain spread elsewhere?
   Are there any other symptoms that seem associated with the pain?
   Is the pain worse at a particular time of day?
   Does anything make the pain better or worse?
   On a scale of 0–10, how severe is the pain, if 0 is no pain and 10 is the worst pain?
(g) What is meant by the term, crepitus?
   Answer:
   Grinding sensation, may suggest damage to articular surfaces or tenosynovitis.

(h) Why do you think that a joint might lock?
   Answer:
   Joint lock suggests a loose body in the joint space, which may be a symptom of
   articular surface degeneration.

Learning Activity 4

(d) What questions would you ask someone with back pain?
Answer:
Where is the pain?
Did the pain come on suddenly or gradually?
How would you describe the pain?
Does the pain spread elsewhere?
Are there any other symptoms that seem associated with the pain?
Is the pain worse at a particular time of day?
Does anything make the pain better or worse?
On a scale of 0–10, how severe is the pain, if 0 is no pain and 10 is the worst pain?

(e) What important points would you note when assessing weakness of the hands?

Answer:
Is the weakness focal or global?
Does the weakness fluctuate?
Is the weakness increasing in severity?
Is the weakness secondary to a painful limb?

(f) What questions would you ask someone presenting with knee pain?

Answer:
Where is the pain?
Did the pain come on suddenly or gradually?
How would you describe the pain?
Does the pain spread elsewhere?
Are there any other symptoms that seem associated with the pain?
Is the pain worse at a particular time of day?
Does anything make the pain better or worse?
On a scale of 0–10, how severe is the pain, if 0 is no pain and 10 is the worst?
Does your knee pain limit your ability to perform typical daily activities?

Learning Activity 5

(d) Using your knowledge of the structures of joints, give some reasons why joints
might swell.
Answer:
The most common reason is arthritis, including rheumatoid arthritis, osteoar-
thritis, gout, psoriatic arthritis, septic arthritis.
(i) A hard swelling
Answer:
Nodal osteoarthritis causes bony, hard swelling.
(ii) A fluctuant swelling (swelling displaced from one part of the joint to another)
Answer:

Joint effusion is a sign of joint inflammation which effusion fluid displaced from one part to another.

(iii) A spongy swelling

Answer:

Ankle swelling is more commonly a spongy swelling due to oedema.

(e) Give two reasons why joints can become deformed:

Answer:

Arthritis and fractures.

(f) What changes are you trying to detect when you inspect and palpate the skin overlying a joint? What is the likely cause of these changes?

Answer:

Skin colour—Bruising: trauma or systemic condition; Red skin: inflammation

Skin temperature increase—Inflammation

Hydration and Texture—Dehydration

Muscles—Always inspect, palpate, and test for muscle power.

Learning Activity 6

(d) Muscle wasting can be a significant finding in joint diseases (e.g. rheumatoid arthritis). Why do you think that this occurs?

Answer:

The exact causes of general muscle wasting are hard to identify. There seems to be a connection with having too much of a protein (cytokine) produced by immune system cells, and because of the pain and difficulty in moving their joints. This lack of activity can lead to muscle wasting.

(e) What is meant by the term, fasciculation? What might be the reason for it?

Answer:

A fasciculation is a spontaneous, involuntary fine muscle fibres contraction.

Causes:

- Certain medications, such as steroid medicines
- Exposure to extreme cold
- Hyperventilation
- Strenuous exercise
- Stress or anxiety
- Tiredness or lack of sleep
- Too much caffeine or alcohol

Fasciculations are a hallmark symptom of diseases that affect the lower motor neurons, like amyotrophic lateral sclerosis (ALS).

(f) What is the significance of muscle cramps?

Answer:

Common causes include forced muscle contraction and dehydration.

Learning Activity 7

(d) Joint disorders are classified into traumatic, infective, inflammatory, and mechanical. Complete the following table using the keywords below:

Inflammatory	Infective	Mechanical

Keywords:

1. Osteoarthritis	2. Tuberculosis	3. Ankylosing spondylitis
4. Gout	5. Pyogenic arthritis	6. Rheumatoid arthritis
7. Systemic lupus erythematosus	8. Reiter's disease	9. Osteochondritis

Answer:

Inflammatory	Infective	Mechanical
Gout Rheumatoid arthritis Systemic lupus erythematosus Reiter's disease Osteoarthritis Ankylosing spondylitis Osteochondritis	Tuberculosis Pyogenic arthritis	Osteoarthritis Ankylosing spondylitis Osteochondritis

(e) Compare and contrast the features of the following joint disorders using the keywords provided:

Rheumatoid arthritis	Osteoarthritis

Keywords:

1. Younger people	2. Middle-aged and older	3. Male & female equally affected
4. Mainly women	5. Symmetrical presentation	6. Asymmetrical presentation
7. Metacarpophalangeal joints	8. Distal interphalangeal joints	9. Proximal interphalangeal joints
10. Mainly affects spine, knees, hips	11. Initially affects fingers, wrists	12. Morning stiffness
13. Later affects large joints	14. Stiffness later in day	15. Systemic involvement

Answer:

Rheumatoid arthritis	Osteoarthritis
Younger people Mainly women Symmetrical presentation Metacarpophalangeal joints Distal interphalangeal joints Proximal interphalangeal joints Initially affects fingers, wrists Morning stiffness Later affects large joints Systemic involvement	Middle-aged and older Male & female equally affected Asymmetrical presentation. Mainly affects spine, knees, hips Stiffness later in day

(f) Two types of hand deformities are associated with rheumatoid arthritis, swan-necked and ulnar deviation. Describe them:

Answer:

Swan Necked characterized by hyperextension of the PIP joint and flexion of the DIP joint due to an imbalance of muscle forces on the PIP.

Ulnar deviation occurs when the joints in the wrist and hand shift so the fingers bend toward the ulna bone on the outside of the forearm.

Learning Activity 8

Look up the definitions of the following:

4. Osteoporosis

    Answer: Osteoporosis is a disease characterized by low bone mass and structural deterioration of bone tissue, with a consequent increase in bone fragility and susceptibility to fracture.

5. Osteomalacia/Rickets

    Answer: Osteomalacia/Rickets is a childhood disease where your child's bones are too soft, causing their bones to warp, bend, and break more easily. It's typically caused by a lack of vitamin D.

6. Paget's disease

   Answer: Paget's disease of bone is a condition that affects the normal recycling of bone tissue, causing bone pain, deformities, and fractures.

Bibliography

1. Welsh, C. (2020). *Hole's essentials of human anatomy & physiology* (14th ed.). McGraw Hill.
2. Dover, A. R., & Innes, J. A. (Eds.). (2023). *Macleod's clinical examination*. Elsevier.
3. Kurtz, S., Silverman, J., Benson, J. & Draper, J. (2003). Marrying content and process in clinical method teaching: enhancing the Calgary–Cambridge guides. *Academic Medicine, 78*(8), pp. 802–809.
4. Miller, S. B. (1990). An overview of the musculoskeletal system. In H. K. Walker, W. D. Hall, & J. W. Hurst (Eds.), *Clinical methods: The history, physical, and laboratory examinations* (3rd ed.). Butterworths.